THE AGED PATIENT
A Sourcebook for the Allied Health Professional

THE AGED PATIENT

A Sourcebook for the Allied Health Professional

NORA S. ERNST, Ph.D.
Assistant Professor
School of Allied Health Sciences
University of Texas Health Science Center at Dallas
Dallas, Texas

HILDA R. GLAZER-WALDMAN, Ed.D.
Assistant Professor
School of Allied Health Sciences
University of Texas Health Science Center at Dallas
Dallas, Texas

YEAR BOOK MEDICAL PUBLISHERS, INC.
CHICAGO • LONDON

Library of Congress Cataloging in Publication Data
Main entry under title:

The Aged Patient: A Sourcebook for the Allied Health Professional

Includes index.
1. Geriatrics. 2. Gerontology. I. Ernst, Nora S.
II. Glazer-Waldman, Hilda R. [DNLM: 1. Geriatrics.
WT 100 G767]
RC952.G447 1982 362.1'9897 82-10917
ISBN 0-8151-3133-X

CONTRIBUTORS

Steven R. Applewhite, Ph.D., Assistant Professor, Center for Studies on Aging, North Texas State University, Denton, Texas

Philip K. Armour, Ph.D., Assistant Professor, School of Social Sciences, The University of Texas at Dallas, Dallas, Texas

Brenda S. Burton, M.S., Center for Studies in Aging, North Texas State University, Denton, Texas

Therese Cristiani, Ed.D., Associate Professor, Department of Behavioral Studies, University of Missouri-St. Louis, St. Louis, Missouri

Carol J. Dye, Ph.D., Research Psychologist, Geriatric Research, Education and Clinical, Veterans Administration Medical Center, St. Louis, Missouri

Seymour Eisenberg, M.D., Chief, Geriatric Medicine, Veterans Administration Medical Center, Dallas, Texas; Professor of Medicine and Chief of the Geriatric Section, Department of Internal Medicine, University of Texas Health Science Center at Dallas, Dallas, Texas

Marvin L. Ernst, Ph.D., Associate Professor, School of Nursing and Gerontology, University of Northern Colorado, Greeley, Colorado

Nora S. Ernst, Ph.D., Assistant Professor, School of Allied Health Sciences, University of Texas Health Science Center at Dallas, Dallas, Texas

Thomas J. Fairchild, Ph.D., Assistant Professor, Center for Studies in Aging, North Texas State University, Denton, Texas

Rickey L. George, Ph.D., Professor, Department of Behavioral Studies, University of Missouri-St. Louis, St. Louis, Missouri

Hilda R. Glazer-Waldman, Ed.D., Assistant Professor, School of Allied Health Sciences, University of Texas Health Science Center at Dallas, Dallas, Texas

Bert Hayslip, Jr., Ph.D., Assistant Professor, Center for Studies in Aging and Department of Psychology, North Texas State University, Denton, Texas

Gail House, Ph.D., Assistant Professor, College of Home Economics, Texas Tech University, Lubbock, Texas

Robert A. Kooken, M.S., Department of Psychology, North Texas State University, Denton, Texas

Roger A. Lanier, Ph.D., Associate Dean, School of Allied Health Sciences, University of Texas Health Science Center at Dallas, Dallas, Texas

Don Mannerberg, M.D., Preventive Medicine Clinic, Richardson, Texas

Leonard Naeger, Ph.D., Associate Professor, St. Louis College of Pharmacy, St. Louis, Missouri

Sharon Young Ward, M.A., Assistant Administrator, The Washington House, Alexandria, Virginia

Sherryl Short Wesson, R.D.H., M.A., Gerodontic Program Coordinator, Dallas City Dental Health Program, Dallas, Texas

Helen L. West, Ph.D., Assistant Professor, School of Allied Health Sciences, University of Texas Health Science Center at Dallas, Dallas, Texas

CONTENTS

PART III HEALTH CARE SCIENCE

FOREWORD

WE ARE EITHER NEARING or have already reached the point at which the supply of health practitioners is in balance with the demand for health care service in this country. While there continue to be sporadic shortages in nursing and some allied health professions, the problem of maldistribution of personnel stands as the major barrier between the public and those prepared to meet its health needs. Great efforts to achieve this state of supply have spanned the past decade.

Almost unnoticed in the push for health care accessibility for all has been a demographic change destined to challenge our present health care delivery system. Our very success in promoting the public health is contributing to rapid growth in the number of individuals over the age of 65, now projected to be 50 million by the year 2000. This expanding segment of the population presents unique needs in such areas as health care and social support services. Failure to plan adequately to meet these needs will result in a serious diminution of the quality of life for this important group of Americans. Moreover, the strength of their numbers will make their voices exceedingly persuasive to elected officials as they present demands for eliminating perceived shortcomings in health care.

Recognition of the needs of the aged is growing, and our government has taken a number of initiatives in this regard. Among them are programs to encourage the development of medical school instruction in geriatric medicine; to provide for the development of educational programs in nutrition with emphasis on the aging; and to support educational programs and centers and institutes for the aging. Slowly but perceptibly, there is appearing an elevated awareness of the general field of gerontology. On all sides we see research, demonstration projects, and service undertakings targeted at our aging population.

Somewhat surprisingly, gerontologic needs have proved to be a powerful catalyst in the development of strong interdisciplinary approaches to health education. The introduction of an identifiable segment of geriatrics into the curricula of many medical schools is just one example. Of even greater importance is the trend toward including gerontology topics in allied health education programs as well as incorporating segments on nutrition, drugs, occupational and physical therapy, and recreational therapy in gerontology curricula. The welcome result has been a growing interaction among various allied health practitioners, where, in the past, the tendency was more in the direction of separate, individual practices.

As increasing attention is directed toward various needs of the aging, there is a pressing demand for more personnel educated in the complexities of geriatric care and the delivery of services to the elderly. Educational institutions have responded by introducing gerontology segments or courses into existing curricula or by launching degree programs that concentrate on the many facets of this discipline. This burgeoning of interest has been accompanied by a concurrent growing wealth of literature that deals with the phenomenon of aging. The collection of readings in this book has been designed to acquaint allied health students with broad aspects of gerontology and geriatric topics. The editors have organized the material so that the student can follow a logical progression through the various topics. This work represents a constructive approach to the presentation of important, practical aspects of services for the aged and will surely constitute a valuable step toward ensuring that our "golden age" is not tarnished by poorly prepared and insensitive health care providers.

JOHN W. SCHERMERHORN, PH.D.
School of Allied Health Sciences
The University of Texas Health
Science Center at Dallas

PREFACE

THE STUDY OF THE AGED revolves around two interrelated disciplines. *Gerontology* is the scientific study of the process of aging, the effects of time on human development. *Geriatrics* refers to medical care of the elderly, and is primarily concerned with medical intervention in the treatment of diseases of the aged. Thus the distinction can be made between changes brought about over time (gerontology) and changes that occur as a result of disease (geriatrics).

Gerontology and geriatrics are interdisciplinary in nature and involve researchers, scientists, and health care practitioners in various fields. The interdisciplinary nature of the field affects patient care for the elderly by emphasizing the benefits of coordinated teamwork and by fostering increased knowledge and understanding of various aspects of the elderly individual.

With the increasing specialization of health care services and the increasing numbers of geriatric patients being treated by various health professionals, there is a need for education in geriatrics and gerontology for the allied health professional. This volume utilizes the interdisciplinary approach to health care for elderly patients. The goal of the book is to provide the reader with increased knowledge and understanding of aspects of gerontology and geriatrics that have direct relevance to interventions for health care of the elderly. Examples and illustrations from a large number of allied health professions have been included to make the book relevant for every allied health professional.

The book is divided into three parts: Social Sciences, Medical Science, and Health Care Science. Part I, Social Sciences, contains chapters on interdisciplinary teamwork, changing roles as a result of aging, communicating with the elderly, public policy and programs, the disadvantaged elderly, and the aged in the year 2000. These chapters present an introduction to gerontology so the reader can appreciate the impact of the elderly population on this era and on the 21st century.

Part II, Medical Science, contains chapters on medical health problems, substance abuse, sensory processes, psychosocial problems, and dental problems. The reader is given an introduction to geriatrics through a discussion of the major health issues facing the aged.

The final part, Health Care Science, includes chapters on the institutionalized elderly, home health services, patient education, and therapeutic interventions—both in general and in the areas of nutrition and mental health. The chapters on intervention are not meant to be inclusive but are intended to provide the reader with a sampling of clinical interventions in a number of allied health disciplines. The final chapter in this section is on humanizing health care for the elderly, which is an issue receiving increased attention by health practitioners.

As discussed in the first chapter, the interdisciplinary team approach is beneficial to the provision of quality medical care for the aged. To function as a productive member of a health care team, it is important for the allied health professional to be aware of the contributions and concerns of the various disciplines available within the team. This volume will help extend the knowledge of allied health practitioners through increased understanding of various aspects of gerontology and geriatrics related to health care of the aged.

NORA S. ERNST, PH.D.
HILDA R. GLAZER-WALDMAN, ED.D.

PART I

Social Sciences

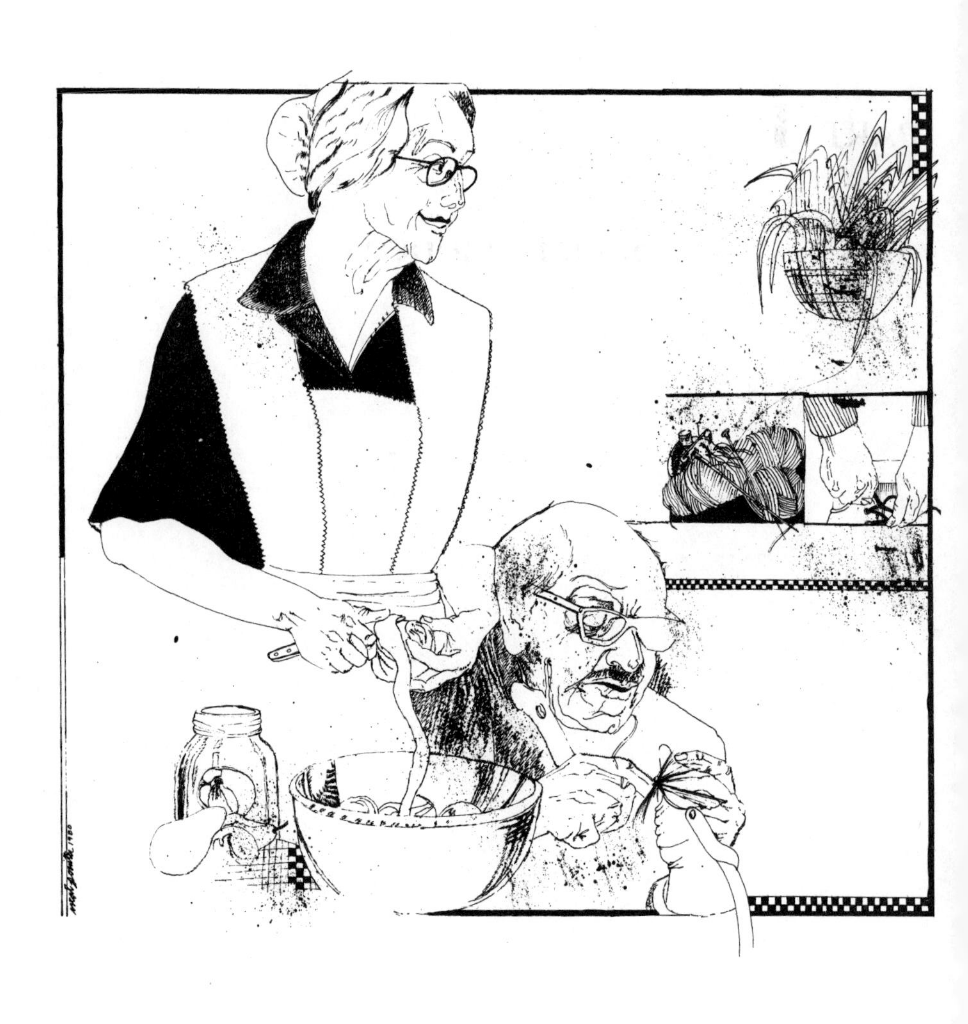

1

INTERDISCIPLINARY TEAM APPROACH TO GERIATRIC CARE

Nora S. Ernst, Ph.D.

"GERIATRICS IS clearly concerned with the whole of the elderly population and is truly a general subject . . . that embraces the whole of general medicine . . . rehabilitation, psychiatry of old age, sociology and gerontology" (Hodkinson, 1975). An aged patient often has multiple chronic conditions and complex health care needs. A variety of health care professionals are necessary, working in a cooperative manner, to meet those needs. The interdisciplinary team is one response to better health provision for the elderly.

The major assumption for the team approach is that an interdisciplinary team will bring together diverse skills and expertise to provide more effective, better coordinated, better quality service—through the performance of similar tasks or of different but interrelated tasks. Team members may have the same kinds and levels of skills or have different kinds or levels of skills (Duncanis and Golin, 1979). An example of this is when the nursing service coordinates the work of the physical therapist. Nursing service is a 24-hour service and involves several levels of providers who perform similar tasks over a time period. When a therapist is brought in, nursing service is maintained but an additional skill is utilized. This can be a health care team.

"A team is a group of people, each of whom possesses particular expertise, each of whom is responsible for making individual decisions; who together hold a common purpose; who meet together to communicate; collaborate, and consolidate knowledge, from which plans are made, actions are determined and future decisions influenced" (Brill, 1976). This definition includes four main components that must be considered before a group can be defined as a work team. First, a team is made up of individuals with inter- and intrapressures. The individual personalities and skills of each team member will affect the group as a whole. Second, a team is a group that constitutes a system and is therefore governed by the basic characteristics of systems. Third, team members have a common purpose that provides focus and direction to the work. All team members must have a clear definition and mutual understanding of this purpose. Fourth, clear communication is essential (Brill, 1976). Involving a number of professionals with a patient does not ensure a team approach; each provider must function as a subunit of the whole in a synergistic relationship (Parker, 1972). Fragmented care does not meet the needs of aged patients. Concern for the patient in medical, social, psychological, and economic terms can be combined with ongoing service delivery but requires coordinated efforts.

There are a number of factors that have influenced the development of the team approach in geriatric care. Areas of primary importance are the structure of the health care organization, health care specialization, internal and external regulations, and communication with the patient. The health problems presented by the aged patient are often interrelated and cannot be adequately treated in isolation. When a number of health services are being received, fragmented and uncoordinated services may cause confusion and apprehension in the older adult.

The older patient must be viewed as an integral part of the team. The health care team needs to be aware of and work with the patient to meet both his perceived needs and his actual needs. Too often, the aged patient enters the health care system seeking relief from one symptom only to receive treatment for another. For example, the aged patient may wish to have relief from a recurring respiratory ailment, but upon presenting the problem to the physician is given a battery of tests and diagnosed as a borderline diabetic. Consequently, efforts to change lifelong diet and exercise behaviors become prominent rather than treatment of the patient's perceived priority problem of a respiratory ailment. The health problem diagnosed by the provider may actually be the one of primary need; but if the older patient does not perceive it as such and chooses a secondary problem as the first priority, the health provider must "help" the perceived priority problem if any treatment is to be successful.

Health Care Organization

The structure of the health care institution is in large part responsible for the creation and maintenance of teamwork. The organization must practice interdisciplinary cooperation and provide opportunities for health care providers to develop team cooperation and collaboration.

Organizations create an atmosphere which pervades everything that happens within them and affects relationships with outside individuals as well. Organizations are required to accomplish their tasks and adjust to the changes taking place in the environment around them, while retaining distinctive characteristics and abilities to perform tasks. The missions of organizations influence both their structure and their climate (Casella, 1977).

Some factors affecting the organization can be modified or influenced by administrative decisions, training, or other actions. These tend to be technical or organizational. *Technical tasks* are those related to the tasks of organization and are activities needed to achieve particular objectives. *Organizational tasks* are internal environmental factors that are designed to support organizational missions. Other variables are outcomes of the above factors. They provide visible evidence of how well the organization is doing (Casella, 1977).

There is evidence that both the structure and the climate of organizations affect staff attitudes and motivations as well as individual functioning. *Organizational climate* includes the intangible aspects of the organization's atmosphere that are sensed directly and indirectly by personnel and that are of great importance in shaping employee attitudes and performance. Climate reflects the internal state of an organization, and the characteristic way in which work is performed.

Organizational goals serve several functions. They indicate the purposes of organizations. They also provide the staff with targets toward which to direct energies and they enhance motivations. It is necessary, however, for the organizational goals to be clear and realistic. *Organizational policies* are general, formal statements of guidelines for staff behavior. These guidelines are spelled out in detail in the form of rules and procedures. Supervision includes leadership practices that are appropriate to the organizational goals, the work to be done, the type of personnel to be directed, and the work methods employed. Staff relations are important indicators of organizational climate (Casella, 1977).

Since most work experiences occur within primary groups, the aspects of *group membership* need to be considered. These aspects include group cohesiveness, group orientation, and group standards and interaction. Group cohesiveness can be considered in terms of the feelings of pride and accomplishment that unite group members. Group orientation is the consistency of work emphasis in stressing rule observance in relation to providing health care, and how each group member views his own position in regard to group work emphasis. Group standards are expectations or goals, while interaction can center on the regard that group members have for one another in the work setting (Casella, 1977).

Organizations require members to perform a wide variety of functions. These functions are assigned to specific positions or jobs. Effective performance demands that these positions or jobs be performed by individuals who have a clear idea of what they are to do and of how others in the organization are expected to behave. The satisfactory performance of role behaviors is a necessary condition for realizing organizational goals.

Individuals, within and outside the organization, expect specific behaviors from the role-holder. However, even the most comprehensive definition of roles will not cover everything that a role-holder must do. The extent to which roles are described is influenced by the functions to be performed. Positions that require professional skill and individual judgment allow wide latitude to role-holders. Faulty identification of roles contributes to many difficulties. *Role ambiguity* occurs in a situation in which role definitions are unclear. The role-holder does not have enough information to perform the role as it should be performed, resulting in partial confusion. *Role congruence* refers to the manner in which the role is performed in relation to formal or informal expectations. *Role conflict* is another difficulty. It is the result of role-holders being subjected to different sets of role assumptions. Satisfying one set makes it more difficult to satisfy the others. *Role overload* is the outcome of role conflict. This occurs when the roles expected of a role-holder are legitimate and compatible, but combine to create demands that are impossible to satisfy. Inability to satisfy the expected role behaviors leads to poor performance and confusion (Casella, 1977).

Role strain in geriatric care is common and can be attributed to several major causes. One cause is confusion and uncertainty within the profession about providing a clear set of defined behaviors. Blurring of roles in the health fields can occur as specialization increases. The need to define new roles as role behaviors are restructured to include additional specializations is important. Role strain is also confusing to patients, who often find it necessary to go from physician to physician to have different medical procedures or examinations performed.

Health Care Specialization

An essential aspect of the interdisciplinary team is the ability of two or more professionals to work together. Potential misperceptions and misunderstandings are usually greater between than within professions because the professional is often not aware of the specific competencies and roles of members of different professions. Overlapping roles, status differences, and differences in viewpoint can easily lead to interprofessional conflict and discord. Conflict and misperceptions among professionals can seriously interfere with collaborative efforts.

Professional ethnocentrism, differences in professional status, and a lack of understanding of other professions were cited as primary barriers to communication among professionals by Haselkorn (1958). Fear of encroachment by other professionals and language barriers can also impede interprofessional collaboration. Health care specialization is a problem in teamwork. Demarcation disputes arising from role overlap are hard to avoid. Professional power and status can impede an interdisciplinary team from developing and functioning (Evers, 1981). The trend toward increasing specialization in health care can create fragmentation of care among types and levels of providers. Each specialist may view the goals, priorities, and definitions of the patient's problem in a singular rather than a multiple manner. "As more and more individuals become involved in providing services to a particular client, the need for clarifying the lines of communication within the agency becomes increasingly acute. Otherwise the organization, like the client, may suffer from the negative effects of fragmentation" (Duncanis and Golin, 1979).

Internal and External Regulations

Organizational constraints define the way in which work is usually performed. Staffs are guided in work activities by the actions of supervisors, rules governing actions, training and orientation procedures, and sanctions to discourage certain practices. Constraints are devised to reduce uncertainty in organizational activities. Since uncertainty cannot be removed entirely, the problem is to determine the level of control that meets organizational needs and also allows staff the opportunity to exercise initiative.

Organizational practices concern two dimensions. The first is whether decisions are made by administrators unilaterally or with the participation of groups. The second is whether emphasis is placed on realizing organizational goals or on strict adherence to organizational rules and procedures. These factors can greatly affect team cooperation. The interdisciplinary health care team can only function in an organization that is flexible enough to allow group decision-making as well as an emphasis on the patient's health care goals (Duncanis and Golin, 1979).

Finally, health care has responded to increasing pressure from local, state, and federal governments to improve its quality and cost-effectiveness. One consequence of these governmental efforts has been an increase in the role of the team in all aspects of health care provision (Duncanis and Golin, 1979).

External regulations can affect teamwork. The elderly are the target population for a myriad of federal, state, and local programs aimed at maintaining independence and promoting health. Often, the health care provider is one of the first persons to come in contact with the aged patient and may be a major source for locating and obtaining services. Conversely, the eligibility requirements and reimbursement regulations may become major impediments to the provision of health care. One example of this is where a third party payee reimburses a health care provider for therapy only as long as the patient shows strong improvement. An aged patient who has suffered a stroke may show excellent rehabilitative potential and enter a therapy program. The dilemma arises when recovery reaches a plateau. The provider may feel that the patient will continue to improve over time but, at the moment, no improvement is shown. What report should the provider make to the payee?

Communication

Communication between patients and providers is an important consideration, as is communication among health care providers. Each provider brings to the team his own unique expertise, resources, philosophies, and biases. There are differences in the amount of contact, decision-making responsibility, and legal responsibility among providers. The primary physician obviously has direct legal and ethical responsibility to the patient, but other team members also have responsibilities and obligations. Different levels of professional responsibility that exist within the team often make team functioning difficult at best. Yet the primary goal should always be to provide quality health care for the patient. The team should orient itself toward this goal.

The physician is usually given ultimate responsibility for the patient in matters of health care and is often designated team leader. With the aged patient, health problems may become more complex. Concurrent problems such as diet inadequacy, loss of social roles and support systems, and loss of independent functioning also become more pronounced. At this point, the physician often becomes dependent on a large number of allied health professionals to provide appropriate care. As the provider group enlarges, problems in communication can arise. Lines of authority, areas of responsibility, and type and quantity of care must be delineated.

As the treatment process becomes more complex, the physician cannot personally oversee every step in the treatment and may not be aware of the community support services available to the aged. Coordination becomes a serious problem as the size of the provider group increases. "The team approach is one way to provide coordination, and the physician may be willing to delegate some responsibility for treatment and decision making to the team itself" (Duncanis and Golin, 1979).

The patient plays a crucial role in the treatment process. First of all, the patient has intimate acquaintance with the problem either on an intellectual basis or on the basis of past experience. Second, the patient's cooperation is necessary if treatment is to be successful. Third, the patient generally has more reason to be concerned about his personal welfare than does any other individual. Finally, it is the patient who will make, or should make, the final decision concerning treatment or nontreatment. The patient should be viewed as an integral and important member of the team.

The aged patient is sometimes not viewed in this light. *Ageism* is a bias or prejudice against the elderly based solely on their age and is often used to describe the discrimination that tends to accompany old age (Levinson, 1981). Such an attitude can result in health care providers viewing aged patients as untreatable or unable to regain total well-being. This is seen particularly in those instances where the patient has several chronic health problems and the prognosis for recovery is poor. Many chronic conditions result in dependency. The aged patient often loses the ability to totally care for his or her daily living activities. The resulting dependency on others can encourage a paternalistic attitude on the part of the health care provider. These attitudes negate positive communication between team members and the aged patient.

The interdisciplinary team deals with the patient differently when the therapeutic situation is primarily a dyadic doctor-patient relationship. Although the health care providers may be expert in only a few areas of the patient's needs, they nevertheless must be concerned with all aspects of the patient and deal with him as a totality. Although the team will emphasize one or another aspect of need at a particular time, it is important that no aspect of the problem be neglected.

People have the right to decide for themselves what they wish to do with their bodies and their lives. This concept is difficult for many health care professionals to accept, since they have, by training and experience, come to expect that once a patient has appeared, he or she will follow any advice or "orders" given by the professional.

Currently, however, it seems that many patients are moving toward a more active role in making decisions about their treatment. Several factors have influenced this trend. One is an increased general awareness of health care as a result of public dissemination and discussion of health-related topics. Secondly, the areas of human rights, patient rights, and rights of the handicapped have been identified and supported by judicial rulings and legislative mandates. Lastly, a general rise in the educational level of the aged population has been noted. As more and more people reach age 65, the level of educational attainment for this group has increased. "The percentage of high school and college graduates has been increasing and the percentage of persons with less than five years of schooling (functionally illiterate) has been declining" (Allan and Brotman, 1981). These individuals are more knowledgeable, and in some cases more skeptical, about the services they receive.

In summary, the characteristics of a team are as follows:

1. A team consists of two or more individuals, since the nature of teamwork requires the action of more than one person.
2. There may be face-to-face or non-face-to-face configurations.
3. There is an identifiable leader.
4. Teams function both within and between organizational settings.
5. Roles of participants are defined.
6. Teams collaborate.
7. There are specific protocols of operation.
8. The team is client centered.
9. The team is task oriented (Duncanis and Golin, 1979).

These characteristics can be used to operationally define the functioning of the team in the health care setting. They can aid in the formation of a new team or the evaluation of an existing one. Obviously, other attributes could be included. Without these basic attributes, however, the team does not exist; rather, there is fragmented service that may or may not meet the overall needs of the aged patient.

Although the problems presented are of major importance in structuring the interaction of the aged patient and the team, other characteristics of the patient also exert an influence. Each patient has a number of traits that do not necessarily relate directly to the problem which led him to seek help from the team. Age, sex, intelligence, personality, and cultural background all influence the way in which the patient will act. The way in which the patient and team interact is a product of the characteristics of the patient, the professionals on the team, and the organizational setting in which the encounter occurs.

The geriatric team is multidisciplinary and varies in scope, focus, and components. The team approach can deliver multiple therapies to relieve the multiple, simultaneous problems of illness often faced by older adults. Services may be administered in the institutional setting (nursing home or hospital), in the community (home health agency), or in a combination of inpatient/outpatient settings (day care center).

Each member of the team must learn to accept and value input from colleagues on the team. Reaching a decision concerning treatment and prognosis requires openness and the ability to be challenged on ideas. Rather than losing professional identity, the health care provider can emerge with a feeling of having contributed to the diminution of suffering and to the improvement of the quality of life for the aged patient.

REFERENCES

Allan C., Brotman H.: *Chart Book on Aging in America*. Washington, D.C., 1981 White House Conference on Aging, 1981.

Brill N.: *Team-work: Working Together in the Human Services*. Philadelphia, J.B. Lippincott Co., 1976.

Casella C.: *Training Exercises to Improve Interpersonal Relations in Health Care Organizations*. New York, Panel Publishers, 1977.

Duncanis A.J., Golin A.K.: *The Interdisciplinary Health Care Team: A Handbook*. Germantown, Md.: Aspen Systems Corporation, 1979.

Evers H.K.: Multidisciplinary teams in geriatric wards: Myth or reality? *J. Adv. Nurs*. 6:205–214, 1981.

Haselkorn F.: Some dynamic aspects of interpersonal practice in rehabilitation. *Soc. Casework* 39:396–400, 1958.

Hodkinson H.M.: *An Outline of Geriatrics*. New York, Academic Press, 1975.

Levinson A.J.: Ageism: A major deterrent to the introduction of curricula in aging. *Gerontology Geriatrics Education*. 1:161–163, 1981.

Parker A.W.: *The Team Approach to Primary Health Care*. Neighborhood Health Center Seminar Program, monograph series no. 3. Berkeley, University of California Extension Berkeley, 1972.

2

CHANGING ROLES AS A RESULT OF AGING

Marvin L. Ernst, Ph.D.

MOST OF US take for granted our involvement with other people. We expect interaction to occur normally within the context of daily living. We relate to other people and transpose our modes of interaction from one social situation to another without reflecting on the various styles and meanings of that interaction. We learn from birth how to get along with other people. From birth to death, social interaction is a constant process of trial and error, success and failure, pleasure and pain.

This chapter explores one aspect of social relations—social roles. It begins by exploring the concept of role and ends with an examination of frequent role losses that occur among the elderly. It should be noted that this is not an attempt to explore or explain the concepts of status or position. Rather, it is to explore social roles as they have meaning for the individuals who play them. While it is true that most social roles are attached to a particular status and position, the premise here is that people have a tendency to internalize the roles they play, and they may continue to identify with them even though the status or position to which those roles were initially attached no longer exists. An individual who occupies a particular position for an extended period of time, such as a business executive, does not easily cast aside behaviors learned while occupying that position. The roles that he or she learned extend beyond the position and may be maintained for years. The crucial factors related to maintenance of role behavior are the extent to which the person identified with the role and the extent to which the surrounding social environment supports that identification. To illustrate, suppose a business executive retires and joins a volunteer organization. This organization, in turn, elects him or her president of the club. The retired executive continues to be rewarded for exhibiting the behavior that was displayed prior to retirement. Hence, a continuation of the executive role is maintained even though the position has changed. If the business executive did not receive the stimuli necessary to perpetuate the role or if his or her involvement with the role was limited, role behavior would change to some new form, depending on the circumstances and needs of the individual.

A second theme throughout this chapter is the concept of loss among the elderly. As an individual ages, there is an increased likelihood of his experiencing a number of losses that may challenge his ability to cope with the surrounding world. It should be noted, however, that losses are highly individualistic in nature. Few, if any, are found to occur among *all* older people. Some people age with a minimum number of losses. Others experience multiple and severe losses at various stages of life. Primary factors in loss are the type incurred, the extent to which the person was able to prepare for it, and the external resources available to help the person adjust to it. The more severe the loss, the less anticipatory adjustment is possible. The fewer the external resources, the poorer the prognosis is for adjustment to the loss.

It must be remembered that differentiation among the elderly is greater than similarity. Not all retired persons are depressed about being retired. Not all widows are unhappy and fearful of their future. The older adult population must be recognized as individuals and responded to as such. Health care providers must learn to identify individual characteristics of older clients and to respond in nonstereotypical ways.

Social Roles

Fundamental to understanding the social nature of aging is the need to comprehend what people mean by the term "social role." Frequently this term has been used to explain various behaviors of individuals without a common, or at least stated, definition of it. While the word "role" is familiar to most of us, we tend to ascribe its meaning to the theatrical world. There is, however, an important distinction between an actor and his or her role. An *actor* is a person. A *role* is a prescribed set of actions and words to be expressed by an actor. In the theatrical sense, a role is independent of any particular actor. The prescription of actions and words would be similar regardless of the individual occupying that role. While certain amounts of latitude are allowed different actors within the role, its essence remains the same. The actor must play the part as prescribed. Too great a deviation from the part will result in rejection of the actor and failure on the part of the audience to legitimate the actor's performance.

Like theatrical roles, social roles allow a degree of independence to the actor performing the role. The behaviors of the occupants of any given position may change the role depending on a number of factors. Some of these circumstances are: (1) the clarity of the role that is to be played; (2) the number and quality of the roles that an individual is expected to perform at any one time; (3) the environmental context in which the role is being performed; (4) the differing motives of both the actor and the audience; and (5) the unique characteristics of the individual playing the role.

Role clarity concerns the degree to which expectations of role performance held by a particular group or society are clear and precise. The greater the unanimity and precision of the role specifications the easier it is for the actor to adapt his or her behavior toward the desired outcome. Thus, if it is obvious within the social context that a particular behavior is both expected and required, the actor has relatively little difficulty performing the role in the way anticipated by the audience. If, however, role clarity does not exist, adjustment of behavior to meet expectations is frequently difficult. In this case the actor may misinterpret the desires of the group and behave in a manner at variance with its expectations.

The above circumstance may occur in a variety of ways. An individual actor may be in a situation where role clarity simply does not exist; the role may not be clearly defined by the social situation. It may be a new or emerging role without a long history of enactment within the group. Perhaps no real definition of the role was ever attained. It is possible that the expectations themselves are in a state of flux due to external or internal causes. Regardless of the case, lack of role clarity can lead to an absence of defined role behavior that results in confusion both for the actor expecting to play the role and for the audience preceiving the role behavior.

For the aging population, role clarity—or the lack of it—has important historical meaning with subsequent consequences for the elderly today. In societies that are more traditional and/or rural, diversification among the group is less. Class structures and social positions are fewer. The length of time particular roles have existed is greater. This means that role expectations are more clearly defined and behaviors that relate to those roles are more stable. The individual can spend years preparing to participate in specific roles, depending on his or her status in life.

Most individuals in past traditional societies did not live to be old, but those who survived were frequently able to view a defined role toward which their behavior could be addressed. While these roles contained both positive and negative elements, the variety of roles was not as great as the number of elderly in modern society. In the United States, for instance, the first generation of retirees occurred during the 1950's. Few persons had retired before them; there were few clear-cut roles to play. Many of these individuals adjusted poorly to the new situation. Traditional societal roles of work were not available, yet new roles for the retiree had not emerged. Thus, forging new roles within the context of the larger society was difficult and confusing to many people; it was not until the 1960's, 70's, and 80's that new roles for retired people began taking shape.

The *number* and *quality* of roles refers to the various positions that an individual may occupy at any one time. Throughout the life span the number of roles an individual is expected to play varies. During early stages of life, the variety and number of separate and distinct roles are relatively small. These are primarily focused on the parent-child relationship.

As one moves from the intimate family surroundings, there is progress through an increasing variety and divergence of roles. The number expands, and questions arise about the compatibility of roles within the context of daily behavior. Role conflict and role strain can emerge when the individual is placed concurrently in two or more positions, each requiring contradictory role enactment. Two types of role conflict are interrole conflict and intrarole conflict. The former occurs when an individual finds that two simultaneous role behaviors have incompatible expectations, such as a friend asking one to help him cheat on an examination. The latter, intrarole conflict, involves contradictory expectations held by others about the same role, such as having a good time and making good grades. The greater the conflict among roles, the more difficult it becomes for the individual to adopt a consistent mode of behavior.

While similar to role clarity, the *number* of roles means that the sheer quantity of roles an individual is expected to play can vary at any one time and over time. One can have a larger or smaller number of roles depending on his or her circumstances. While variance among individuals occurs at all times and at all ages, deviation over time for the individual can have serious consequences. The later years are fraught with the possibility of a decline in the number of roles a person is expected to play. As Rosow (1973) states: "Role loss generates the pressures and sets the conditions for emerging crises, and taken together, these delineate the social context of the aging self." These challenges to role involvement are crucial to an individual's well-being. The ability and/or opportunity for individuals to maintain "normal" role involvement, based on previous patterns, is crucial to adjustment in old age. If roles are lost and not replaced, serious consequences can ensue for the individual.

In addition to the quantity of roles, quality of the roles played is also important. Not all roles have equal meaning for the person. The greater the importance of the role, the greater the hardship when the role is lost. Some persons, for instance, experience a considerable amount of role loss when their children leave home; for others, this is a relatively mild loss. The crucial variable is the centrality of the role. In the first instance, parenting was a central, important role and the loss of it required considerable adjustment. In the second instance, parenting was not the central role. The greater the centrality of a particular role, the more difficult the adaptation to its loss.

The environmental circumstances in which the roles are enacted is also important to understanding role losses and changes. Crucial to the enactment of any role is the social and physical environment in which that role exists. It is within this confluence that the individual has an audience for whom the role is played and the physical attributes necessary for adequate role enactment. In essence, "roles are social entities that define a certain range of behaviors for their occupants. To people both in and out of roles, these definitions are expectations that publicly locate their selves" (Gubrium, 1976). Roles do not exist in a vacuum, nor are they completely independent of the surrounding environment. There exists a person-environment transaction that involves transmitting environmental expectations of particular role behavior, individual perception and interpretation of these environmental conditions, and subsequent action and reaction to the process. To use the theatrical analogy, the actor is to play a defined role as prescribed by the author and director. The audience has expectations about how that role is to be played. As the actor portrays the role the audience reacts to his effort. The actor, in turn, responds to these reactions and he may or may not adjust the performance. Any break in this system, such as unclear roles, changes in audience expectations, or inaccurate assessment of audience reaction, can lead to a lack of "fit" between the actual performance and the reception of that performance. Agreement on the performance and accurate interpretation of it act to reinforce future aspects of the transaction.

For the aged, the conditions under which the roles are played may change as a result of variations in expectations. Societal expectations are not static. While some changes occur more rapidly than others, individuals are affected by subsequent variations. If the roles were static, then individuals could prepare themselves fully for future role occupancy. As new generations of elderly play out the roles and as external pressures exert themselves, future role participation will remain unclear.

In addition, it is possible for the interpretation of the audience reaction to break down. During the intake and interpretation phase of role enactment a considerable amount of emphasis is placed on accurate transmission of expectations. Some aging adults experience physical and mental conditions that inhibit the accurate interpretation of audience reactions. Changes in vision or hearing, or drug interactions, may impede accurate interpretation of the presenting stimuli. While the person would like to respond appropriately, failures in transmitting action often result in inappropriate responses. This breakdown causes consternation for the actor and for the audience. The actor may have assumed that the response was appropriate, only to discover that it was interpreted as inappropriate.

Finally, the context of role enactment can change. High mobility rates and changing neighborhoods cause variations in the environment in which the actor is located. Relocation, however slight, creates new social contexts; the transportability of one set of roles to a new situation may be questionable. New social groups may have differing prescriptions for behavior. Behavior appropriate in one group may be inappropriate in the new environmental context.

Even if the individual does not move, the conditions under which he or she plays the roles may change. Often, the aged live in transitional neighborhoods that experience an out-migration of peers and an in-migration of new and differing types of people. For many years the older person was integrated into his neighborhood, but changing circumstances now make him or her only the "old man" or "old lady" who lives down the street. The new neighbors judge them on the basis of new circumstances and new expectations and not upon the older, established roles and behavior.

Differing motives of the actor and the audience can also have an important influence on role behavior. A common assumption is that the motivational components of the interaction are similar. While in most cases this is probably true, in some instances the motivation of the two central actors is not only different, but is in opposition. *Role enactment* is overt social behavior of a person in a social setting. Covert reasons, however, influence the type of behavior that a person displays. For instance, an older adult may approach a health care provider with a specific request for treatment. The health provider judges this request based on the patient's actions. The presenting condition may indicate a particular illness or disablement for which a specific treatment is prescribed. Yet, upon further analysis, it is revealed that the underlying patient motivation is to receive the attention of the health care provider, not to achieve resolution of the condition. The extent to which underlying motivational components of behavior are understood and diagnosed is crucial to effective interaction with the elderly.

Unique characteristics relate to the fact that not all individuals react to the same set of role expectations in a similar manner. Role skills are characteristics possessed by the individual that result in effective and convincing role enactment. Like other skills, there is wide diversity among individuals in the enactment of particular roles. There are two main components of role skills: (1) cognitive abilities and (2) motor abilities.

In general, cognitive skills facilitate or retard role enactment. The ability of the individual to infer future reactions from available cues affects subsequent role response. Difficulty in processing cues, as noted earlier, is one problem; failure to be socialized to divergent situations is another. If the individual is unable to adopt the position of another person, participation is limited. If, however, the actor brings a wide diversity of response patterns, interaction within new and differing circumstances is enhanced.

The motor skills component is related to the expressive nature of the roles. Accurate portrayal of the role requires distinct vocal responses and precise motor responses. Posture, body movements, facial expressions, vocal tone, and amplitude are all important sources of information to the observer. As age intervenes, the physical ability to respond within the role context may decline, thus affecting subsequent judgment in the individual's role performance. While the roles themselves may change with age, so too may the individual's ability to perform them. Since these changes are highly individualistic, the behavior of any single person must be judged in the light of changing circumstances and individual limitations.

Major Role Changes

With this basic understanding of the concept of role, attention will now be focused on four major contexts within which role changes are likely to occur: the family, social relations, work groups, and societal involvement. These are considered to be the major areas of transition for the aging adult.

Changing Family Roles

Throughout life, involvement with the family both expands and contracts. Variables related to expansion include such things as marriage, and having children and grandchildren. Variables related to contraction include children leaving home, widowhood, and death of parents, siblings, aunts, and uncles. While not connected to age, many of these events occur at similar ages for most people. At age 20, it is typical to marry and have children. Around age 40, the children leave home. At ages 50 and 60, there is an increased likelihood that some family members will die.

Adjustment to changes and losses and the subsequent role changes is highly individualistic. The adjustment depends on the way the loss is perceived and on the ability to modify behavior to compensate for the loss. For some people, the fact that the children have grown and left home can be traumatic. The "empty nest," as it has been called, is difficult for those who oriented their life around the care and nurturance of their children. When the family role is very focused, such as the woman who does not work in order to care for the children, the burden of finding alternate meaningful activities can be difficult, particularly if no compensating role is developed.

It may be that the role of grandparent can replace some of the lost parental role. Work outside the home or accentuated emphasis on the couple relationsip can be used to fill the gap. However, with the current trend toward smaller family units and highly mobile offspring, the empty-nest reaction can be quite severe for some people.

The loss of family members due to death can be extremely difficult. When parents die, the grown child may feel alone in the world; no longer are the parents available for advice and counsel. The death of brothers, sisters, aunts, and uncles causes a shrinkage in the family world of aging individuals. The death of each family member causes the diminution of a number of family roles.

The most significant loss is that of a spouse. While remarriage in old age is becoming widely accepted, it is difficult to reestablish the same type of relationship that the person enjoyed for many years. This is particularly true for the widow. Longer life expectancy for women can mean that many older women will live the rest of their lives without the husband-wife relationship.

While the number of family roles differs according to individual circumstances, it is possible to at least partially list the major family roles that most people play throughout life. Table 2–1 depicts differing family roles at various ages and typical events which may occur that affect the number and quality of each set of roles. The roles reflect a hypothetical person who lives beyond the age of 80. Major life roles at each stage of life are italicized.

The table illustrates the range of roles that a person might play and the relative importance of different sets of roles. It is important to note that it is unlikely that a person would play the exact roles as portrayed. Roles are highly varied according to individual circumstances. There are differing roles at different ages and the importance of any *one* role must be judged in relation to other role involvements. It is also possible for the roles to place competing demands on behavior. It is highly likely that when the husband and wife are facing the financial crisis of sending a child to college, they

TABLE 2–1.—POSSIBLE CHANGING FAMILY ROLES

AGE	ROLES	EVENTS
Birth–20	*Son/daughter**, brother/sister, grandchild, niece/nephew	Birth of siblings
21–40	Son/daughter, brother/sister, grandchild, niece/nephew, aunt/uncle, *husband/wife*, *parent*	Marriage; children
41–60	Son/daughter, brother/sister, niece/nephew, aunt/uncle, *husband/wife*, parent, *grandparent*	Death of grandparent; children leave home
61–80	*Husband/wife*, parent, *grandparent*, aunt/uncle	Death of parents, aunt/uncle, brother/sister
81+	Parent, *grandparent*, *great-grandparent*, aunt/uncle	Death of spouse

*Roles shown in italics represent main differing family roles at various ages.

are also faced with the crisis of retiring parents. The competing demands in such a situation place a great deal of strain on family relationships and on the individual.

Understanding changing family roles, both from a current and from a historical perspective, can assist health care providers in working with older adults. The meaning attached to the role and the subsequent adjustment to this role change may have a long-lasting influence on the person's life. It is thus necessary to discuss the changing roles with the older adult to determine their influence on him. A good social history is, therefore, the key. A history that takes various stages of the person's life and tracks role changes and subsequent adjustments is crucial; this history delves into the meaning of the role for the individual and his feelings regarding changes in it.

Social Relations

Throughout life, people are involved with other people. Ranging in nature from close, intimate relationships to simple contact with other people, these relationships have considerable meaning for the people involved. It has been found, for instance, that people who lack social relationships are frequently depressed and have low morale. On the other hand, people who are able to maintain contact with others tend to be more cheerful and to feel better about themselves.

Not all social relationships have the same meaning, nor do all people have the same need for relationships. Some people are quite satisfied to have one or two persons with whom they share activities and interests, while others need a wide variety of people and numerous social activities. Early experiences in social relationships tend to influence our lifelong patterns. The child who learns early to depend on himself for entertainment may not need as many friends or acquaintances as the child who had early contact with a wide variety of people. This does not mean that the former does not need social relations, but rather that the breadth of relationships may be somewhat narrower.

The literature on social relationships typically distinguishes between intimate, close relationships on the one hand, and more distant, less intense relationships on the other. The most intimate type of relationship is with the *confidant*—one whom the individual trusts and with whom secrets are shared. Some evidence suggests that the number of confidants a person has is relatively small in number, but great in meaning. Various authors have noted that a confidant relationship is more closely related to good mental health and high morale than is high social interaction with many different people. For many people, the confidant is the spouse. For others, the confidant is one who has been a friend for a long time—long enough for a sense of trust to be built between the persons concerned.

The second type of relationship is *friendship*. People tend to have a number of close friends with whom they share activities and experiences, but where the relationships are not as intimate as with a confidant. Most friendships are among people who have similar characteristics. They tend, for instance, to be of the same sex, of similar age, and of approximately equal socioeconomic conditions.

When people are asked to state how many friends they have, they often list a large number of individuals; it is suspected that they frequently fail to distinguish between friends and acquaintances. The difference, however, is that friendship is based on a more personal and intimate level of interaction than acquaintanceship. Friends interact with each other over time and tend to perceive the relationship similarly. There is less formal involvement with friends than with acquaintances, and both participants receive some type of benefit from the interaction.

Not all friends supply the same needs for people. Some friendships may exist because they provide a particular type of stimulation to the person. One may have friends with which to share different experiences: friends who play bridge, friends who go to ball games, friends to have fun with, and friends with which to be serious. Typically, friends are people who are compatible with each other, who provide mutual aid and support. While the number of friends a person has may vary over time and geographic location, most people seek out friendship. Without friends, many people feel lost and lonely; they try to fill the void by seeking new friends to replace lost ones.

The third type of relationship is that of *acquaintance*. Most individuals have many other people whom they know and who know them. Based on a number of roles and interaction formalities, acquaintanceship is less personal and involves considerably less sharing. Acquaintances may include neighbors, fellow club members, and people at work. Whereas friendship and confidant relationships are based on intimacy and sharing, acquaintanceship is based on recognizing that various persons play a particular role within a social context.

Social Relations and Aging

The evidence on confidants, friendships, and acquaintanceships is mixed. Some authorities have contended that there is a shrinkage of the social world as one gets older, others have found a relatively similar pattern of social relationships at each stage of the life cycle. It seems to be apparent that people will maintain approximately the same number of social contacts throughout life if those social relationships are available. A reduction in the social world can ensue if the person is unable to continue previous activities or if there are fewer possible people with whom to engage. In the former case, serious illness, lack of transportation, or lack of motivation may affect the individual, limiting the ability to "get out" and make friends. The bedridden individual, for instance, may be unable to attend a monthly club meeting. This can cause a reduction in the overall amount of interaction that is undertaken. It is a highly individualistic occurrence, but tends to be found more often among the aged, particularly the very old. Within this group the possibility of accumulating various impediments to interaction is increased and the likelihood of a reduced social world is enhanced.

Where a reduction in the number of possible people with whom to form relationships has occurred, shrinkage of the social world is external to the individual. The death of friends, neighbors, siblings, and spouse can limit the person's social world. If one is unable to reestablish meaningful social contacts, there can be a reduction in overall social involvement. Most of the time, new friends and acquaintances can be made; however, there are occasions when the person simply is unable to find someone to take the place of someone who died. High school friends, for instance, who continue a close personal relationship throughout life can never be replaced. For the individual this means a loss of one source of emotional release and support.

Both the inability of the person to relate to other people and the absence of people with which to relate are closely associated. Illness in the older person may be accompanied by the death of a friend. These multiple losses increase the probability that the social world of the older adult will shrink, and even when new relationships are formed, they may not fulfill the needs of the individual. If a person had a few very good friends who died, a large number of acquaintances may not have the same meaning in his life.

Reduction in the number of contacts can have serious consequences for an individual. Isolation and loneliness may ensue. While isolation is not always accompanied by loneliness and loneliness is not always accompanied by isolation, the two tend to be found together. It is possible for an isolated person not to be lonely. Some people relish the opportunity to be away from people; they may be "loners" whose need for social interaction is relatively small. It is also possible to be among people and be lonely. Loneliness stems from the desire of the person to have social contact that is perceived as meaningful. Someone who desires a confidant, but only has a large number of acquaintances, has a need that is not being met.

The separation of a person from others can often have serious consequences for all relationships. As noted earlier, one learns how to be a sociable adult. It is theoretically possible that lack of practice in social skills can cause a diminution of these skills, which may result in an inability to participate socially when the opportunity arises. Take, for instance, the cues that people give each other through conversation. If one person is boring another, there is a well-developed system to indicate boredom such as looking at a watch, giving a pained expression, closing the eyes, yawning, and perhaps even leaving. All cues are transmitted to the person talking. A fully socialized individual can regularly pick up transmitted cues and act accordingly; the conversation can be changed, the other person can be encouraged to communicate, or the cues can be ignored. Individuals who have lost some of their interactive skills, such as an extremely isolated person, may not perceive the transmitted cues and thus continue to bore the listener. Or personal concerns can be so preemptive that cues are ignored. Whatever the case, this behavior soon destroys the possibility of future interaction and can cause increasing isolation because other people avoid individuals who exhibit such social behavior.

In addition to the isolation and loneliness that result from the loss of social involvements, other losses occur. Since confidants, friends, and acquaintances frequently assist each other in normal activities and crises, the loss of these relationships may mean that no one is available to assist the older person in a time of need. Much national attention has been focused on the formal and informal support networks that surround the elderly. The informal support system is typically composed of family members, friends, and neighbors who assist the elderly in various ways. Loss of the social network challenges the resources of older persons and seriously jeopardizes their adaptive ability. What can an older person do if there are no friends or acquaintances around to assist him in obtaining needed help? The result is that already taxed resources may be strained to the breaking point.

Finally, the absence of friends, confidants, and acquaintances may result in detachment of the person from the society at large. Without social interaction and communication, it is quite possible that a person will become increasingly introspective. Concern over bodily functions can become important. Total withdrawal from society may occur.

Work Groups

Throughout the major portion of adult life, most people are involved in some type of gainful employment. This employment dominates life for 40 to 50 years. The main portion of working hours during the week are spent either directly at work or indirectly thinking about it. An individual's job can define time and set a structure to his life pattern. Vacation time is determined by the constraints of work. Lifestyle is directly related to the amount of money earned through work efforts. Conversations among strangers usually begin with the question, "What do you do for a living?"

While attachments to a job are not always of the same intensity, the domination of work over various other aspects of life is evident. A worker may not feel emotionally involved in the work he does, but it does require him to be present at a certain time and to leave when the work day is over. Because financial reimbursement is at a set level, the amount of money available is necessarily limited. Even if the worker is totally enamored with the job, the constraints, though perceived differently, are still there. Certain times must be set for work-related activity; certain expectations of employment must be met.

As a person ages, a number of changes take place in his means of making a living. New employees rarely start out at the top of a profession. After a period of service, advancement may come. Peak earnings, responsibility, and authority may be reached by midlife. Later, retirement occurs. Each of these transitions represents changes in income, responsibility, and work roles. As a person gains authority, he or she may be more widely respected, move into different circles of employee relationships, and, in general, perceive the work role as central to his life.

With the growing establishment of private and public pension plans, an increasing number of people are able to retire from an active work role. Before these pensions became widely available, most people continued a pattern of work until their physical state precluded continued employment. Today, more and more people are able to retire and to spend a number of years not monetarily employed or having life oriented toward a job structure. In recent years, the average age for retirement has declined to about 60 years of age. This means that an ever-expanding number of people must redirect their lives and spend considerable time out of the work environment.

The meaning of a lost work role is, of course, different for different people. Some people react to retirement with anticipation; others reject even the possibility that they may have to retire. Various individuals adjust to the postretirement period quite well while others never adjust. Some people involve themselves in alternate activities; others simply sit out their retirement years.

The adaptation to retirement appears to be related to a number of variables. One such variable is the decision to retire. Contrary to popular belief, most people retire voluntarily from active employment. Contingent on the perception that they will have enough income to provide a satisfactory lifestyle after they retire, many people look forward to doing so in order to have more free time. A number of people retire because of poor health.

Frequently, the myth that retirement "kills" people is related to the fact that people with poor health retire. Retirement is not the precipitator of death; the ill health that forced the retirement is the major factor. Preretirement planning is also related to the decision to retire. The greater the amount of planning, the more likely it is that a person will retire voluntarily. With more favorable predisposing factors influencing retirement, the greater the probability of adjustment to that role. Those who look forward to retirement are generally better adjusted when they do so than persons who reject the idea.

The process of retirement may have a number of serious consequences for the person involved. First, there is a reduction in the amount of money available for spending; the greater the disparity between preretirement and postretirement income, the greater the difficulty in adaptation. People who are able to maintain an income close to that previously obtained suffer only minor alterations in lifestyle. Available funds can continue to be spent on activities and interests that have been a lifelong pattern, thus decreasing the possibility of curtailing activities. People who experience a drastic reduction of income must redefine their spending priorities and, as a consequence, must alter their lifestyle.

Second, because work frequently defines the manner in which time is distributed throughout the week, retirement means a restructuring of time spent on various activities. No longer is time spent on the job, preparing to go to the job, or relaxing after the work day. The emphasis on alternate activities forces the individual to gain gratification from non-work-related activities, similar to that obtained from work. Evidence indicates that most people are able to do this, particularly if they have preretirement activities in which they can continue to engage.

Third, retirement affects the manner in which a person perceives himself, especially when he had strongly identified with the work role. Individuals who gain a great deal of personal satisfaction from being the "boss" or from being "in charge" may not have this role after retirement. If such a person is unable to achieve a similar feeling of importance from retirement activities, questions about feelings of worth can affect the way he feels about himself.

Loss of Work Group

A final factor in the retirement process is loss of involvement with people in the work world. Regardless of occupational status, many people form interpersonal relationships within the work environment that may be difficult to replace after retirement. While such relationships are not always friendships, people can become used to having others around with whom they share experiences. The mutual sharing that occurs, particularly when they have worked together for a long time, may establish a bond among work mates that is difficult to replace.

Loss of the work role means curtailed involvement with the work group. No longer does the retiree share work experiences with fellow workers; upon visiting the place of work after retirement, he may not be able to actively engage in work-related conversation. Other workers may retire or move on so that the retiree is no longer familiar with all the faces in the work environment.

The loss of interpersonal involvement can have a major impact on subsequent adjustment. If the individual is unable to develop a new circle of individuals with mutual interests, he or she may feel lonely and detached from the surrounding social world, and may feel that there is no one around who can discuss common issues—no one who is stimulating. Regret at the loss of social involvement at the work site can create depression and the belief that no one is really interested in his or her knowledge or experience, any longer.

The retiree must also alter the focus of his or her own behavior. For many years, the employee orients existing behavior toward what is acceptable to the work situation; if the job requires wearing a suit and tie, the worker wears a suit and tie, or if the job requires cocktails at five, one has cocktails at five o'clock. When the work role is lost, these expectations of work-related behavior are no longer in force. The social group is no longer available to guide individual behavior. Is a suit and tie to be worn? Do cocktails start at five? Without the reinforcement of a group consensus regarding behavior, the individual must develop his or her own mode of action—sometimes in a deviant manner.

Societal Involvement

Throughout life, behavior is patterned toward other human beings, both through intimate personal relationships and through less intimate, more formal relationships. As noted previously, one of the principal elements in structuring life is work involvement. There are, however, additional activities that influence the manner in which one conducts daily living. For the most part, these are other associational involvements contracted at various times such as social or recreational clubs, organizational membership, church and religious activities, or political participation.

These associations tend to be composed of individuals who share common interests; they are often focused toward achievement of a particular goal or activity. People join these groups for various reasons, but usually they share the motivation of other group members for the accomplishment of a goal. For instance, one joins religious groups for the purpose of sharing faith and participation in religious rituals. The degree to which the organization is active in achieving the group goal and satisfying its membership often determines whether or not individual participation is maintained. Failure to achieve the goal or lack of consensus about what the goal should be often causes disillusionment with the group.

While motivation to join groups often comes from perceived similarity between individual goals and group goals, many other things happen within the group that enhance participation. Frequent social interactions with members may lead to a commitment to group participation. It is possible that the overall group goal that led to initial membership becomes secondary to the desire for interaction with group members. Mutual sharing that occurs may lead to a feeling of camaraderie among group members that transcends the initial motivation for joining the group. The group may become an anchor by which behavior external to the group is determined.

Group membership may provide the member with a number of motivators that enhance continued participation. First, belonging to the group may give the individual a sense of being somebody, of having a place in society. While not all group members participate at the same level, identification as a member often enhances the individual's sense of self-worth.

Second, continued interaction can lead to a sense of mutual sharing. The reciprocity that evolves provides the individual with a feeling that he or she has something important to contribute to the group, even if it is only attending group functions. The role or roles that the individual plays within the group frequently heightens the members' self-interest.

Third, through participation within the group, communication on various topics is often improved. Many organizations have newsletters in which important events that are meaningful to group members are shared. Often, people look forward to this form of communication. Checking the mailbox for important communications can become a daily ritual.

Fourth, for many group members the organizational attachment becomes a vehicle for sharing ideas without fear of harsh sanctions. Since most groups narrow their conversational range, members soon learn which topics are acceptable to the group and which are not. Knowledge of the range of topics appropriate to the group increases the probability that the member can express his or her views on a particular issue. For instance, participation in a conservative political group will enhance the likelihood that members will express conservative political opinions without fear of criticism by nongroup members. This can give the person an avenue of release for many ideas without the subsequent embarrassment of being out of place.

Finally, groups and organizations frequently create identifiable symbols that members share. These can range from badges to identification cards to secret signals that transmit to other members a sense of mutual sharing. By knowing about these shared symbols, the group member can show that he has a broader attachment to the world beyond himself. This can be reinforced by participation in group meetings, travel to other chapters, or sharing of mutual ideas when two members meet outside the group context.

Of course, not all groups have a highly developed set of external norms, internal communications, or other more formal activities. Some organizations tend to be rather loose confederations of people with similar interests who may not even meet formally. These groups do, however, contribute to the individual's sense of participation in the larger society. Perhaps a good example of this type of affiliation would be a group of people who share a common hobby. While they may not get together for meetings, they perhaps read the same journals and attend the same conventions. When chance meetings occur, there is a common focus of attention and acceptance based on shared knowledge.

Loss of Social Involvement

Research evidence suggests that attachments to informal and formal organizational groups constitutes a pattern established very early on that tends to be maintained throughout life. Some people join a large number of organizations; others, relatively few. The principal voluntary association is church-related with the majority of people having some type of religious affiliation. Other affiliations tend to be related to work, hobby groups, or social-oriented organizations.

The typical pattern of participation appears to be that while the organization is available and one has the ability to continue contributing, participation will continue. When the organization is no longer available to the member or when environmental factors restrict his ability to participate, organizational attachments are lost. It is possible that a group will disband after the accomplishment of its stated goal. Unless a new goal can be substituted for the one accomplished, there is no real purpose for continued association with the group and it usually dissolves.

If the person cannot continue participation, perhaps due to physical or financial limitations, active involvement in the group may dissipate. Attachment may continue, such as watching religious programs on television, but the reinforcement of the group is not available. Internal motivation must be maintained by the individual. The positive rewards of mutual discussion and recognition of individual worth provided by group members must be intrinsically satisfied by the individual's self-satisfaction and internal rewards.

Departure of a group member is also affected by the way that participation is terminated. Voluntary dissociation is much more satisfying to the individual than involuntary dissociation; the group member who decides not to participate in the group believes that the decision is correct.

Involuntary group withdrawal can seriously affect the individual's feelings about himself or herself and others. Unable to participate with other group members, the individual may feel detached from the larger society. No longer receiving positive group reinforcement, feeling cut off from participation, the individual can become isolated and withdrawn.

Typically, in the aging population, social contacts and group participation are maintained until the person can no longer actively participate. Breakdowns in physical health, transportation resources, and financial stability can cause increasing numbers of elderly to withdraw from group participation. Since these tend to be involuntary actions, withdrawal can be traumatic. A sense of loss may ensue. They may feel that no one really cares about or is interested in them. Time can weigh heavily on them since no one is available with whom to discuss issues of concern.

Conclusions

The importance of understanding role changes and role losses among the elderly is twofold. First, by recognizing common role changes that occur as individuals age, the health care provider can gain a heightened awareness of the changing environmental and individual circumstances of the elderly for whom care is to be provided. This, in turn, can help the provider to understand the context in which care is provided. Knowledge of the patient's history and an understanding of individual motives and motivations can aid in developing appropriate intervention techniques that can be adjusted to individual circumstances. This enhances the probability of effective rehabilitation.

Second, through knowledge of the changing situations of the elderly, the health care provider can work toward the resolution of current problems and the prevention of future ones. Frequently, health care providers fail to consider the future circumstances of the older population. In an attempt to address the immediate medical crises, the need for future and long-range health care is often overlooked. Through the use of information about situations that may arise, patients can be helped to anticipate and prepare for the future through rational planning.

Finally, it is important to remember that diversity among the elderly is greater than homogeneity. All elderly patients are individuals with historical roots; they must continue to be perceived as such and responded to appropriately. Stereotypical responses will not help achieve better living conditions for ourselves and for the elderly.

REFERENCES

Atchley R.C.: Issues in retirement research. *Gerontologist* 19(no.1):44–54, 1979.

Atchley R.C.: *The Social Forces in Later Life*. Belmont, Calif., Wadsworth Publishing Co., 1972.

Breytspraak L.M.: *Self-Concept in Adulthood: Emergent Issues and the Response of the Symbolic Interactionist Perspective*. Gerontological Society Annual Meeting, Louisville, October 1975.

Burnside I.M.: Loss: A constant theme in group work with the aged. *Hosp. Community Psychiatry* 21:173–177, 1970.

Cameron P.: *Self-Centeredness in Adulthood*. Gerontological Society Meeting, Portland, Ore., October 1974.

Carroll K. (ed.): *Compensating for Changes and Losses*. Minneapolis, Human Development in Aging Project, NIMH Grant No. 23924, 1978.

Friedmann E.A., Orbach H.: Adjustment to retirement, in *American Handbook of Psychiatry*, vol. 1. New York, Basic Books, 1974.

Gubrium J.: *Time, Roles, and Self in Old Age*. New York, Human Sciences Press, 1976.

Hunter S., Powers E.A., Bultena G.: The confidant: An anchor in a problematic world? *Sociology Report* 95. Ames, Iowa State University, 1972.

Lowenthal M.F., Thurnher M., Chiriboga D.: *Four States of Life*. San Francisco, Jossey-Bass Publishing Co., 1975.

Peretti P.O., Wilson C.: Voluntary and involuntary retirement of aged males . . . . *Int. J. Aging Hum. Dev*. 6(2):269–275, 1975.

Powers E., Bultena G.L.: *Sex Differences in Intimate Friendships in Old Age*. Gerontological Society Meeting, Portland, Ore., November 1974.

Rosow I.: The social context of the aging self. *Gerontologist* 13(No. 1):82–87, 1973.

Shanas E.: Social myth as hypothesis: The case of the family relations of old people. *Gerontologist* 19(No. 1):3–10, 1979.

3

IMPROVING COMMUNICATION WITH OLDER ADULTS

Rickey L. George, Ph.D.
Therese Cristiani, Ed.D.

THOSE WHO WORK frequently with older adults often fail to remember that they share with other humans the need to be recognized as being important. Like everyone else, they have two basic self-concept needs that may appear contradictory: (1) the need to be seen as being different, as having unique qualities that make them worthy of some kind of special recognition; and (2) the need to be seen as being the same, as having feelings, attitudes, and beliefs that are acceptable and normal. Everyone has fears that result from these two needs, although the fears may intensify in reaction to the aging process. Such fears generally revolve around two main insecurities:

1. Am I becoming just another older person, with nothing to offer and nothing to give and, therefore, of little importance to others?
2. Am I becoming "strange" as I grow older, with abnormal feelings and reactions to events and situations?

Older adults share with all of us the dual needs of feeling important and feeling acceptable. Whether or not these needs are met is largely a result of the quality of interpersonal relations that older adults experience on a day-to-day basis. Unfortunately, the psychological stress that typically accompanies the aging process makes it more difficult for these needs to be met.

Increasing physical changes often cause older adults to feel "left out," as they miss more of the interactions that occur. These changes often begin with a slowed pace, with movements frequently limited by stiffening in the joints. This slower pace is then intensified by a slower reaction time so that the elderly often become slower in responding to a stimulus, which makes the timing of the response a little late and thus sometimes inappropriate.

A slower reaction time also generalizes to communication, when the older adult may be slow in responding to verbal stimuli. Added to this difficulty is a decline in hearing and sight that usually accompanies the aging process. Since humans normally depend a great deal on their visual and auditory functions to interpret messages sent to them by others, sensory losses of aging greatly interfere with the communication process.

These physical changes that result from aging often cause a feeling of being handicapped or different, and lead to a greater sense of loneliness. At the same time, the aged often believes that because of the slower pace and the difficulties in communication, others consider him a burden or obligation. In response, the older adult may withdraw, thus incurring greater loneliness.

Changes in social roles resulting from job retirement and an accompanying "retirement" from active roles in churches and other organizations often have an immense impact on the older adult's self-concept. This role change seems to have a more serious impact on men, who no longer are "breadwinners" and who feel they have nothing to contribute. Women frequently experience a similar change when their children grow up and leave home. However, retirement usually does not have quite as great an impact on women since their traditional roles are not altered as much. Houses still must be cleaned, meals must be cooked, and laundry must be done. If the grandchildren live close enough for occasional babysitting, the woman's retirement role can be perceived as meaningful. At the same time, the role of the older adult—for both men and women—is changing and these changes often concern the individual's feeling of diminished importance, of having less and less to offer. Chapter Two on role changes provides an in-depth analysis of this issue.

Accompanying these physical and social role changes are great losses for the elderly. Their hopes and aspirations for success, for leaving legacies to society, and perhaps for leaving a comfortable inheritance to their families may no longer be realistic. At the same time, their loss of income may intensify the fear that their savings will not last long enough, and cause them to be a burden to their families. These losses, along with a loss of meaning and purpose to their lives, generally have much less impact than the loss caused by the deaths of spouses, siblings, and close friends. The grief generated by such losses is often intensified by various other emotional responses, such as anger, guilt, and fear.

As older adults face these increasingly difficult situations, they are often losing the source of emotional support they need. The deaths mentioned above often isolate them. In their desire both to be independent and to avoid being a burden to their families, older adults may discourage their families from too much contact, leading to a greater sense of isolation and loneliness; or they may react to their situation by whining or complaining. Thus, at the time they desire and need their families most, the elderly may push them away. Emotional problems of the elderly can become greater because they lack someone with whom to talk. In some cases, the health care provider may be one of the few individuals available with whom the older adult can talk about his fears and anxieties, his loneliness and depression. Helping professionals who work with the elderly have an important responsibility to establish meaningful communication to alleviate the psychological stress being faced and thus reduce its effect on physical problems.

Barriers To Communication

Effective communication occurs when the intent and the effect of interpersonal interaction are identical, for the meaning of a message to be perceived as it was intended requires that the two individuals involved must have similar perceptions regarding the message. Unfortunately, some verbal responses made by practitioners actually block communication, since these responses are usually interpreted differently than intended and because these responses often act as barriers to further communication. Gordon (1974) identified a number of response patterns that serve as barriers to communication. A few of these are particularly important to those who work with older adults.

Giving Advice

Offering older adults advice often has the effect of making them feel that they are no longer capable of coping with their own problems, thus serving to increase their dependence on others.

Moralizing and Preaching

When moralizing or preaching, the health care provider is evaluating the older adult's behavior and indicating what he "ought" to do or how he "should" feel. The effect of moralizing is often guilt, which frequently makes the older adult feel as if he or she is no longer capable of making moral decisions. By attempting to alter the aging person's behavior in the direction of the practitioner's value system, the health care provider is failing to understand the older adult's world from his perspective.

Analyzing and Diagnosing

Analyzing and diagnosing a problem may easily be an example of ineffective and nonaccepting communication because it also puts the practitioner in the position of viewing the older adult's problem from an external, objective frame of reference.

Judging or Criticizing

When a health care provider judges or criticizes the older adult, the person typically withdraws and withholds further information or feelings. Also, further guilt is often induced.

By working to avoid responses that block communication, the health care provider is able to establish a more open psychological environment where older adults are willing to discuss the fears and anxieties that are central to their lives. By not shutting off the older adult, a more understanding attitude is conveyed and the older person is likely to feel accepted as a normal human being.

Skills For Improving Communication

It has been demonstrated that certain skills are clearly associated with effective communication. These skills, frequently used in close relationships, are often ignored when helping professionals work with older adults. Although not highly sophisticated, these skills are very important if communication with older adults is to be improved.

Warmth and Positive Regard

Warmth, defined interpersonally, simply means showing an interest in others. At a more effective level, warmth refers to the importance of the helper's ability to genuinely prize the older adult as a person of worth and dignity. This appreciation is demonstrated by the way the helper interacts with the older person both verbally and nonverbally.

Nonverbally, warmth may be communicated by:

Turning toward the speaker
Ceasing an activity
Showing interest by facial expression
Moving toward a speaker
Appropriate eye contact
Appropriate voice tone
A touch on the hand, arm, or shoulder

Although most people have some awareness of the impact of their nonverbal behavior, health care practitioners must constantly review their own actions to determine if they are conveying what they wish to convey. Good attending behaviors (those used when listening to another) are one example. These behaviors—such as eye contact, posture, facial expression, and body movements—are typically carried out without much forethought. Yet they make a powerful impression on the listener. When a person communicates genuine interest by giving another his undivided attention, the relationship is greatly strengthened. Since older adults often feel that others have no time for them, using good attending behavior helps to counteract this negative attitude.

Many health care providers would benefit from experiencing firsthand both the negative reactions to poor attending and the positive reactions to good attending. Note the next time you talk to someone who continues to read or doodle or look around the room. You are likely to feel annoyed, disgusted, or frustrated, but, most important, you will probably feel that the other person is uninterested in you. Perhaps you would talk louder or softer, faster or slower, as a way to capture the other's interest. Another situation that can be disconcerting is when someone talks to *you* while looking around the room, or at least does not look at you. The reaction again is likely to be that the other is really not interested in talking to you.

Care must also be given to facial expression. Social psychologists have accumulated considerable evidence suggesting that listeners respond more often to our facial expression and voice inflection than to the words spoken. One way to check this is to say "yes" while shaking your head from side to side; you could also try determining the feeling the other is expressing and then show that feeling in your facial expression. Check the results by noting how this affects the speaker or by asking the speaker for her or his reactions. By experiencing firsthand their own reactions to certain behavior, health care providers may become more careful in utilizing attending behaviors to convey genuine interest in the older adult.

Good attending behaviors have many benefits. They make it easier to listen and remember since you focus all your attention on the person. These behaviors facilitate self-exploration by older adults through reinforcing their openness and self-disclosure. They enhance the self-respect of older adults, encouraging them to feel better about themselves because the health care provider is giving them energy, time, and attention. In addition, use of good attending behaviors models appropriate behavior. As a result, older adults can become better listeners and thus be more helpful to each other.

Warmth can also be shown by asking leading questions (especially if such queries are followed by listening to the answers) and by using encouraging actions, such as head nods, "hmm hmm," "Really," or "Tell me more." Basically, then, warmth is a way of telling the older adult, "Hey, I have time for you." Sometimes practitioners will *tell* older adults they are interested in listening. However, their nonverbal expressions of uninterest, impatience, or concern with time say otherwise. In interpersonal relationships, too, actions speak louder than words.

It can be difficult to communicate warmth toward some older adults. The whining, complaining, criticizing older adult is not easy to approach. However, communicating warmth to such an individual may bring about behavior change, since that person's irritating behaviors may result from feelings of being unwanted and unimportant. By communicating warmth, the health care provider may contribute a more positive self-image, and, therefore, a more positive attitude.

It is unlikely that older persons could get too much attention and caring communicated by "warmth" behaviors. More likely, there are many times when professional responsibilities cause the practitioner to be too busy or in too big a hurry to spend much time with the person. By combining warmth with self-disclosure, however, it is possible for the practitioner to communicate caring and still move on to other activities. For example:

Older adult: "Can I talk to you now?"
Practitioner: (turning toward the person, smiling, looking directly into the other's eyes) "I can't right now, Mrs. Jones. I have this job to do. But I"ll be happy to talk with you later."

By combining positive nonverbal behaviors with a negative verbal message, the health care provider is still able to communicate warmth and caring. The basic message is still "You're important, but I must do other things right now." Of course, if the practitioner is *always* too busy, the positive nonverbal behavior will soon be meaningless. Unless the nonverbal messages are perceived as real and genuine by the other person, no warmth is communicated.

Genuineness and Self-disclosure

When communicating with older people, a high level of trust is critical to the relationship. While several factors influence the development of trust in any helping relationship, the ability of the practitioner to be open, honest, and direct in communicating with the elderly is of utmost importance. In other words, the practitioner must appear as a concerned person who is not hiding behind a "helper role." The ability to relate without this professional front or facade is what is meant by the practitioner's *genuineness*. Health care providers who are genuine do not hide behind a mask. They can communicate a "realness" in the relationship with an older adult that facilitates the development of trust.

What does it mean to be honest and direct in our communication with others? Primarily, it means that we present our communication directly and unambiguously. We are more self-disclosing than self-concealing (Combs, 1971). We share ourselves openly and honestly, allowing others to see us as we truly are—to know our feelings, thoughts, and reactions. This type of communication is typically characterized by a degree of spontaneity. Thoughts and feelings are shared as they are experienced; our verbal responses match our internal feelings.

This process of being open and direct in communication, revealing feelings and reactions to events and people as they occur, has been referred to as *self-disclosure*. Self-disclosure, from this definition, means sharing intimate details of one's past only as this information is relevant to a clear understanding of the present. Thus, it is not necessary for the practitioner to make personal confessions related to past experiences unless the information will clarify present behavior and feelings.

Self-disclosure is dependent on the practitioner's self-awareness and self-acceptance (Johnson, 1972). In other words, we cannot share our experiences in the present if we are not in touch with our feelings; we must have a high level of self-awareness to be able to share spontaneously. Likewise, we must not only be aware of internal reactions, feelings, and thoughts, but also must not be threatened by them. We must be accepting of ourselves, our thoughts and feelings, if we are to share them with others.

What role does practitioner genuineness and self-disclosure play in work with older adults? We have mentioned that genuineness and self-disclosure are fundamental to the establishment of trust in the relationship. As elderly people seek help for the various difficulties associated with aging, they need someone with whom they feel safe and secure. They need to be able to reach out and share the intimate details of their experiences. They must feel that the person who listens to their concerns is someone they can trust with those parts of themselves that are most difficult to share. The practitioner's security with himself or herself allows the older adult to experience the same sense of security in the relationship.

The health care provider's ability to be honest and direct with the older person promotes greater depth in the relationship by encouraging closeness and intimacy. In other words, through self-disclosure the helper may share honest reactions with the older adult. This type of positive confrontation can greatly facilitate personal growth, since it encourages the older person to explore personal issues and behaviors that may be hindering other relationships. This risk-taking behavior promotes intimacy and moves communication to a new level (George & Cristiani, 1981).

Another reason self-disclosure is important in working with older people is that some may be hesitant to share very personal matters such as those related to sexuality or financial difficulties. It is often helpful in these instances for practitioners to communicate acceptance and understanding by sharing brief personal examples from their own lives that involve similar reactions and feelings. For example, a widow in her mid-60s might present the following situation:

Older adult: My husband passed away a few years ago. We had been married for 25 years. Sex was never a big part of our relationship. Now I'm starting to date and I'm just not feeling very comfortable. It's so awkward to be with another man.

Practitioner: (a remarried divorcee): I remember the struggles I had after my divorce, before I remarried. I felt so awkward dating and yet I had so many physical needs. I found it so difficult to cut off my sexuality, yet I just couldn't get involved without experiencing so much guilt.

In this example, the practitioner uses self-disclosure to relate a similar experience. In so doing, the client is made to feel more comfortable because the health care provider has acknowledged similar feelings and experiences. Additionally, the helper has discarded a professional role or facade and has become a real person in the relationship—one who engenders trust, safety, and security. Since the older adult's level of risk-taking has been reciprocated, the relationship can move forward and greater emotional risks can be taken.

Self-disclosure, while highly effective in promoting the helping relationship, should be used carefully. It can be difficult for two reasons: the practitioner's experience must closely resemble that of the older adult's and the practitioner must disclose enough information to draw the similarity, but not so much that focus of the discussion shifts to the helper (George & Cristiani, 1981).

Empathic Understanding

As human beings, we all experience the need to be completely understood. It seems that we rarely experience that moment when another person has so carefully listened to our feelings, thoughts, and perceptions that we feel totally understood. At this moment in a relationship our unique experience has been clearly understood by another person and we feel we are not alone. *Empathy* is this ability to adopt another's internal frame of reference so that his or her private world and its meanings are accurately understood and can be communicated back clearly.

In order to respond empathically, the health care provider must be both sensitive to the older adult's feelings and able to identify reasons for those feelings. In other words, empathy concerns the ability to hear and respond to another's feelings of depression, loneliness, fear, isolation, joy, excitement, relief, and so on. The ability to accurately identify another's feelings increases the individual's feeling of being understood. As others listen to us, as our feelings are heard and responded to, we are more capable of accurately "hearing" ourselves.

Empathy also involves a nonevaluative attitude on the part of the health care provider. If we listen carefully enough to adopt another's internal frame of reference, we are forced to suspend judgment and criticism of their thoughts, feelings, attitudes, values, and behaviors. We are more capable of viewing another's world as it appears to them, and we are thus less likely to evaluate the "rightness" or "wrongness" of their experiences. The most powerful factor in empathic understanding is thus the communication of acceptance of the other person in the relationship.

The therapeutic value of acceptance cannot be overstated. If we risk sharing the most intimate and threatening aspects of ourselves and share feelings and thoughts that have been unacceptable to us and perhaps denied awareness, this risk needs to be met with unconditional acceptance and understanding. We will then be free to grow and change. Rogers (1961) has described very clearly the therapeutic value of acceptance in his formulation of an "If—Then" hypothesis: He stated that if the helping professional could establish a relationship characterized by genuineness and transparency, by warm acceptance and prizing, and by empathic understanding of the other's world, then that other individual would experience and understand aspects of self that previously had been repressed, leading to greater self-direction, self-confidence, self-understanding, and self-acceptance. As a result, the person would be able to cope with the problems of life more adequately and more comfortably.

As noted in this hypothesis, acceptance on the part of the practitioner frees the client to grow and change. We must fully accept ourselves before we can move in a more positive direction.

While empathy is most fundamentally an *attitude* of understanding and acceptance, it is also a *skill* that can be learned. An example of an empathic response follows:

Older adult:	"Jim Patterson died last Friday. I just don't understand it. Just the other day, he was out mowing the lawn and now he's gone. He was only 73."
Health care provider:	"It must make you feel really sad and depressed to watch friends die. It must be kind of scary, too, to realize you're not getting any younger."

In this response the practitioner identified several feelings the older adult was experiencing—sadness, depression, and fear. As shown in this example, the feelings were not expressed directly; rather, the practitioner inferred them from the content of the response, as well as the nonverbal communication of the client.

Learning to respond empathically involves several steps. First, the health care provider must identify the primary feeling the older adult is expressing, verbally and nonverbally. Second, the content of the statement made by the older adult must be accurately paraphrased. This normally involves listening to several sentences and then summarizing the most important points in one sentence. The final step is to identify the stimulus for the feeling. In other words, an empathic response is an attempt to respond accurately to the *reason* the person is experiencing the expressed feeling.

In summary, empathic responses are very powerful facilitators of communication. Older adults do not differ from the rest of the population in their need to be clearly and accurately understood, and to be prized and valued for being who they are.

Summary

Health care practitioners for the elderly must recognize the importance of communication in health care delivery. Older adults must be handled in a caring manner in which they feel respected as human beings if they are to respond most fully to the health care provided.

The communication process can be improved by establishing trust and by accepting the older adult's feelings without judgment or denial. Most important, the practitioner must communicate genuineness and empathic understanding. The result is that older adults retain a sense of personal worth, feel they are not alone in handling the stress from changes that accompany the aging process. Rather, they can be given the feeling they are important enough that others will take the time and care to help them explore and accept their fears, anxieties, loneliness, and depression.

REFERENCES

Combs A.W., Avila D.L., Purkey W.W.: *Helping Relationships*. Boston, Allyn & Bacon, 1971.

Gazda G.M., Walters R.P., Childers W.C.: *Human Relations Development: A Manual for Health Science*. Boston, Allyn & Bacon, 1974.

George R.L., Cristiani T.S.: *Theory, Methods, and Processes of Counseling and Psychotherapy*. Englewood Cliffs, N.J., Prentice-Hall, 1981.

Gordon T.: *T.E.T.: Teacher Effectiveness Training*. New York, David McKay Co., 1974.

Johnson D.W.: *Reaching Out: Interpersonal Effectiveness and Self-Actualization*. Englewood Cliffs, N.J., Prentice-Hall, 1972.

Rogers C.: *On Becoming A Person*. Boston, Houghton Mifflin Co., 1961.

4

PUBLIC POLICIES FOR THE AGED

Philip K. Armour, Ph.D.

Social Change and the Aging Society

THE GROWING POPULATION of older Americans poses particular and painful problems for policymakers in all modern societies. This aged population, as measured by the percentage of people 65 and over, has grown steadily as birth rates have fallen in nations that have experienced the interrelated social and economic processes of urbanization and industrialization. Old people have become a population in need in modern societies and have become the force for expansion of health and welfare services and income security programs (Wilensky, 1975). For example, during the past decade in the United States, the population 65 and over grew by 20%, while the overall population grew by only 13%; as a percentage of the U.S. population, persons 65 and over increased from 3.1% in 1900 to 11% in 1978. Other industrial societies have surpassed this percentage; for example, in Sweden 14% of the population is 65 and older. Projections are that the United States will probably achieve the Swedish level of 14% in 2015 (Schulz, 1980).

Examination of these trends in the aging population in terms of percentage of increase from 1977 through 2000 suggests that there will be significant increases in the very old among all persons 65 and over. From 1977 to 2000, the 65 and over age group will increase by 35%; but within that age group, persons 65 to 74 will increase only 19.6% while persons 75 to 84 will increase 56%, and persons 85 and older will increase 84%. The 1978 report to the U.S. Senate Committee on Aging concluded that:

> The increasing number and proportion of older persons reflects both the impact of longer life expectancy and the movement of the post-World War II baby boom through the population pyramid. Projections based on lower fertility rates also show a much slower rate of growth of the older population after 2030 when today's babies and youngsters start reaching age 65. (U.S. Senate, Special Committee on Aging, 1979).

Changing Dependency Ratios

These demographic shifts will result in an increase in the ratio of persons dependent on the working-age population and in shifts in the composition of that dependent population. When the United States was a young frontier society in which most persons were employed in agriculture and other primary extractive work activities, most of the dependent population was composed of persons 14 years and younger. In 1880, 38% of the population was 15 years and under and only 3.4% was 65 and older; by 1970 the percentage of 15-year-olds and under had dropped to 28.5% while those 65 and over had increased to 9.8% (U.S. Bureau of the Census, 1970). Thus, there are more elderly in the population of nonworking persons dependent on the working-age population for financial and other forms of support. Because of the complex and expensive needs of an increasingly frail and chronically ill segment of that aged population (persons 75 and over), policy-makers are concerned about how the United States will meet the costs of an aging society.

Stranding of the Aged

These demographic facts of life are connected with the changing family system in all urban, industrial, modern societies. Urbanization and industrialization have significantly modified the extended kinship system of traditional societies; the nuclear family of parents and children has replaced the family household made up of parents, grandparents, and other relatives. As a consequence, the aged do not have the traditional social role of community elders as repositories of knowledge and skills to be passed on to the next generation. In fact, census data show that the nuclear family in which the husband works and the wife stays home to tend the children is a minority of all U.S. households. In 1955, 65.3% of families were headed by men whose wives did not work; by 1978, such households were only 44.5% of all families; and families with a wife working increased from 21.5% to 38.3% from 1955 to 1978. Most significantly, women heading households jumped from 9.4% to 14.4%. Thus, the traditional family system has clearly been modified by urbanization and industrialization (U.S. Bureau of the Census, 1980).

Associated with this decline of the extended family system is increased geographic mobility and dispersion. The working-age population must be free to move where the jobs are; such recent trends explain the rise of Sunbelt cities in the South and West and the decline of the old centers of urban-industrial America (Kasarda, 1980). The elderly who remain behind in decaying city centers are obviously stranded. However, the retired themselves have joined this "move to the sun," forming new households in retirement communities and cities that offer a less harsh climate than north central and northeastern cities. These mobility trends can further exacerbate the social and psychological isolation of the elderly. Also, given that the risks of a spouse dying and ill health are much greater in old age, the retired person today is much more likely to find himself or herself alone. The result can be diminished resources to support oneself when confronted with failing health and rising costs for food, energy, transportation, and housing.

In sum, a complex set of interconnected social, economic, and demographic forces has created a mix of social problems associated with old age in modern societies. Though the aging population and declining birth rates are measures of the success of the modernization processes, these very advances create problems for society and its political leaders that will not be solved easily or inexpensively. The problems of funding for adequate old age pensions; provision of housing, nutrition, transportation, and related needs; and financing and distribution of health services all require policy solutions. The solutions arrived at and the new proposals being contemplated are subjects of concern for analysts of public policies for the aged.

Public Policies and the Aging

The plight of the elderly has captured the attention of political leaders in modern societies. Governments have realized that many older persons run a greater risk of poverty. Through no fault of their own, elderly citizens are more likely to suffer from chronic illnesses, social isolation, and psychological disorders. Even the crudest and earliest public policies attacking the problem of widespread poverty (associated with the initial phases of European and American industrialization and urbanization) recognized that the elderly ran a greater risk of poverty. The 17th-century Poor Laws, promulgated in England and other nations, tried to distinguish among the broad and diverse group of people seeking public assistance; only persons deemed as deserving and as meeting local residency requirements were eligible for poor relief from frugal Poor Law officials. However, the methods of these early antipoverty, public assistance programs were inadequate. A rise in the dependent population of all ages, associated with dislocations from the transformation of the rural-agricultural society, ultimately overwhelmed the officials of Poor Law programs, making reform of these programs inevitable. Further, the stigmatizing label "on public relief" was increasingly perceived as grossly unfair. Nineteenth-century students of poverty began to rethink the causes of economic dependence—ill health, industrial accidents, overpopulation, urban decay, illiteracy—and began devising more humane solutions to this pressing social disorder (Trattner, 1979).

For example, the late-19th-century leadership of Imperial Germany pioneered the concept of governmentally administered, universally financed retirement programs; the conservative government of Chancellor Otto von Bismarck also developed the model for modern health insurance and work injury laws. These three pieces of legislation, enacted in the 1880s, were based on the notion that society has the responsibility of assisting persons to plan for old age and of insuring persons against risk of illness and unemployment due to work injury.

Following the German lead in policy innovation, other nations have adopted similar legislation and have extended the scope of government social insurance programs to cover risks such as unemployment (unrelated to work injury), large family size (by means of family allowance programs), and disability (due to mental defects, illnesses, and nonwork-related injuries). These programs thus constitute the array of programs considered as social security (Wilensky, 1975). It is interesting to note that the first modern social security concepts were enacted by a conservative monarchy that valued a strong military and pursued an aggressive expansionist foreign policy. The explanation for the German innovations is that Bismarck feared the consequences of an increasingly militant, socialist-oriented, trade union movement. By stealing a plank from the platform of his political opposition, Bismarck hoped to coopt the working class supporters of socialism. Bismarck also sought to increase social control by his military-minded, conservative aristocratic class by giving the lower classes a stake in the industrializing German society; he reasoned that with investments in old-age pension schemes, workers would feel like part of the social system and would be less likely to rebel against it (Briggs, 1961; cf. Janowitz, 1976).

While most developed nations followed Germany's lead in instituting social insurance programs that benefited the aged and other dependent persons, the United States lagged behind in initiating these public policies. Though unemployment insurance and veterans' benefit programs predated the Social Security Act, it was not until 1935 that the United States passed national old-age and survivors insurance legislation; it was not until 1965 that limited national health insurance was passed for the elderly and the poor. The failure to follow social policy innovations in other comparable industrial societies testifies to the intense American hostility to welfare and social programs. Thus, the current suspicion of government policy-making innovations and spending programs is not new; recent revolts by property tax payers and political campaigns that attack welfare corruption are only contemporary manifestations of a long-standing American antagonism toward government (Wilensky and Lebeaux, 1965; Wilensky, 1975; Coughlin, 1979).

Policy Design and Implementation

The discussion thus far has begged important questions: What is a public policy? What differentiates a policy from a program? What is program implementation? How is program implementation related to the processes that cause policies to be enacted? For a more complete understanding of the aging policies and programs in the United States and other modern societies, it is crucial that these questions be answered and that some clear concepts be brought into the discussion of policies and programs on aging.

In this chapter *public policy* will be defined as the broadest statement of a decision to act or not to act to solve a social problem. Embedded in this policy statement is a mechanism for dealing with that problem; or, in other words, a policy statement contains or is based on a theory, an understanding that if certain actions are taken (or not taken) then definite, measurable results will flow from those actions. Thus, a policy statement by federal, state, or local government is the most general statement of how political leaders will solve a social problem based on an understanding of the mechanisms that cause that social problem and the methods that can help to alleviate the collective disorder (Heclo, 1974).

Such policies may be enacted by legislative bodies (Congress, state legislatures), or they may be issued by a chief executive of a government (a presidential executive order), or they can be promulgated by federal, state, or local court decisions and orders (U.S. Supreme Court decisions). The crucial point is that in the complex web of the U.S. federal governmental system with its separation of powers, policymaking is rarely confined to one branch or level of government. The sharing of policymaking responsibilities requires concerted and coordinated activities by governmental officials to achieve a policy goal (Ripley, 1974).

Program Implementation of Social Policies

Social programs can be analytically separated from social policies. Programs are the specific methods used by different policy makers in the process of realizing the often broad and sometimes vague policy goals. Programs specify which governmental agents will be involved in policy enactment, determine how money will be spent, and provide guidelines for accountability of program managers, participants, and related activities. Thus, program activities are ways in which the policies of public officials are to be implemented. Like the policy enactment process, program implementation is a political process (Pressman and Wildavsky, 1979).

Since public policy often emerges from a highly charged political decision-making process, implementation of programs will also be politicized. Of course, not every program is highly controversial and the subject of intense political struggle; some programs may engender little public debate. Everyone—from elected official to uninterested voter—may generally agree that the particular policy and its program are necessary, are administered competently, operate cost-effectively, and require only customary review by policymakers. City sanitation services are an example of such generally noncontroversial, nonpoliticized public programs, though creating such services in the polluted and epidemic-ridden 19th-century cities was highly political; and current debates over locating a new water-treatment plant can embroil local officials in political turmoil that may endanger a city council member's career (Bardach, 1977).

Reform Movements and Interest Groups

Policy adoption and program implementation are highly politicized processes precisely because of the strength and vigor of organized groups that try to influence the formal policymakers—elected officials, bureaucrats, judicial authorities, and the like. The U.S. tradition of active reform movements and interest group organizations ensures that principal policymakers will be monitored closely. Thus, the interest groups and reformers who may have called for the adoption of the policy and worked for its enactment will continue to play a role in the implementation process to achieve the original policy goal. Conversely, interest groups and reformers who oppose a policy and fail to block its enactment or promulgation will try to kill the policy at the implementation stage. In either case, reformers and interest groups surround the policymaking processes and ensure that program implementation is politicized (Alford, 1975; Armour, 1981).

Implementation Pitfalls

In some cases, programs may be so poorly designed that well-meaning implementors cannot effectively realize the policy objectives. Even with the aid of reformers and interest groups, some government officials cannot overcome the barriers to effective implementation created by the policy designers. Sometimes the policy meets with such hostility and resistance by government officials and interest groups that it cannot be implemented; it is captured, neutralized, and destroyed by its opponents. In still other cases, the original policy concept is substantially altered by amendments to the policy act and by additions to the program elements so that the current program bears little resemblance to the original concept. Such amendments, in some ways, represent a measure of success for a policy concept: the idea is so appealing that related policy concepts are attached to it. Thus, the very success of a policy concept can lead to diffusion of the policy goal. As will be shown, incremental additions to the U.S. Social Security Act of 1935 have ensured that social security is a central feature of American policy concepts and have also resulted in a complex web of social insurance programs that almost defy reform (cf. Aaron, 1973).

Thus, the public business of policymaking is highly political and fraught with dangers for policymakers and program implementors. One thing is certain: An original policy concept will never be fully or completely realized as originally intended. There are too many policymakers and implementors interested in modifying the policy or destroying it outright for it to survive unaltered (Bardach, 1977; cf. Moynihan, 1969).

Different Policy Approaches to Aiding the Elderly

Since enactment of the Social Security Act of 1935, the United States has adopted a variety of policy approaches to the financial, social, and physical problems of the aged in modern society. There are several distinct policy theories embedded in each of these legislative actions that can be classified into several broad groups. The first of these policy concepts is transfer of income to the elderly through the government insurance program. Principal among these *income transfer insurance programs* is the Old-Age, Surviviors, and Disability Insurance (OASDI) of the Social Security Act in which payroll taxes paid by employers and employees are collected and paid out to eligible retirees who have participated in this tax-collection insurance scheme. A second policy of insurance involves the *transfer of in-kind benefits* instead of cash, although such benefits have a cash value. The health insurance program for the elderly, Medicare (passed in 1965), transfers hospital benefits and related health benefits to the elderly; funding is by a payroll tax and is disbursed from a specific health insurance trust fund. A third concept utilizes the notion of *noninsurance income transfer* of cash from the working-age population to the nonworking population, but does not employ the contributory insurance principle as in OASDI or Medicare. The Supplemental Security Income (SSI) program uses general government revenues received from income tax and other federal taxes to support the aged and other dependent adults with no means. A fourth concept is based on providing in-kind benefits that are noninsurance financed. An example of a *noninsurance financed in-kind benefit* is the food stamp program that helps many senior citizens living below the poverty level to supplement their incomes and diets. Medicaid, food stamps, subsidized housing, and other transfer programs (in-kind benefit and noninsurance income) are *means tested* or *income conditioned*. That is, the staff of an administering agency requires senior citizens to reveal their income and assets to become eligible for these income and benefit programs. The basic concept of a means tests is that only persons in need who lack income and assets will be supported by programs like SSI and food stamps. A fifth concept that guides the formulation of social policies of the aged is *direct services*. Rather than providing income or benefits, rendering services is a way of directly meeting the older person's transportation, nutrition, medical, recreational, and other needs. While these direct services have a cash value, they are not purchased with vouchers as food is purchased in the food stamp program, nor are these services counted as income supplements the way that OASDI, SSI, or Medicare programs are. Let us consider how each of these strategies assists the elderly.

Income Transfer Insurance Programs

The Social Security Act of 1935 is a landmark piece of policy legislation, establishing the concept of income security programs for the aged and other dependent persons. This act also illustrates the incremental growth of public policies. The current array of programs that make up "social security" reflect additions to and expansions of this primary policy concept; now social insurance is provided to millions of people who were not originally intended to be program recipients. The 1935 act created the old age pension plan (old-age insurance) and the federal-state system of unemployment insurance; the legislation also contained a title that provided limited support to families with dependent children (AFDC). In 1939, survivors' and dependents' benefits were added to the original policy mandate. By 1956, disability insurance to protect the severely disabled from the risks of poverty was added; hence, the current name of Old-Age, Survivors, and Disability Insurance (OASDI) for nonhealth functions of this transfer program.

Further, federal legislation has placed an increasing number of occupational groups under the OASDI programs: some farm and domestic workers (1950), the self-employed (1954), members of the armed forces (1956), U.S. citizens working for international organizations (1960), physicians (1965), and ministers (1967); and the railroad retirement programs were integrated into OASDI in 1974. There are current proposals to require federal, state, and local government employees not enrolled in OASDI to contribute to payroll taxes. Historically, federal employees and many other public servants have had separate pension programs because of the relatively lower annual pay for government service and the inability to participate in private corporate pension plans.

The *indexing* of OASDI payments to the Consumer Price Index (CPI) was an important innovation in policymaking for the elderly. This 1972 legislation required that OASDI monthly payments to recipients be increased automatically with increases in the "market basket" of goods and services represented by the CPI. Justification for these annual increases tied to CPI increases was that the aged were hardest hit by inflation; people living on fixed incomes were less able to adjust their household spending patterns to compensate for the relentless rise in costs of basic goods and services.

Old-Age, Survivors, and Disability Insurance is the oldest and the largest insurance principle, income support program. Payroll taxes collected from employers and employees are pooled in an OASDI trust fund administered by the Social Security Administration. These taxes are only for use in making payments to persons eligible for the expanded benefits of this income maintenance program. The OASDI expenditures have increased dramatically since the benefits were first paid out in the 1940s (Table 4–1). In 1945, $265 million was expended from the trust fund; in 1965, $15,660 million was distributed to beneficiaries; and by 1975, $64,294 million was being transferred from the trust fund—a 24,162% increase from 1945 to 1975.

The monthly benefits of OASDI vary, depending on the average annual earnings of persons who have paid into the trust fund, the age at which a person retires, the sex of the beneficiary, marital status, and employment status. Table 4–2 reveals the complexity of OASDI payments; benefits ranged

TABLE 4–1.—OASDI TRUST FUND STATUS 1940–1975
(IN MILLIONS OF DOLLARS)

	NET INCOME	NET EXPENDITURES	ASSETS
1940	$ 550	$ 29	$ 1,745
1945	1,432	265	6,613
1950	2,362	783	12,893
1955	5,525	4,436	21,141
1960	10,359	10,869	20,828
1965	16,443	15,660	19,698
1970	31,745	29,024	32,616
1975	58,757	64,294	39,947

Source: Table M–5, *Social Security Bulletin*, October 1976.

TABLE 4–2.—EXAMPLES OF MONTHLY SOCIAL SECURITY PAYMENTS
(EFFECTIVE JUNE 1977)

	AVERAGE YEARLY EARNINGS COVERED BY SOCIAL SECURITY AFTER 1950						
Earnings	$923 (or less)	$3,000	$4,000	$5,000	$6,000	8,000*	$10,000
Benefits can be paid to:							
Retired worker at 65	114.30	236.40	278.10	322.50	364.50	453.10	502.00
Worker under 65 and disabled	114.30	236.40	278.10	322.50	354.50	453.10	502.00
Retired worker at 62	91.50	189.20	222.50	258.00	291.60	362.50	401.60
Wife or husband at 65	57.20	118.20	139.10	161.30	182.30	226.60	251.00
Wife or husband at 62	42.90	88.70	104.40	121.00	138.80	170.00	188.30
Wife under 65 with one child in her care	57.20	125.00	197.20	272.60	304.20	339.80	376.60
Widow or widower at 65 if worker never received reduced benefits	114.30	236.40	278.10	322.50	364.50	453.10	502.00
Widow or widower at 60 if sole survivor	81.80	169.10	198.90	230.60	260.70	324.00	359.00
Widow or widower at 50 and disabled, if sole survivor	57.30	118.30	139.20	161.30	182.40	226.60	251.10
Widow or widower with one child in care	171.50	354.60	417.20	483.80	546.80	679.80	753.00
Maximum family payment	171.50	361.40	475.30	595.10	668.60	792.90	878.50

*Maximum earnings covered by social security were lower in past years and must be included in figuring average earnings. This average determines the payment. Because of this, amounts shown in the last two columns generally will not be payable until future years. The maximum retirement benefit generally payable to a worker who was 65 in 1977 was $437.10.

Source: Department of Health, Education, and Welfare, Social Security Administration, Washington, D.C., 1977.

from $114 to $878 in 1977; however, these figures do not reflect current benefit levels, adjusted by cost-of-living increases since 1977.

Initially, contributions to the old age insurance and the other trust funds greatly exceeded expenditures, but beginning in the 1970s, payments exceeded income. There are a number of explanations for these excess expenditures since 1975: the old age dependency ratio was lower in the 1940s and 1950s, meaning that there were plenty of working-age persons to contribute to the trust funds; the aged population now is increasing the percentage of people dependent on the working-age population; benefit program rolls were greatly expanded in the 1960s and 70s by persons who had paid little into the trust funds (disabled persons, the very old) and who became entitled to lifetime benefits; life expectancies increased with declining birth rates and improved medical care for the elderly, thus increasing the life span of beneficiaries; the high unemployment in the 1973–75 recession reduced payroll taxes paid into the OASDI trust fund; and indexing of payments to the Consumer Price Index in 1972 (implemented in 1975) raised payments from the fund.

Policymakers have continued to act to stem the excess flow of funds from the trust fund and to ensure that payments can be continued to the expanding population of persons with lifetime entitlements linked to rises in the cost of living. Social Security payroll taxes were increased in 1977. Retirement Security and Disability Insurance taxes (RSDI) were increased from 4.95% in 1977 to 5.05% in 1978 (by 1990, the tax rate will be 6.20%); corresponding increases were made in the Health Insurance (HI) tax rates (Table 4–3). This tax increase, largest in the nation's history, was felt to be a political necessity; no politician wanted to take the blame for the social security system "going broke." Yet, there remains considerable public doubt

TABLE 4–3.—CHANGES IN SOCIAL SECURITY CONTRIBUTION RATES

WAGES RECEIVED DURING CALENDAR YEAR	RSDI RATE %	HI RATE %	COMBINED RATE %	TAX BASE*
1977	4.95	0.90	5.85	$16,500
1978	5.05	1.00	6.05	17,700
1979–80	5.08	1.05	6.13	22,900
1981	5.35	1.30	6.65	29,700
1982–84	5.40	1.30	6.70	36,000
1985	5.70	1.35	7.05	38,100
1986–89	5.70	1.45	7.15	40,200
1990+	6.20	1.45	7.65	42,600

*Estimated.
Source: Calculated from Table M–5, *Social Security Bulletin*, vol. 40, no. 10, October 1977.

about long-term solvency of the OASDI trust funds. And politicians continue to confuse the complex issues—economic, demographic, social, and political—in their attempts to make political gains from the justified confusion over the viability of a system of income security that over 33 million households depend on (Heffernan, 1979).

Other Earned Income Maintenance Programs

Besides OASDI transfer programs there are several other contributory pension programs that directly benefit the elderly. As mentioned, the federal government, and many state and local governments and their agencies, maintain pension programs for their employees. Many of the same concerns that plague the OASDI programs plague these plans: rising inflation rates, growing number of entitled beneficiaries, and increased unemployment rates. For example, the indexing of federal workers' pensions to the CPI is the subject of a current budgetary debate. The Reagan administration has proposed reducing the inflation adjustments for federal workers, along with raising the retirement age, and other changes, in order to control the increase in government's mandated, but uncontrollable expenditures. Whether Congress will institute such changes and will suffer the wrath of federal employees is unclear at this time.

Veterans' benefits are another crucial package of payments that are disproportionately benefiting the elderly. As such, Veterans Administration expenditures should be considered part of the income support system that sustains the retired person at a time when inflation and budget cuts are eroding the life-support systems of the retired (Schulz, 1980).

In-kind Benefit Insurance Programs

A major policy breakthrough occurred in 1965 when health insurance for the elderly was passed by Congress. A powerful interest group, the American Medical Association and its allies in the private insurance industry and in hospital associations, had opposed such legislation since the early 20th century when the first efforts to pass government-sponsored health insurance were made at state and federal levels. The policy precedent for federal health care assistance was provided by a 1950 amendment to the Social Security Act that granted assistance for medical care to indigent recipients of public assistance. In 1960 another amendment authorized federal matching funds to make medical care payments for indigent recipients of Old Age Assistance (OAA was a grant program to support persons not eligible for OASDI). After an intense political struggle in which two presidents employed the maximum amount of executive influence possible, national health insurance for the elderly (Medicare) was passed and signed into law as Title XIX of the Social Security Act (Marmor, 1973).

The hospital insurance program of Medicare provides benefits financed by a compulsory payroll tax collected along with the OASDI tax. The program of hospital benefits and other health insurance benefits covers all persons 65 and over entitled to OASDI, those in the railroad retirement system, and most disabled beneficiaries under the age of 65. Medicare provides a variety of hospital and posthospital benefits, subject to deductibles. Included in this group are persons suffering from chronic renal failure or kidney disease; this new group of dependents is covered by 1972 amendments to the Social Security Act under which the federal government now pays for hemodialysis or renal transplantation for persons suffering from end-stage renal disease. 1980 estimates suggest that $1.2 billion was spent to maintain just under 60,000 persons who otherwise would have died of chronic renal failure (U.S. Department of Health and Human Services, 1980). In addition, a supplementary insurance program is subsidized by the government to help Medicare recipients pay for all medical care not covered by Medicare's basic plan.

If one examines the ten-year period since Medicare was enacted, it can be seen that it has changed the health care industry in the United States. Seventy-five percent of all health care expenditures were from private sources (private health insurance, patient fees, and the like); federal expenditures were negligible. By 1965, the federal share had jumped to 11.9% while the private share remained at about 75%; however, in 1967, when Medicare began to be implemented, the federal share of health expenditures grew to 20.5% and the private share declined to 67%. By 1975, the private share was down to 57.8% and the public share had grown to 42.2% with the federal government's share of total expenditures at 28.6%. Other expenditure increase data show that since the introduction of Medicare the annual average rate of increase in all health-related expenditures was 14.5%—outstripping increases in the Consumer Price Index for most years since 1965. Not surprisingly, total health expenditures have risen too: in 1965, the U.S. spent $38,892 million on health; in 1967, the amount had grown to $47,879 million; and by 1975, the figure was $118,200 million. As a percentage of gross national product, total health expenditures were 5.9% in 1965, 6.2% in 1967, and 8.3% in 1975; today, both public and private health expenditures are nearly 10% of the gross national product (Klarman, 1977). Clearly, the introduction of Medicare has had a dramatic impact on the country's health care budget. The federal government has increased its share of an ever-increasing health expenditure budget that is consuming an ever-larger share of the gross national product.

At the same time, studies demonstrate that Medicare represents a transfer of health benefits to that segment of the population, the elderly, who run the greatest risk of suffering from disabling and financially crippling diseases: heart diseases, cancer, stroke, diabetes, and other degenerative diseases (Klein, 1973). In this sense, Medicare may have achieved its goals (transferring health care resources to the aged), but at a cost that the policymakers of the 1960s did not anticipate.

Noninsurance Transfer Payment Programs

The insurance concept is not the only one employed to devise transfer payment programs for the elderly and other dependent populations. These financial assistance programs that aid the poor are the oldest of the social welfare policies and programs. They have their origins in the late-medieval-era Poor Laws that differentiated among various categories of the poor, seeking to aid only the deserving poor who could pass *means tests* (i.e., demonstrate they lacked the means to support themselves) and could meet residency requirements (Piven & Cloward, 1971; cf. Polanyi, 1957; Marshall, 1970). The most controversial and politically explosive U.S. noninsurance transfer payment program is Aid to Families with Dependent Children (AFDC). However intriguing the AFDC program is for purposes of policy analysis, an assessment of it is beyond the scope of this chapter. Fortunately, there are several income transfer programs that do directly benefit the elderly that must be considered in this evaluation of aging policies and programs (Aaron, 1973).

Supplemental Security Income (SSI) is one such program that millions of retired and other dependent persons rely on for income support. SSI is a 1974 amendment to the Social Security Act that consolidates and federalizes a group of aid programs for the aged, disabled (physically and mentally), and blind. Unlike OASDI, SSI is funded from general federal revenues and establishes uniform national eligibility requirements and benefit levels. In addition to federalizing welfare for the most needy of the dependent—persons not qualified for OASDI or those receiving minimal OASDI payments—SSI legislation encourages (and in some cases requires) states to supplement SSI payments. Like other noninsurance principle programs, SSI has income and financial assets tests, and benefits are reduced when the income of SSI recipients increases. While half of the 5 million persons receiving a total of $7 billion in annual SSI payments are disabled, not aged, this program is a crucial safety net for the aged drawing social security monthly benefits (Schulz, 1980).

Further evaluation of SSI recipients shows they greatly favor this relatively new welfare program; persons expressed pleasure at the higher level of benefits, the lack of degrading welfare-department evaluations, and the new approach to assisting the aged and disabled poor that established national entitlement to minimum income supplements.

Besides SSI there are other noninsurance principle programs that help the aged. The main program is General Public Assistance. These state and local public assistance programs are highly variable; benefit levels and means tests differ considerably from authority to authority. In general, these assistance programs are short-term relief measures, designed to aid a person or family in an acute financial crisis until they can enroll in SSI, AFDC, or another program for which they are eligible.

Noninsurance, In-kind Benefit Programs

The elderly are beneficiaries of several noninsurance, in-kind benefit programs. Chief among these are Medicaid, food stamps, and housing subsidies. Medicaid was passed along with Medicare in 1965. It represents a federalization and expansion of a 1961 program of medical assistance for the indigent aged and the 1950 Social Security Act amendments that provide benefits for the dependent, blind, and disabled not qualified for Medicare. Low-income persons that pass income and assets tests can receive medical care from state-administered programs, which share costs with the federal government—expenses that range from 50 to 80%, depending on state per capita income. In this way, low-income states are assisted by federal payments and the inequalities in states' ability to pay for in-kind benefits are thus reduced.

Medicaid and many of the other noninsurance, in-kind benefit programs do not assist the elderly exclusively. All states provide Medicaid to AFDC families; about 30 states cover all aged, blind, and disabled SSI recipients; other states have restrictive medical standards that limit SSI recipients' access to Medicaid benefits; and persons ineligible for cash assistance and who are aged, blind, or disabled may also receive Medicaid if they cannot meet medical expenses. A 1970 survey found that only 39% of people using Medicaid were aged (65 and over); yet this program is a crucial benefit for the millions of aged receiving its assistance and must not be overlooked when considering programs for the elderly.

The national food stamp program also must be included in the income and in-kind benefits that sustain the elderly. Begun in the 1960s as part of President John F. Kennedy's efforts to combat pockets of poverty and expanded in the Great Society period of policy innovations under Lyndon B. Johnson, food stamps are currently available without the controversial purchase requirement to aged couples with assets of less than $3,000 (excluding their home) and gross annual income of $4,000. Such a household was entitled to $300 per year. As with other benefit programs and transfer payments, food stamp allocations are increased in January and July to reflect increases in the consumer price index. This indexing of benefits provides the aged with some insurance against inflation that would otherwise rapidly erode the value of food stamp allocations. With about one million persons aged 60 and over using food stamps, this program, as well as SSI payments, OASDI checks, Medicare, and Medicaid, are the income and health support systems for the elderly.

In addition to medical and food benefits, senior citizens receive assistance with housing costs. Federal programs, dating from the 1937 Federal Housing Act, have assisted the aged with the costs of rent and home loans. The National Housing Act of 1959, based on the 1937 policy precedent, authorized a program of loans to nonprofit agencies (e.g., churches) to develop housing for the aged and handicapped. Estes (1979) notes that although this 1959 act was popular with politicians anxious to enhance their election prospects, only 45,000 housing units were actually built in the first decade of the legislation's life. In the 1970s the Nixon administration impounded funds for this program but they were released again under the Carter administration. In 1977, $630 million was awarded to sponsors of 24,000 housing units; and, of the nearly identical amount authorized in 1978, $562 million was allocated exclusively for the aged.

In Estes' view the allocations were inadequate; studies have shown that in Los Angeles alone there are 100,000 elderly persons who need adequate housing. As a result, there are five applicants for each available housing space (cf. Butler, 1975). Other federal housing legislation stemming from the Great Society era of social legislation has set national housing goals that include statements of plans to meet the special housing requirements of senior citizens. The Housing and Urban Development Act of 1964 and the Demonstration and Metropolitan Development Act of 1966 (the so-called Model Cities Act) expanded on earlier local, state, and federal urban renewal and housing programs that included rehabilitation of housing and rent subsidies for low-income persons. The 1974 Housing and Community Development Act was accompanied by a Ford administration program of rent supplements intended to ensure that the poor, including the elderly, be required to pay only one fourth of their income on housing. This program of rent supplements also fell short of its goal; instead of reaching the targeted 400,000 families, only 76,900 were participating in the program in 1976. Thus, housing support efforts have been launched under both Republican and Democratic administrations, and households that would not otherwise have been aided were assisted by these various programs. In Estes' view, however, the federal housing effort has not met the need of hundreds of thousands of senior citizens who could benefit from these programs; and it has not made up for the disasters associated with ill-conceived urban renewal programs and interstate highway construction projects that destroyed many inner-city neighborhoods, displacing elderly residents and reducing the stock of low-income housing (cf. Estes, 1979).

Finally, transportation benefits are an integral part of the in-kind benefits that many aged draw upon to sustain themselves when they face income reductions associated with retirement, but also must meet increased costs associated with ill health. National transportation programs have recognized senior citizens' need for accessible, affordable public transportation. In-kind benefits have been provided under the Older Americans Act programs that transport the elderly to meal centers and to other places for medical and shopping needs. More important, operating subsidies from the federal government to local transportation services (for both capital expenditures and operating costs) stipulate that municipal and regional transportation systems must provide lower fares to senior citizens and handicapped persons. The Urban Mass Transportation Act requires that the elderly and handicapped be charged no more than half the normal fare, except during rush-hour periods. This lower-fare program is a benefit to the aged who would otherwise have to limit their transportation expenditures and thus reduce the number of necessary as well as recreational trips that they take. As such, these federal requirements have enhanced the lives of senior citizens, but at a cost to transportation services when federal subsidies do not make up for the loss of full fares.

Direct Services

Estes (1979) has noted and assessed some 80 federal programs for the elderly. A chief source of direct-service funding can be found in the programs of Title XX of the Social Security Act. Title XX illustrates the incremental growth of public policies and programs. The framers of the 1935 legislation did not envision that additions to this landmark act would mandate federal support of social services such as adult day care, home-delivered meals (or so-called meals on wheels), homemaker services, and home-management assistance. In 1976, in fact, $117.5 million was spent on these programs that help maintain senior citizens in their homes and that reduce the need for institutionalization in a nursing home.

Title XX is an example of the *block-grant* method of funding federal government services. In contrast to *categorical* grants, in which fund expenditures are specified for government units, the block-grant method is used to determine only the broad outlines of a program and then allocates funds for that program (e.g., social services for the elderly, handicapped, and others on AFDC, SSI, and other programs). Actual implementation of block-grant expenditures is left to the states (Schram, 1981). States have broad powers to decide which of the services available under Title XX will actually be provided. One of the problems with the block-grant concept as applied in Title XX is the issue of age discrimination. While the states that administer Title XX funds intend to address the social service needs of all their citizens who meet income and other means-test requirements, the aged find they are unable to receive service dollars in proportion to their segment of the population or in line with the growing needs of this most rapidly increasing segment of the dependent population in America. State and local social service agencies have been locked into spending commitments on children and others among the poor and needy, but another federal aging program has sought to alter the priorities of state and local governments so that senior citizens receive their appropriate share of social-service allocations. This advocacy and planning program is contained in the Older Americans Act (OAA).

In 1965, Congress passed, and President Johnson signed into law, the Older Americans Act. The 1970s amendments required that planning be added to the OAA service-delivery activities. OAA created state agencies on aging (SUAs) to plan for state service needs and local area agencies on aging (AAAs) to plan for services at the local level (regional and municipal); AAAs coordinate service delivery at the local level, pool resources for senior citizens, and work with state offices on aging (SUAs) to implement this coordination activity at that level. In addition to these goals, the Older Americans Act authorized the creation of federally funded senior centers and the establishment of regional nutritional programs and transportation services to support these meal services. In sum, the Older Americans Act provided the nation with area planning agencies for senior service needs under Title III, with senior day-care centers under Title V, and with nutritional and transportation services under Title VII.

In 1978, amendments and reauthorization of this Great Society program consolidated the three strategies of the OAA under one new Title III. Other OAA services (model projects in research and training and an employment program) were continued with new title numbers. Since the 1978 reorganization and reprioritization of functions, the Title III services of the OAA have played a crucial role in some communities. The 1978 amendments required that 50% of the Title III-B funds be expended for access (transportation), in-home, and legal services for the elderly, in addition to the nutrition and recreational services at meal sites and senior centers. Critics of the OAA strategy argue that there is an inherent contradiction between the federal requirements for fund accountability and the mandate that services be developed by local agencies to meet local needs; further, the OAA, even in its 1978 amended form, is flawed by the tension between planning and advocating senior citizen services while providing the services (cf. Armour et al., 1981). Given the Reagan administration's intent to cut social service budgets and given the financial crises of many midwestern and northeastern city and state governments, the OAA may not survive to resolve these dilemmas created by contradictions within the policy mandate. However, the small size of OAA (e.g., $245 million in 1975 for OAA compared with $2.5 billion for Title XX services in the same year) may mean that the withdrawal of funds may not have a great impact on senior citizens, though the loss of OAA staffer's jobs will create some political disquiet.

In sum, there is a wide range of policies and programs for senior citizens. Ranging from insurance principle income programs to direct-service delivery strategies, the federal, state, and local governments have assumed an increasing burden of maintaining the U.S. aged population, from enactment of the Social Security Act of 1935 to the present. As has been suggested in this discussion, the burdens have increased in recent years. The rise in the number of old persons, expanded entitlements of many income maintenance programs, inflation and unemployment, taxpayer revolts, and other forces have altered the environment for policy creation and implementation in the 1980s.

Fiscal Crisis of the Welfare State: The Case of Social Security

Recent accounts have alarmed the public by predictions that the centerpiece of U.S. income maintenance policy, Old-Age, Survivors, and Disability Insurance, is going broke. In 1977, Congress passed legislation that raised payroll taxes to offset cash shortfalls in the trust funds of retirement, disability, health, and other funds of the Social Security system. But in 1980 it became clear that these massive tax increases would not forestall a temporary deficit in 1982—before the retirement trust funds are replenished by the 1977 tax increase. A long-term shortage looms on the policy horizon. Members of the post-World War II baby boom will retire in the early decades of the 21st century, and analysts raise questions about the ability of trust fund revenues to cope with the demands for retirement income for this generation that has been disrupting social institutions since the 1950s and 1960s. Specifically, dependency ratios will drastically change in the next century. Currently there are 100 workers for every 31 beneficiaries; by the year 2010 there will be 70 dependents per 100 contributors, requiring a 40% OASDI tax increase just to meet current levels of transfer payments (Myers, 1981).

Social Security's problems stem not only from the demographic forces that will transform the age profile of U.S. society in the next 30 years; policymakers of both parties in Congress and the Executive Branch have employed incremental and ad hoc adjustments of the 1935 Social Security

Act. This tinkering with the original simple concept of old age insurance has transformed the program into a complex array of income maintenance plans that seem to defy rational consideration.

In 1972, Congress voted to raise benefit levels 20% and linked the OASDI transfer payments to increases in the consumer price index. Congress' generosity is understandable: the U.S. Social Security system is a very popular program; politicians that propose to substantially modify the plan have been rejected by the electorate (e.g., Senator Barry Goldwater in the 1964 presidential race; Ronald Reagan in the 1976 contest for the Republican party's presidential nomination). In fact, social insurance schemes for the aged, along with national health insurance, are the most popular social programs in all modern, urban industrial societies. Coughlin's (1979) cross-national analysis of public opinion data reveals the deep, widespread support for old age pensions and health care plans in Europe, North America, and Australia. Thus, congressional expansion of OASDI benefits in an election year is understandable: politicians believe that increasing OASDI benefits will ensure their reelection.

Further, Congress has done more than increase benefits to current recipients; benefits were extended at the program's margins to upgrade payments to persons at the lowest levels of the plan's payment schedule. The so-called minimum benefit payment (currently $122 per month) was instituted to provide income support, regardless of how little a person might have contributed to the OASDI trust fund in his working career. Currently, three million persons draw this minimum benefit.

These increased expenditures, growth in the population of persons dependent on OASDI, and higher payroll taxes were based on assumptions that the United States would experience sustained economic growth (with high levels of employment) and reduced levels of inflation. Neither assumption has proved valid. As a result of chronic levels of unemployment and continuing high inflation rates, the OASDI trust fund is being drained by ever-increasing payments and is not being replenished by payroll taxes at rates fast enough to accumulate a surplus so that the system can cope with the enormous increase in payments that will be required after the year 2010. In 1981 and 1982, relatively small deficits of $6 billion to $9 billion per year will develop in the Old Age insurance fund, and these will be offset by accumulated surpluses in the disability insurance fund. However, by 1985 and 1986, estimates place the OASDI deficit at approximately $30 billion per year until the 1990s, when the trust fund will begin to grow again as a result of 1977 tax increases. This late-1980s crisis is termed the medium-term cash shortage to differentiate it from the long-term funding disaster supposedly facing the system in the 21st century. Unless birth rates and migration swell the ranks of the working-age population that contributes payroll taxes, and unless "stagflation" (cycles of slow growth, high inflation, and concomitant high unemployment) is broken, OASDI will face staggering burdens that will necessitate massive tax increases (cf. Aaron, 1981).

There are several proposals to deal with these medium-term and long-term cash crises. First, Congress is considering legislation to permit borrowing among the formally separated OASDI trust funds. Proponents of the borrowing concept suggest that the medium-term crisis can be averted by authorizing OASDI funds to borrow from the health insurance (HI) fund of Medicare; these borrowings will be replaced when the OASDI fund receives added tax revenues in the 1990s. Second, there are proposals to reduce benefit levels to retirees, from the current rate of 42% of preretirement income to 39% in 1987. Related to this proposal is one that raises the age at which workers could draw full benefits. The retirement age for full benefits would be raised to 68, and persons who retire at 62 would have their benefit levels reduced from 80% to 55% of age-65 retirement income. Third, annual inflation adjustments could be raised at a rate lower than the CPI rate of increase; and the formula used to calculate the CPI could be modified to deflate the CPI inflator, reflecting more closely expenditure patterns of retired persons. Fourth, the OASDI trust funds could be authorized to borrow from general tax revenues to get the fund over the medium-term cash problem or to pay benefits to persons that now receive minimum payments. Proponents of this view argue that the welfare-income maintenance functions of OASDI could be segregated from the old age insurance functions originally intended for the plan. Fifth, taxes can be raised, a prospect that all politicians of all parties dread. But if such taxes were the less-visible sales tax or national value-added taxes (VAT) (developed and widely used in European nations), then the electorate would feel the tax pinch less acutely. Finally, the number of persons eligible for benefits could be cut. For example, college-age dependents of OASDI beneficiaries could be cut from the rolls; stricter standards could be set for disability-status determination.

The Political Process and Policymaking

Analysts of the social security policymaking process are not confident that presidents and Congress will deal rationally and dispassionately with these painful policy choices. Given the high political risks associated with modifying the Social Security system, politicians are likely to avoid the tough and necessary options. In the early 1981 round of budget cuts proposed by the Reagan administration, Congress adopted the Reagan proposal to cut the minimum benefit from the federal budget. The Reagan administration argued that this welfare activity was not envisioned by the original policy framers of OASDI and should be eliminated to save money at a time when budget deficits at the national level were estimated to be $45 billion for fiscal year 1981. But when these deficit estimates were raised to $65 billion or even higher, Congress voted to reintroduce the minimum benefit payments. The political backlash—real and imagined—associated with this cut in Social Security was too great for both Republican and Democratic members of Congress. With all House of Representative members and one third of the Senate up for reelection in 1982, no one wanted to be blamed for slashing income assistance programs to old people, even a marginal area like minimum benefits of OASDI.

Thus one can predict without too much difficulty that the policymaking process in this crucial area of social insurance, affecting over 30 million household incomes and one fourth of the federal budget, will continue to be highly politicized. Rational judgments and detached evaluation of these policies and programs will probably not be made by partisan policymakers. The prospects are great that decision-making will take place in an ideologically charged atmosphere at various points in the crises of the OASDI trust fund. Ad hoc, incremental adjustments will be made in this crisis environment, and decisions that could remove the OASDI trust fund debate from the political arena for the next several generations will not be made. In a word, short-term crisis management of the OASDI fund will be the rule; long-term policy planning and implementation will not occur.

Summary

This chapter has attempted to give students of aging and gerontology insights into the policymaking process and its outcomes. As our society continues to age, with persons 65 and over growing in numbers and as a proportion of the population, policy decisions affecting the aged will be even more critical and costly. Students need to be aware that the complex array of aging programs almost defies reform by well-intentioned policymakers. As a consequence, the nation faces recurring crises, both financial and political. These crises might result in a new form of intergenerational conflict. Increasing heavy taxation of the working-age population might cause them to rebel against tax burdens associated with supporting the growing aged population dependent on pay-as-you-go income transfer plans. Given that any one individual is powerless to change the course of these events, it is hoped that students can at least gain some understanding of the dangerous social, economic, and political course we have undertaken.

REFERENCES

Aaron H.: *Why is Welfare So Hard To Reform?* Washington, D.C., Brookings Institute, 1973.

Aaron H.: Salvaging Social Security. *Brookings Bull.* 17:13–16 Spring, 1981.

Alford, R.: *Health Care Politics*. Chicago, University of Chicago Press, 1975.

Armour P.K.: *The Cycles of Social Reform: Mental Health Policy Making in the United States, England, and Sweden*. Washington, D.C., University Press of America, 1981.

Armour P.K., Estes C.L., Noble M.L., et al. (eds.): *The Aging in Politics*. Springfield, Ill., Charles C Thomas, Publisher, 1981.

Bardach E.: *The Implementation Game*. Cambridge, Mass., MIT Press, 1977.

Briggs A.: The welfare state in historical perspective. *Arch. of Eur. Sociol.* 11:221–258, 1961.

Butler R.N.: *Why Survive: Being Old in America*. New York, Harper & Row, 1975.

Coughlin R.M.: *Ideology, Public Opinion, and the Welfare State*. Berkeley, Institute of International Studies, University of California,1979.

Estes C.: *The Aging Enterprise*. San Francisco, Jossey-Bass Publishers, 1979.

Heclo H.: *Modern Social Politics in Britain and Sweden*. New Haven, Conn., Yale University Press, 1974.

Heffernan J.: *Introduction to Social Welfare Policy*. Itasca, Ill. F.E. Peacock, 1979.

Janowitz M.: *The Social Control of the Welfare State*. Chicago, University of Chicago Press, 1976.

Kasarda J.D.: The implications of contemporary distribution trends for national urban policy. *Soc. Sci. Quar.* 61:373–400, 1980.

Klarman H.E.: Financing Health Care. *Daedalus* 106:215–234 (Winter), 1977.

Klein R.: Policy Problems and Policy Perceptions in the NHS. *Policy and Politics* 2:3, 1973.

Marmor T.: *The Politics of Medicare*. Chicago, Aldine Publishing Co., 1973.

Marshall T.H.: *Social Policy in the Twentieth Century*. London, Hutchinson, 1970.

Moynihan D.P.: *Maximum Feasible Misunderstanding*. New York, Free Press, 1969.

Myers R.J.: *Social Security*. Homewood, Ill., Richard D. Irwin, 1981.

Piven F.F., Cloward R.: *Regulating the Poor*. New York, Random House-Vintage Books, 1971.

Polyani K.: *The Great Transformation*. Boston, Beacon Press, 1957.

Pressman J., Wildavsky A.: *Implementation*. Berkeley, University of California Press, 1979.

Ripley R.: *American National Government and Public Policy*. New York, Free Press, 1974.

Schram S.E.: Title XX Implementation and the Aging, in Hudson R. (ed.): *The Aging in Politics*. Springfield, Ill., Charles C Thomas, Publisher, 1981.

Schulz J.: *The Economics of Aging*. Belmont, Calif., Wadsworth Publishing Co., 1980.

Trattner W.L.: *From Poor Law to Welfare State*. New York, Free Press, 1979.

U.S. Department of Commerce, Bureau of the Census: *United States Population, 1970*. U.S. Government Printing Office, 1970.

U.S. Department of Commerce, Bureau of the Census: *Social Indicators-II*. U.S. Government Printing Office, 1980.

U.S. Department of Health and Human Services, Health Care Finance Adminis-

tration: *End-Stage Renal Disease, Second Annual Report to Congress*. U.S. Government Printing Office, 1980.
U.S. Senate, Special Committee on Aging: *Developments in Aging, 1978*. U.S. Government Printing Office, 1979.
Wilensky H.L.: *The Welfare State and Equality*. Berkeley, University of California Press, 1975.
Wilensky H.L., Lebeaux C.: *Industrial Society and Social Welfare*. New York, Free Press, 1965.

5

DISADVANTAGED ELDERLY

Steven R. Applewhite, Ph.D.

THE EXAMINATION of ethnicity and aging begins with the fundamental principle that aging is a universal process. Gerontology, the study of aging, attempts to explain this process as a complex interaction of biologic, psychological, and sociological changes. Although it is acceptable to consider aging as a common phenomenon, it is inappropriate to assume that there are no discernible distinctions within population structures (Decker, 1980). Indeed, Cowgill and Holmes (1972) identified both universal elements and distinct variations in the aging process across different cultures and subcultures. Likewise, it is unreasonable and misleading to assume that in the United States all elderly share the same experiences of aging. Since this nation is composed of distinct racial and ethnic groups, the study of aging must be tempered with the cultural uniqueness of identifiable racial and ethnic groups, including blacks, Hispanics, native Americans, and Pacific-Asians.

This chapter discusses general concepts, characteristics, and issues related to elderly minority groups in the United States. While there are numerous definitions of minority populations, this discussion considers data specific to the four major minority groups, with emphasis on the black and Hispanic aged. Further, this chapter describes situational variants that may help to explain the differences as well as similarities among the divergent elderly groups. The tendency to make sweeping assumptions about elderly minority groups always severely limits such discussions. Therefore, the emphasis of this chapter is primarily on the demographic variables related to black and Hispanic aged. While the plight of native Americans and Pacific-Asians is no less significant, discussion of these two groups will be more cursory.

Developments in Aging

In the last decade, the problems of the aged in general have emerged consistently in the gerontologic literature. Among the prime forces behind the surging interest are two major factors. First, a shift in the population structure, resulting from the postwar baby boom that lasted from 1947 to 1957, indicates that the aged will represent the population wave of the future. For instance, between 1970 and 1980, the population aged 65 and over increased by 23.2%, compared to 6.3% for the under-65 age group and 9.1% for the total general population. This trend is expected to continue, and it is anticipated that by the year 2030 the percentage of the population 65 or over will have reached an estimated 18.3% of the total population in this country, as shown in Table 5–1.

The second factor is an economic one. Today's economy delivers less income and higher inflation rates for the average elderly. Consequently, it subjects the aged to greater social and economic stress and dramatically threatens their sense of contribution and their psychological well-being. It is abundantly clear that the population transformation, commonly referred to as the "graying of America," has been turned from the natural process of aging into the national "problem" of old age. Accordingly, the U.S. Select Committee on Aging has determined that the growing number of senior citizens in America, which should be considered a triumph, has come

TABLE 5–1.—PERCENTAGE OF POPULATION 65 OR OVER AND MEDIAN AGE OF TOTAL U.S. POPULATION, 1900–1980, AND PROJECTIONS, 1990–2040

YEAR	PERCENTAGE OF TOTAL POPULATION AGED 65 OR OVER	MEDIAN AGE OF TOTAL POPULATION
	Estimates	
1900	4.1	22.9
1910	4.3	24.1
1920	4.7	25.3
1930	5.5	26.5
1940	6.9	29.0
1950	8.2	30.2
1960	9.3	29.5
1970	9.9	28.1
1980	11.2	30.2
	Projections	
1990	12.1	32.8
2000	12.2	35.5
2010	12.7	36.6
2020	15.5	37.0
2030	18.3	38.0
2040	17.8	37.8

Sources: U.S. Bureau of the Census: *Historical Statistics of the United States, Colonial Times to 1970;* and *Current Population Reports,* series P–25, no. 704, *Projections of the Population of the United States: 1977–2050.*

to be viewed as "a burden, a drain on the economy, and a menace to our well-being" (U.S. Congress, House of Representatives, 1980).

In view of such harsh realities, Tate (1979) sees the devastating effects of aging on many of our elderly as a crisis that must not go unchallenged. Tate emphasizes, however, that beyond the global nature of the problems experienced by the general population, there is a particular need to focus on the minority aged. The minority elderly experience the major social, health, and economic problems experienced by the elderly population in general, but these problems are too often exacerbated in later years as a result of a lifetime of discrimination, underemployment, impoverishment, and social indignities (Levkoff et al., 1979). It is no surprise, then, that poor health, deplorable housing, and the lack of vitally needed services continue to serve as reminders of the "differential structure of opportunities for minority groups" (Hendricks and Hendricks, 1977).

Minority Group Status

In order to understand minority aging, we must first define the concept of minority status. Drawing on the early writings of Young (1932), Wirth (1945), and Barron (1953), Rose (1965) defined minority groups as

> those groups whose members share certain racial and ethnic similarities which are considered to be different from or inferior to the traits of the dominant group and who are thereby "singled out for differential and unequal treatment."

In a similar vein, Cuellar and Weeks (1980) add that:

> because of physical characteristics, color, language, or culture, [minority groups] are treated as objects of collective prejudice and discriminated by the dominant majority in society. By definition . . . *minorities do not enjoy a full share of society's benefits when compared to the majority*. (Emphasis added.)

More recently, Jackson (1980) has concluded that the unequal treatment experienced by minority populations has extended beyond race or language and now includes discrimination by sex and national origin—all harmful effects of "institutionalized victimization" and "systemic discrimination."

To illustrate the influence of these circumstances, the aged in minority groups have been described as experiencing double, triple, or multiple jeopardy (Benedict, 1972; Dowd and Bengtson, 1978; Fujii, 1976; Hill, 1972; National Urban League, 1964). This thesis maintains that minority elderly are jeopardized and truly disadvantaged as a result of old age, poverty, and minority status. One must add that minority aged experience the multiple effects of discrimination based on physical, cultural, and political conditions, including differential statuses related to wealth, power, and prestige (Harris and Cole, 1980).

Minority Gerontology

The concept of minority aging has a distinct place in the field of gerontology. As previously mentioned, minority elderly are victims of multiple jeopardy. To better understand the problems experienced by minority aged, empirical research and critical knowledge of subpopulations are necessary. Moreover, there is an apparent need to examine critical issues *within* and *across* minority aged communities, as well as *in comparison to* the dominant elderly population.

As indicated by Bengtson (1979), "most of the research in social gerontology, at least until 1972, has been undertaken on respondents who are middle-class, white, predominantly native-born Americans, resulting in inadequate information concerning the wide diversity among the over-65 population." This view has been affirmed by a number of researchers (i.e., Eribes and Bradley-Rawls, 1978; Moore, 1971a; Solomon, 1974), who have called attention to the paucity of valid and reliable data on minority elderly. Furthermore, studies on minority aged that consider ethnicity as a constant variable have been proposed on the basis that, while minority status yields shared experiences and problems, diversity among minority groups lies in the distinctive patterning of life (Kent, 1971).

The lack of reliable data for comparative purposes has limited our comprehension of the elderly in minority groups. More critically, the absence of such studies has often led to false generalizations about minority aged groups in this country. Cuellar (1980) stresses the need to pursue *minority gerontology* in order to make "systematic, comparative analysis of the aging process, age stratification, and status of older persons in national minority communities in order to draw implications for addressing their needs over time." Fandetti and Gelfand (1976), Woehrer (1978), and others have pursued the issue still further, suggesting a need for a sociocultural approach to the study of diverse ethnic groups beyond those in minority positions (Sanchez-Ayendez, 1981).

Finally, in order to better understand minority elderly, Moore (1971b) listed five propositions he considered essential in the analysis of such groups:

1. Each minority group has a special history and collective experience.
2. Each group has experienced within its special history a pattern of discrimination and negative stereotyping.
3. Within each group, variant subcultures have developed with distinct value sets, statuses, and behavioral norms.

4. For each group, cultural coping mechanisms have developed and become institutionalized.
5. For each minority group, there is a constant subjection to change taking place rapidly as history is continuously being rethought and rewritten.

Against this background on theoretical perspectives in minority aging, the next section examines briefly the demographic, socioeconomic, and related characteristics of four aged minority groups: black Americans, Hispanics, Pacific-Asians, and native Americans.

Minority Elderly

The Black Aged

The largest elderly minority group in the United States is the black population. In 1978, there were approximately 25.5 million blacks in the United States, constituting 12% of the total population. The Bureau of the Census also estimates that there are slightly less than 3 million elderly blacks aged 60 and over, representing 11.2% of the total black population, or 8.4% of all senior citizens in the United States. By the turn of the century, the black population aged 60 and over will reach an estimated 4.1 million, with more than 3 million blacks aged 65 and over.

Proportionately, the elderly black population is increasing at a faster rate than elderly whites and younger blacks. Similarly, the proportion of black elderly women is increasing faster than the black male population. For example, in 1978, more than 57% of the over-60 black population was female, a 73% increase since 1960, or 27 percentage points more than that of black males (U.S. Department of Health and Human Services, 1980).

Geographic Distribution

Geographically, black aged are more likely to live in the South (60.2%) and are least likely to live in the western states (8.1%). In addition, the largest concentration of elderly blacks lives in the central cities (58%) or the nonmetropolitan areas (24%). A significant change in residential patterns has occurred since 1960 (Table 5–2). Essentially, a white exodus from the central cities within the last two decades has left the inner cities with a lower tax base—a key problem in social service provision (Hendricks and Hendricks, 1977).

Labor Force Participation

Rates of labor force participation for elderly black and white men, as well as women, have remained similar over the last 20 years. However, when

TABLE 5–2.—U.S. OLDER POPULATION BY REGION, MARCH 1978*

REGION	BLACK		WHITE
	Total	65 Plus	65 Plus
Total	24,710	1,930	20,316
Percent:†			
Northeast	17.7	15.3	25.5
North Central	20.0	16.4	28.0
South	53.3	60.2	30.7
West	9.1	8.1	15.8

*Data exclude persons in institutions.
†Percentages may not total 100 because of rounding.
Source: Bureau of the Census, *Current Population Reports*, series P-60, no. 119, in U.S. Department of Health and Human Services, *Characteristics of the Black Elderly, 1980*, by Williams B.S., DHHS Publication no. (OHDS)80–20057.

one combines the variables of income, sex, and unemployment rates, black men are twice as likely to be jobless or, if working, earning approximately 70% of the wages of their white male counterparts (Hendricks and Hendricks, 1977). Older blacks are also overrepresented in lower-paying, less desirable jobs. Atchley (1980) adds that, in 1970, 44% of employed blacks aged 55 to 59 were service workers, laborers, and janitors, compared to 9% for elderly white men. For older women, 67% of black women, compared to 21% of white women, occupied lower-status menial jobs. Atchley concludes that "this cohort difference in the occupational distribution is the result of discrimination many years ago, but older blacks are still paying for it, particularly in terms of their ability to generate adequate retirement income."

Income and Poverty Distribution

A serious difference between black and white elderly is also reflected in the income and poverty distribution. According to 1977 U.S. census figures, the blacks aged 65 years and older were concentrated more at the lower end of the national income scale than were elderly whites. For example, the median income of black families headed by persons 65 years or older was $6,066, compared to $9,458 for corresponding white families. Within the same family category, the percentage of families with incomes below $3,000 was 11.6 for blacks, compared to only 2.8 for whites. Similarly, the median income of unrelated individuals 65 years or older was $2,804 for blacks, compared to $3,947 for whites. Also within this category, the proportion of individuals whose income fell below $3,000 was 56% for blacks and 27.1% for white elderly. Black men aged 60 to 64 years had median incomes of $7,172, compared to $4,401 for blacks aged 65 to 69 years. For black women in these age categories, the median incomes were $2,706 and $2,618, respectively (Department of Health and Human Services, 1980).

In 1980, similar trends continued for older blacks. Approximately 800,000 blacks 65 years and older were impoverished (an annual income of $3,941 for unrelated individuals or $4,954 for a couple). These data apply to about 38.1% (two in every five) of the over-65 black population, compared to 13.6% of whites over 65. Black men were 3.5 times more likely than whites to live in poverty. Among those identified as marginally poor (annual income between 100% and 125% of the poverty threshold), 1.1 million blacks 65 and over were poor or nearly poor; 65% of black elderly women lived in poverty, and 80% were poor or marginally poor (Bureau of the Census, 1981).

Health Status and Life Expectancy

Jackson (1978) suggests that few health problems, if any, are racially unique. Still, more older blacks suffer chronic health problems than do elderly whites. For example, more than half (51%) of blacks 65 or older were victims of chronic health conditions, compared to slightly over one third (36%) of whites in the same age group. Hypertension, neoplasms, and some forms of heart or cerebrovascular diseases were the leading causes of death (Table 5–3). Presumably, many of the elderly suffer from un-

TABLE 5–3.—DEATH RATES FROM SELECTED CAUSES FOR WHITE MALES AND FEMALES AND BLACK MALES AND FEMALES AGE 65 AND OVER, 1973, PER 100,000 POPULATION

	WHITE		BLACK	
	Men	Women	Men	Women
Diseases of the heart	5,447	4,055	3,814	3,125
Cancer	1,584	875	1,450	735
Cerebrovascular diseases	1,656	1,587	1,388	1,326
Influenza and pneumonia	566	369	422	236
Arteriosclerosis	395	377	243	222
Accidents	134	95	108	61
Diabetes mellitus	162	171	154	232

Source: Siegel J.S., *Demographic Aspects of Aging and the Older Population in the United States, Current Population Reports,* series P-23, no. 59, Washington, D.C., U.S. Government Printing Office, 1976.

treated illnesses as a result of poverty, malnutrition, and inadequate medical care.

Other indicators of disability, self-care maintenance, and injury were also greater for blacks. For instance, restricted activity, disability (bedridden), and lost work days per person per year were all greater for noninstitutionalized blacks age 65 and over. Also, the frequency of physician visits per person is lower for elderly blacks, whereas they have greater average lengths of hospitalization. The latter is attributed to the belief that blacks postpone seeking medical attention until major health problems develop.

Average life expectancy is considered to be shorter for blacks (and other races) than for whites. In 1977, black life expectancy at birth was 64.6 years for men and 73.1 years for women, compared to 70.0 years for white men and 77.7 years for white women. The differential life expectancy is thus approximately 5.4 years greater for white males and 4.6 years greater for white females (Table 5–4).

The Hispanic Aged

Hispanics constitute a highly diverse community, much like that of the Pacific-Asian or native American groups. Next to blacks, people of Spanish heritage represent the second-largest minority group in this country. Of the many studies that have been done on Hispanic elderly, the majority have focused primarily on the Mexican-American population (i.e., Camarillo, 1974; Carp, 1968; Clark, 1969; Eribes and Bradley-Rawls, 1978; Maldonado, 1975; Sotomayor, 1975; Torres-Gil, 1975). As a result, less is known about other Hispanic groups such as Puerto Rican, Cuban, and other groups

TABLE 5–4.—AVERAGE LIFE EXPECTANCY AT SPECIFIED AGES BY RACE, 1977

	AVERAGE NUMBER OF YEARS OF LIFE REMAINING					
	Blacks and others			White		
Age	*Total*	*Male*	*Female*	*Total*	*Male*	*Female*
At birth	68.8	64.6	73.1	73.8	70.0	77.7
45 years	29.3	26.3	32.4	32.1	29.0	35.2
50 years	25.5	22.7	28.3	27.7	24.7	30.7
55 years	21.9	19.4	24.5	23.6	20.8	26.4
60 years	18.7	16.5	21.0	19.8	17.1	22.3
65 years	16.0	14.0	17.8	16.3	13.9	18.4
70 years	13.1	11.4	14.5	13.1	11.1	14.8
75 years	11.2	9.7	12.5	10.3	8.6	11.5

Source: Bureau of the Census, *Current Population Reports*, series P-60, no. 119, in U.S. Department of Health and Human Services, *Characteristics of the Black Elderly—1980* by Williams B.S., D.H.H.S. Publication no. (OHDS)80–20057.

of Spanish origin from Central or South America. In this section the primary emphasis is on the Mexican-American elderly, while realizing the heterogeneity that exists in the Hispanic culture.

Population Estimates

In 1980, the Spanish-origin population was estimated to be 14.6 million. Of this total, about 7.9 million (59.9%) were of Mexican origin; 1.8 million (13.8%) of Puerto Rican origin; about 830,000 (6.3%) of Cuban origin; about 1 million (7.7%) of Central and South American origin; and approximately 1.6 million (12.3%) of other Spanish origin. The Hispanic elderly population 65 years and older represents 4.2% of the total Hispanic population; and about 1.1 million, or 9.6%, of all Hispanics are 55 years of age and older (White House Conference on Aging, 1978).

Primarily as a result of high fertility rates, the Hispanic population is considerably younger than the white population. By comparison, the median age of Hispanics is 23.2 years, compared to 31.3 for whites and 24.9 for blacks (Bureau of the Census, 1981). The lower proportion of older Hispanics is also attributed to the fact that Hispanics have shorter life expectancies; they die at earlier ages, thereby skewing age structures toward the earlier years. Second, immigration and repatriation patterns have occurred over the last 60 years, with massive deportation of Mexicans during the 1920s, 1930s, and again in the 1950s. Conversely, the Cuban exodus in the 1960s and, more recently in the 1980s, has affected the age structure of Hispanics. Finally, the voluntary migration of middle-aged and older Mexican Americans to Mexico has contributed to the younger population structure (Hendricks and Hendricks, 1977).

Since Hispanics are a highly heterogeneous group, differences in nationalities and background make generalizations about the total group difficult. Caution must be observed in interpreting population statistics for two reasons. First, the Bureau of the Census has historically mislabeled Hispanics as either *white* or *Caucasian* and *nonwhite*. Estimates cannot be accurate unless separate categories are established for the various Spanish-heritage groups. A second problem results from sizable undercounting because the census is avoided by undocumented workers, persons who speak English poorly or not at all, illiterates, and other Hispanics suspicious of census-takers. The effects of mislabeling and undercounting have resulted in "constantly shifting census populations" (Cuellar, 1980).

Geographic Concentration

Data indicate that over 50% of Hispanics aged 65 and over are concentrated in five southwestern states—Arizona, California, Colorado, New

Mexico, and Texas. Other states that have significant Hispanic populations include Florida, Illinois, New York, Ohio, and Pennsylvania. Mexican Americans are more clustered in the southwestern states; Puerto Ricans, along the Eastern Seaboard and in the Commonwealth of Puerto Rico; and Cubans, mostly in Dade County in southern Florida. Other states such as Michigan, New Jersey, and Washington have also absorbed Hispanic populations, largely as a result of early migrant labor patterns and heavy industrial work (Administration on Aging, 1977).

By 1978, more than 80% of older Hispanics lived in metropolitan areas in the Southwest and on the Eastern Seaboard. However, in comparison to other Hispanic groups, a higher proportion of Mexican Americans lived in rural areas (Torres-Gil and Negm, 1980; Lacayo, 1980).

Language and Culture

Perhaps more than any other factor, the Spanish language has been a unifying theme among Hispanic populations. The elderly members, more than the younger cohorts, have retained their native language and preserved their culture. Like other groups, the Hispanic elderly are viewed as repositories of cultural traditions, values, and history. Linked closely to this fact is the view that the Hispanic elderly are highly respected and thus represent the bond among family members, friends, and other integrated members in the extended family network. More recently, a conflicting view has emerged, suggesting that the revered status of Mexican-American aged may be jeopardized as extended family structures break down and nuclear families become more common. The automatic guarantees of emotional and financial support are threatened as the matriarchal and patriarchal roles of the Hispanic elderly are slowly abandoned (Maldonado, 1975). Although debatable, at least in the present generation, there is still consensus that most Hispanic elderly maintain a relevant position in intergenerational family activity.

Income and Poverty

The proportion of older Hispanic persons with adequate incomes continues to lag behind the rest of the population in this country. In 1978, 23.2% of Hispanic elderly had incomes below the poverty level, compared to 14% of all persons in the United States. The median income of Hispanic families where the head of the household was 65 or over was $7,538, compared to $9,110 for non-Hispanic families. In addition, the unemployment rate for elderly Hispanics 55 years of age and over was 5.3%, compared to 3.0% for whites (Torres-Gil and Negm, 1980).

Data from the Bureau of the Census (1977) also indicate that two thirds of Hispanic elderly living alone were either poor or marginally poor. Other statistics demonstrate that only 55% of Hispanic aged, compared to 75% of all aged, receive Social Security benefits (Lacayo, 1980).

It can be assumed that a large number of Hispanics do not receive old-age entitlement benefits since many (e.g., farm laborers, service workers, private household workers) have not been in covered employment for the required number of quarters. Moreover, the issue of life expectancy, which is lower for Hispanic elderly than for the general population, precludes their eligibility for various types of age entitlement benefits. Stated differently, because life expectancy for Hispanics is measurably lower (e.g., 56.7 years for Mexican Americans and 47 years for Mexican-American migrant farm workers) than it is for white elderly, many Hispanics do not live long enough to collect their benefits after a lifetime of contribution to medical and Social Security trust funds.

In terms of regional differences, Bell, Kasschau, and Zellman (1976) state that 46.7% of Mexican-American elderly, 60 years of age and living in the South were impoverished, compared to 26.9% of whites in the same region. By contrast, the level of poverty was lower in the western region, where 28% of elderly Mexican Americans were poor, compared to 16.8% of whites. Bell suggests that the interregional patterns between Mexican Americans and whites are similar to those of elderly blacks and whites. Therefore, it may be assumed that "intra-racial differences across regions are as great as interracial differences within regions."

Housing Patterns

The 1979 Census Bureau estimates indicate that, in 1978, there were 195,000 Hispanic families who had heads of households 65 years of age and over; 454,000 families were headed by persons over 55 years (Torres-Gil and Negm, 1980). In 1978, the U.S. Department of Housing and Urban Development noted that only 71% of Hispanics were able to maintain adequate housing without spending more than 25% of their income for it (U.S. Department of Housing and Urban Development, 1978). Cuellar (1980) concludes that Hispanic elderly experience greater housing problems related to (1) cost of rent or mortgage payment, home maintenance, and repair; (2) vulnerability to crime and fear of victimization; (3) distance from family, friends, and necessary goods and services; (4) narrowly defined and often inappropriate program eligibility requirements; and (5) traumatic forced relocation. Finally, according to the National Association for Hispanic Elderly, physical adequacy and affordability of housing are of paramount concern to the Hispanic aged, the latter directly related to income. Moreover, inadequate housing is highest in the West and lowest in the north central areas (Lacayo, 1980).

Health

There is a serious lack of literature on the health status of elderly Hispanics. Bell et al. (1976) suggest that Mexican Americans of low socioeconomic status have needs for medical care that are similar to (if not greater than) those of other ethnic groups.

Among the leading health problems of older Hispanics generally are arthritis, high blood pressure, heart trouble, and circulation problems. The high rate of illness is largely due to poverty, inadequate health care, and, to a lesser extent, lack of familiarity with health care practices.

According to Cervantes (1972), medical folklore is an alternative system of health care delivery in the face of high-cost medical care. Therefore health care, with its highly depersonalized and bureaucratic approach, also acts as a barrier to health care service utilization. Bell affirms this view and adds that utilization differentials are due to language and cultural barriers, high costs of physician and hospital services, lack of transportation, inaccessibility of health care facilities (due to location problems), and inadequate information regarding available services.

There are other significant and numerous factors that describe the overall position of aged Hispanics. There is an appreciable amount of evidence to support the view that social and economic factors impact heavily on the lives of Hispanic elderly.

The Pacific-Asian Aged

The Pacific-Asian aged constitute a highly diverse segment of the population that includes two primary groups: Pacific Islanders and Asian Americans. The former includes persons of Fijian, Guamanian, Hawaiian, Micronesian, Samoan, and Tongan descent; the latter includes Burmese, Cambodian, Korean, Malayan, Filipino, Thai, and Vietnamese individuals (Kamikawa, 1981). The vast differences among these groups are significant and should constantly be kept in mind in our discussion (Kim, 1973; Munoz and Murase, 1973; Valle and Mendoza, 1978; Guttman, 1980; Cuellar & Weeks, 1980). However, Bell et al. (1976) see some similarities in immigration histories, social and economic conditions, and racial persecution.

This section provides only a brief review of the population characteristics of Pacific-Asian elderly. It is also limited mostly to present data on Chinese and Japanese Americans in the United States.

Historical Antecedent

The Pacific-Asian population, like other minority groups, have been victims of racism and discrimination, ranging from indentured servitude in this and previous centuries (i.e., Chinese) to internment in war camps during World War II (i.e., Japanese). Other forms of discrimination and hostility were evident from such laws as the Chinese Foreign Miners Tax of 1850, the Chinese Exclusion Act of 1882, the Japanese Alien Land Law of 1913, and the Filipino Exclusion Act of 1934. For the most part, such laws restricted immigration and travel and prevented these population groups from becoming citizens of this country. Prejudicial legislation also denied Chinese men the right to bring their wives and families to the United States. The Japanese were also subjected to harsh treatment, although they were less regulated than the Chinese. One form of discrimination was the denial of land ownership to first-generation Japanese, called Issei. It was later overcome as second-generation Japanese, Nisei, were allowed to buy land and housing legally. The Alien Exclusion Act of 1924 also reflected racist practices in this country since it barred Japanese immigration from 1924 until 1965 (Levkoff et al., 1979).

Other groups of Pacific-Asian heritage such as Filipinos and Indo-Chinese refugees also experienced similar forms of denial in American society. Yet, through the years, the Pacific-Asian communities have been able to survive such hardships because of their value orientation, interdependence or mutual help, and strong sense of self-reliance and ethnic pride.

Population Estimates

Census Bureau reports indicate that in 1970 there were 1.9 million Pacific-Asians, of whom 203,000, or 12%, were aged 60 and older. More recent estimates (1977) show that the total Pacific-Asian population has increased to 2.5 million, with 250,000 elderly aged 60 and over. Included in this figure are 533,000 immigrants from South and East Asia, of whom 24,000 were elderly (Kamikawa, 1981).

According to Fowles (1977), the majority of the aged live in urban areas (87%), with the greatest concentration of Pacific-Asians in California. Cities with the largest Pacific-Asian populations include Honolulu, Los Angeles, San Francisco, New York, Chicago, Oakland, Boston, Seattle, Philadelphia, Denver, Washington, Stockton, Norfolk, Fresno, San Jose, and San Diego.

In 1980 there were approximately 435,000 Chinese Americans, of whom 6% were over 65 years of age and 57% of that age group were men. By comparison, approximately 600,000 Japanese Americans live in this country. Nearly 8% of this population are over 65, and over two thirds (67%) of this group are women (Levkoff et al., 1979).

According to the Administration on Aging (1977), most Pacific-Asians are concentrated in California, Hawaii, New York, Illinois, and Washington.

TABLE 5–5.—PACIFIC-ASIAN ELDERLY POPULATION DISTRIBUTION BY STATE

STATE	NUMBER OF APIA'S*	PERCENTAGE OF ALL APIA'S IN U.S. AND PACIFIC TERRITORIES
California	67,245	33.2
Hawaii	47,591	23.5
New York	19,591	9.5
Illinois	6,248	3.2
Washington	5,777	2.8
Trust Territory of the Pacific	4,816	2.4
Pennsylvania	4,246	2.1
Massachusetts	3,945	1.9
New Jersey	3,818	1.9
Ohio	3,565	1.8
All other states and territories	35,994	17.8

*APIA = Asian and Pacific Island Americans.

Although exact numbers of Pacific-Asian elderly are difficult to obtain, Kamikawa (1981) provides a population distribution estimate of Pacific-Asian elderly by states (Table 5–5).

Employment and Income

Historically, few Pacific-Asians have held white- or blue-collar positions, most occupying low-paying jobs and positions not covered by Social Security. The median income of Pacific-Asian elderly has also been about $400 less than for all elderly men, and for women it was approximately $200 less (Fowles, 1977). Kamikawa (1981) adds that labor force participation was greater for Chinese, Japanese, and Filipino elderly, compared to the older population in general, in blue-collar jobs as service and farm workers.

Of the two major subgroups in the Pacific-Asian population, the median income of elderly Chinese men 65 years of age and over was $1,943; for women, this figure was $1,188. The average income of elderly men was $3,348. Median income for Japanese American men was $2,482 and the average income was $3,984 (Bell et al., 1976).

This section was a limited examination of the conditions of Pacific-Asian elderly. The omission of other potentially significant demographic data should not serve to underrate the severity of the situation experienced by this minority community. Above all, assumptions and major conclusions can only be measured if there are comprehensive, accurate, and relevant data.

The Native American Elderly

Of the four minorities, native Americans are perhaps the most identifiable disadvantaged group in this country. Ironically, less is known about this group's health conditions, socioeconomic status, and life experiences in different environmental settings. Because of their history of subjugation and forced displacement, native Americans have lost many of their political and economic rights. Past relationships between the federal government and Indian tribes have also led to the loss of sovereignty for many Indian nations. These inequities, in addition to social isolation, have resulted in deprivation unequaled among other minority groups.

Population Characteristics

According to the U.S. Department of Commerce, Bureau of the Census (1981), the Indian population (American Indian, Eskimo, and Aleut) as of 1980 reached 1,418,195. Of that total, approximately 75,000 were 65 years and older. According to Levkoff et al. (1979), the belief that all Indians live on reservations should be dispelled. The authors indicate that the majority of American Indians live off the reservation and in urban areas. However, the aged, for the most part, do continue to live on reservations or in rural areas.

By geographic distribution, five states accounted for about 53% of the elderly population 55 years and over. Eight states had populations with at least 1% or more of Indians 55 years or older. The greatest proportion of Indians live in the West and are less likely to live in the Northeast. In 1970, Oklahoma had the largest Indian population, followed by California, Arizona, New Mexico, and North Carolina (White House Conference on Aging, 1978).

Employment and Income

Employment rates for older native Americans on reservations are virtually nonexistent. Unemployment figures for elderly Indians is over 80%. The effect of such high unemployment is that a large proportion of elderly American Indians are ineligible for Social Security benefits. Harris and Cole (1980) point out that the Indian elderly cannot turn to their children for economic support, since many of them also have woefully inadequate incomes. Per capita income of the total Indian population was $1,573 in 1970 and $1,520 in 1975 for Indians living on reservations.

The high incidence of poverty is reflected in the fact that 45.6% of older Indians live below the poverty level. In terms of employment opportunities, the native American population as a whole is economically more disadvantaged than the total general population. In particular, the Indian population in the western United States is poorer (46.7%) than populations in the rest of the country (Levkoff et al., 1979). Moreover, the plight of the Indians has been aggravated by a host of other factors, including lower mean levels of education, extreme health problems and shorter life expectancy, deplorable housing, limited access to social service programs, and stringent government controls.

Conclusion

This chapter has attempted to describe the problems of the disadvantaged minority aged populations. Unfortunately, for the minority elderly as for the larger population, the prospect of significant increases in benefits and services in the future appears doubtful.

Ostensibly, there is need for coherent and foresighted policy on aging that will address the unique problems and needs of minority aged. The wholesale attack on existing programs and services, coupled with a bewildering maze of government policies and regulations, increases the lamentable circumstances of our minority aged. In order to establish an equitable network of services and benefits for the elderly, social policy and social ethics must receive greater consideration. Organizational needs, research interests, and a system of negotiations are necessary if the network of aging programs and services is to survive to meet the needs of the disadvantaged elderly in the coming years. A continuum of services that considers the social, psychological, health, financial, and cultural characteristics of minority aged must be advocated to promote the greatest social benefits for the disadvantaged elderly. As proposed by Rawls, "Differences in life prospects are just if the greater expectations of the more advantaged improve the expectations of the least advantaged and . . . the basic structure of society is just throughout provided that the advantages of the more fortunate further the well-being of the least fortunate" (Lowy, 1980).

The challenge is not solely one of service to the community and political expediency. Rather, the greatest challenge is to eliminate the problems of scarcity and major misery in a nation of surplus resources.

REFERENCES

Administration on Aging: *Fact Sheet on the Pacific-Asian Elderly*. Grant 90-A-980/1. U.S. Government Printing Office, 1977.

Atchley R.C.: *The Social Forces in Later Life*. Belmont, Calif., Wadsworth Publishing Co., 1980.

Barron M.L.: Minority group characteristics of the aged in American society. *J. Gerontol*. 8:477–482, 1953.

Bell D, Kasschau P., Zellman G.: *Delivering Services to Elderly Members of Minority Groups: A Critical Review of the Literature*. Santa Monica, Calif., Rand Corporation, 1976.

Benedict R.: A profile of Indian aged, in *Minority Aged in America*. Ann Arbor, Mich., Institute of Gerontology, University of Michigan, 1972.

Bengtson V.L.: Ethnicity and aging: Problems and issues in current social science research inquiry, in Gelfand D.E., Kutzik A.J. (eds.): *Ethnicity and Aging*. New York: Springer Publishing Co., 1979.

Camarillo M.: Areas for research on Chicano aging, in Stanford E.P. (ed.): *Minority Aging: Institute on Minority Aging Proceedings*. San Diego, Calif., San Diego State University, 1974.

Carp F.: *Factors in Utilization of Services by the Mexican American Elderly*. Palo Alto, Calif., American Institute for Research, 1968.

Cervantes R.A.: Urban Chicanos: Failure of comprehensive health service. *Health Serv. Rep*. 87:932–940, 1972.

Clark M.: Mexican American aged in San Francisco: A case description. *Gerontologist* 9:90–95, 1969.

Cowgill D.O., Holmes L.D. (eds.): *Aging and Modernization*. New York, Appleton-Century-Crofts, 1972.

Cuellar J.B.: An expanded outline and resource guide for teaching introduction to Hispanic aging, in Sherman G.A. (ed.): *Curriculum Guidelines in Minority Aging*. Washington, D.C., National Center on the Black Aged, 1980.

Cuellar J.B.: El senior-citizen's club: The elder Mexican American in the voluntary association, in Myerhoff B., Simic A. (eds.): *Life's Career—Aging: A Cross-Cultural Investigation of Growing Old*. Beverly Hills, Calif., Sage Publications, 1979.

Cuellar J.B., Weeks J.: *Minority Elderly Americans: A Prototype for Area Agencies on Aging*. Washington, D.C., Executive Summary, AoA Grant No. 90-A-1667(01), 1980.

Decker D.L.: *Social Gerontology*. Boston, Little, Brown & Co., 1980.

Dowd J.J., Bengtson V.L.: Aging in minority populations: An examination of the double jeopardy hypothesis. *J. Gerontol*. 33:427–436, 1978.

Eribes R., Bradley-Rawls M.: The underutilization of nursing home facilities by Mexican American elderly in the Southwest. *Gerontologist* 18:363–371, 1978.

Fandetti D.V., Gelfand D.E.: Care of the aged: Attitudes of white ethnic families. *Gerontologist* 16:544–549, 1976.

Fowles D.G.: *Asian and Pacific Island Americans 60+ Report*. Washington, D.C., Administration on Aging, 1977.

Fujii S.M.: Older Asian Americans: Victims of multiple jeopardy. *Civ. Rights Dig*. 9:22–29, 1976.

Guttman D.: *Perspective on Equitable Share in Public Benefits by Minority Elderly*. Washington, D.C., Executive Report, AoA Grant No. 90-A-1671, 1980.

Harris D.K., Cole W.E.: *Sociology of Aging*. Boston, Houghton Mifflin Co., 1980.

Hendricks J., Hendricks D.C.: *Aging in Mass Society*. Cambridge, Mass., Winthrop Publishing Co., 1977.

Hill R.: A demographic profile of the black elderly. *Aging* nos. 287–288:2–9, September/October 1978.

Hill R.: A profile of black aged, in *Minority Aged in America*. Ann Arbor, Mich., Institute of Gerontology, University of Michigan, 1972.

Jackson J.J.: *Minorities and Aging*. Belmont, Calif., Wadsworth Publishing Co., 1980.

Jackson J.J.: Special health problems of aged Blacks. *Aging* nos. 287–288, 15–20, 1978.

Kamikawa L.: The elderly: A Pacific/Asian perspective. *Aging* nos. 319–320:2–9, July/August 1981.

Kent D.P.: The elderly in minority groups: Variant patterns of aging. *Gerontologist* 11:26–35, 1971.

Kim B.C.: Asian Americans: No model minority. *Soc. Work* 18:44–53, 1973.
Lacayo C.G.: *A National Study to Assess the Service Needs of the Hispanic Elderly*. Final Report. Los Angeles, Calif., National Association for Hispanic Elderly, 1980.
Levkoff S., Pratt C., Esperanza R., et al.: *Minority Elderly: A Historical and Cultural Perspective*. Corvallis, Oregon State University, 1979.
Lowy L.: *Social Policies and Programs on Aging*. Lexington, Mass., D.C. Heath & Co., 1980.
Maldonado D. Jr.: The Chicano aged. *Soc. Work* 20:213–216, 1975.
Moore J.W.: Mexican Americans. *Gerontologist* 11:30–35, 1971a.
Moore J.W.: Situational factors affecting minority aging. *Gerontologist* 11:88–93, 1971b.
Munoz F.V., Murase K. (eds.): *Asian American Task Force Report: Problems and Issues in Social Work Education*. New York, Council on Social Work Education, 1973.
National Urban League: *Double Jeopardy: The Older Negro in America Today*. New York, 1964.
Rose P.I.: *They and We*. New York, Random House, 1965.
Sanchez-Ayendez M.: Puerto Rican elders: Adaptations to aging in an ethnic minority group in the United States. Unpublished paper. Amherst, Mass., University of Massachusetts, 1981.
Solomon B.: Growing old in the ethnosystem, in Stanford E.P. (ed.): *Minority Aging: Institute on Minority Aging Proceedings*. San Diego, Calif., San Diego State University, 1974.
Sotomayor M.: Social change and the Spanish-speaking elderly, in Hernandez A., Mendoza J. (eds): *Proceedings of National Conference on Spanish-speaking Elderly*. Kansas City, Kans., National Chicano Planning Council, 1975.
Tate N.P.: Ethnic considerations in service delivery to the minority aged, in Colen J.N., Soto D.L. (eds.): *Service Delivery to Aged Minorities*. Washington, D.C., Administration on Aging, 1979.
Torres-Gil F.: Concerns of the Spanish-speaking elderly, in Stanford E.P. (ed.): *Minority Aging: Second Institute on Minority Aging Proceedings*. San Diego, Calif., San Diego State University, 1975.
Torres-Gil F., Negm M.: Policy issue concerning the Hispanic elderly. *Aging* nos. 305–306, 2–5, 1980.
U.S. Congress, House of Representatives. Select Committee on Aging: *Future Directions for an Aging Policy—A Human Services Model: A Report by the Subcommittee on Human Services*. U.S. Government Printing Office, 1980.
U.S. Department of Commerce, Bureau of the Census: *Current Population Reports*, Series P-20, no. 361. *Persons of Spanish Origin in the United States: March, 1980*. Advance Report. U.S. Government Printing Office, 1981.
U.S. Department of Commerce, Bureau of the Census: *Current Population Reports*, Series P-23, no. 59. *Demographic Aspects of Aging and the Older Population in the United States*, by Siegel J. U.S. Government Printing Office, 1978.
U.S. Department of Commerce, Bureau of the Census: *Current Population Reports*, Series P-25, no. 704. *Projections of the Population of the United States: 1977–2050*. U.S. Government Printing Office, 1977.
U.S. Department of Commerce, Bureau of the Census: *Historical Statistics of the United States: Colonial Times to 1970*. U.S. Government Printing Office, 1975.
U.S. Department of Commerce, Bureau of the Census: *Supplementary Reports: 1980 Census of Population*, Series PC80-S1-1. U.S. Government Printing Office, 1981.

U.S. Department of Health and Human Services: *Characteristics of the Black Elderly—1980,* by Williams B.S. DHHS publication no. (OHDS)80–20057, 1980.
U.S. Department of Housing and Urban Development: *How Well Are We Housed?* September, 1978.
Valle R., Mendoza L.: *The Elder Latino*. San Diego, Calif., Campanile Press, 1978.
White House Conference on Aging: *Fact Sheet on the Hispanic Elderly*. Washington, D.C., 1978.
Wirth L.: The problems of minority groups, in Linton R. (ed.): *The Science of Man in the World of Crisis*. New York, Columbia University Press, 1945.
Woehrer C.E.: Cultural pluralism in American families: The influence of ethnicity on social aspects of aging. *Fam. Coord*. 27:329–339, 1978.
Young D.: *American Minority Peoples*. New York, Harper & Row, 1932.

6

AGING IN THE YEAR 2000

Thomas J. Fairchild, Ph.D.
Brenda S. Burton, M.S.

The world of the year 2000 has already arrived, for in the decisions we make now, in the way we design our environment and thus sketch the lines of constraints, the future is committed.

Daniel Bell

CURRENT INTEREST IN the social, political, and economic natures of our society in the 21st century has been stirred by popular movies such as "Star Wars" and books like *The Third Wave* by Alvin Toffler. In addition to this popular interest, academic literature has focused more and more on examining the changes that will occur in the 21st century, and on the implications of these changes for our society.

The dynamics of population change is one such area that has been recognized and given priority in academic literature and by policymakers. The purposes of this chapter are to highlight changes that will occur in the absolute and relative numbers of the aged by the year 2000, and to suggest some of the potential impacts of these changes on the health care needs of the elderly and on the health care professionals who meet these needs.

Before we can discuss the future, a clear appreciation of the past is necessary. Therefore, this chapter will first review the position of the aged in our society from the turn of the century to 1980, and will then deal with changes that will occur in this segment of the population between 1980 and 2000. Finally, the impact of these changes on the health of elderly Americans will be discussed. Health is viewed not only in terms of the well-being of the older person but also from the perspective of the training given to, and the services delivered by, health and allied health care professionals.

For practical reasons, age 65 and older will be used as the criterion for identifying and describing the elderly population. Although this definition of the elderly is convenient, it is used with a strong caveat. Although the segment of the population over 65 is different from the group under 65, the elderly as a group are extremely heterogeneous. "If anything, the accumulation of life experiences accentuates rather than diminishes differences between one older person and another" (Soldo, 1980). Just as it is unreasonable to expect homogeneity in attitudes, beliefs, and service needs from a group of people that we label middle-aged, so, too, it is unfair and equally as inaccurate to assume that all older people share the same attitudes and beliefs and have the same health, economic, or social needs. If we treat the elderly as a homogeneous group, we not only do a tremendous disservice to the aged by perpetuating a myth, but we also distort our ability to accurately plan for the wide range of needs of this segment of the population.

Current Demographics

The 20th century has witnessed a dramatic increase in the number of Americans age 65 and older. In order to better understand the aged population of the 21st century, it is enlightening to first trace the changes that have occurred since the beginning of the 20th century. Preliminary reports from the 1980 census show that the number of people over 65 has grown 27% since 1970, from 20 million to 25.5 million. The elderly now represent approximately 11.3% of the total population. The impact of these numbers is even more significant when we realize that in 1900 there were only 3 million people 65 years and older, or 4.1% of the total population (see Table 5–1).

As can further be seen from Table 5–1, the population of the United States has been getting progressively older. This increase in the proportion of elderly has helped push the U.S median age—the age at which half the population is younger and half is older—to 30 from 28 in 1970. This compares to a median age of 23 in 1900.

Not only are we older as a population, but we are living longer now than at any previous time in history. A child born in 1900 could anticipate living 47.3 years. In 1950, life expectancy had increased to 68.2 years. Today, the average life expectancy at birth is 73.3 years. The near elimination of deaths from infectious disease in the period from 1900 to 1950 increased average life expectancy about 20 years. Subsequent increases in average life expectancy have lessened somewhat in the past three decades.

While dramatic changes have occurred in the overall age structure of the population, the most significant patterns of change have taken place within the aged population itself. Table 6–1 illustrates the changes that have occurred within the older population from 1900 to the present. The population experiencing the most profound change since the beginning of the century is that which Neugarten (1975) called the "old-old" (i.e., 75 years and older). Those aged 75 and over are the most rapidly growing segment

TABLE 6–1.—TOTAL POPULATION IN THE OLDER AGED AND DECENNIAL INCREASES: 1900 TO 1980*

	65 YEARS AND OVER		75 YEARS AND OVER		85 YEARS AND OVER	
Year	Number	% Increase	Number	% Increase	Number	% Increase
Estimates:						
1900	3,099	N.A.†	899	N.A.†	122‡	N.A.†
1910	3,986	28.6	1,170	30.1	167‡	36.9
1920	4,929	23.7	1,449	23.8	210‡	25.7
1930	6,705	36.0	1,945	34.2	272‡	29.5
1940	9,031	34.7	2,664	37.0	370	36.0§
1950	12,397	37.3	3,904	46.5	590	59.5
1960	16,675	34.5	5,621	44.0	940	59.3
1970	20,085	20.4	7,598	35.2	1,432	52.3
1980	25,544	27.2	9,967	31.2	2,240	56.4

*Numbers in thousands; estimates and projections as of July 1, 1975.
†N.A. = not applicable.
‡Estimates for 1900–1930 as of April 1, 1975.
§Pertains to 10¼-year period.
Source: U.S. Department of Commerce, Bureau of the Census. *Current Population Reports,* series P-23, no. 59. *Supplementary Reports,* PC80-S1-1, 1981.

of the population, having increased from 900,000 in 1900 to 9.9 million in 1980. The most significant growth has occurred in the 85-plus age group, which experienced a 56.4% increase between 1970 and 1980.

The 85 and over group now constitutes about 8% of the population over 65, compared to 4% in 1900. The 65–74 age group has decreased slightly as a proportion of the total aged population. In 1900, this group constituted 71% of the total aged population; by 1975, the percentage had dropped to 62.

In comparison to the white population, in which the elderly account for 11.8% of the total white population, the black elderly represent 7.9% of the total black population, while the elderly of Spanish origin account for about 4% of that total population. Between 1970 and 1975, the Hispanic aged population grew by 23%. This difference in age structure is clearly reflected in the 1980 census, where whites had the highest median age—31.3—compared to blacks, with a median age of 24.9, and people of Spanish origin, with a median age of 23.2 years. The differences between the age structures of the white and black populations are accounted for primarily by the higher fertility of the black population, the relatively greater declines in mortality rates among younger blacks, and the large immigration of whites prior to World War I (Bureau of the Census, 1978). A similar explanation may apply to the population of Spanish origin with the additional factor of large numbers of young men of Spanish descent immigrating to the United States.

The disparity in the numbers of men and women is a relatively modern phenomenon that is reflected at most age ranges in the population. In 1900, there were 102 men over the age of 65 for every 100 women. As a result of significant reductions in maternal mortality rates, we have witnessed a reversal in this ratio, particularly over the last 40 years (Table 6–2). Based on preliminary data from the 1980 census, there were three women for every two men over the age of 65. For the 85-and-older group, there were 1,558,293 women and 681,428 men—a ratio of more than 2 to 1 (Bureau of the Census, 1981).

The primary reason for the imbalance in the numbers of aged men and women is the differential impact of sex on life expectancy. Women, on the average, outlive their male counterparts by 8 years. In 1978, the average life expectancy at birth for women was 77.2 years and for men, 69.5 years. The results of this difference are clearly mirrored in the fact that 41% of women between 65 and 74 are widows while 69% of women over 75 have lost a spouse (Bureau of the Census, 1978).

The dramatic growth of the aged population has been caused by interaction of the basic demographic functions of fertility and mortality. The decrease in mortality rates, coupled with a declining fertility rate, has resulted in changes in the age structure. While decreases in mortality rates have been fairly steady, fertility rates have tended to fluctuate. A high level of fertility at the beginning of the century resulted in many people aged 65 and over today. Fertility then began to decline until the high birth rates of the 1950s, the baby-boom decade. The birth rate has been steadily declining since the end of the 1950s and is currently at a below-replacement

TABLE 6–2.—SEX RATIOS OF AGE GROUPS: 1900 TO 1975*

AGE	1900	1930	1960	1970	1975
All ages	104.4	102.5	97.8	95.8	95.3
Under 15	102.1	102.8	103.4	103.9	104.1
15–24	98.3	98.1	101.4	102.2	102.2
25–44	109.1	101.7	96.9	96.9	97.3
45–54	113.9	109.4	97.2	93.3	93.6
55–64	106.5	108.3	93.7	89.7	89.6
65–74	104.5	104.1	86.7	77.7	76.8
75–84	N.A.†	N.A.	77.4	65.9	61.5
85 and over	N.A.	N.A.	63.8	53.2	48.5
65 and over	102.0	100.4	82.6	72.0	69.3
75 and over	96.3	91.8	75.0	63.3	58.4

*Men per 100 women as of July 1, 1975. Figures for 1960 and later years include armed forces overseas.

†N.A. = not available.

Source: U.S. Department of Commerce, Bureau of the Census. *Current Population Reports,* series P-23, no. 59, p. 13. U.S. Government Printing Office, 1978.

level, or approximately 1.7 births per woman (Bureau of the Census, 1975).

Since 1900, there have been dramatic drops in the mortality rate for the total population. The age-adjusted death rate has decreased significantly since the turn of the century, from 17.8 deaths to 8.4 deaths per 1,000 population in 1977.

The main reasons for this changing mortality rate are (1) reductions in deaths from infectious diseases and (2) the shift in death rates from infectious causes to chronic illnesses such as heart disease. Of all deaths, those among the aged account for two thirds of the total. Seventy-five percent of deaths in the 65-and-older population are the result of three major killers: heart disease, cancer, and stroke. Deaths from heart disease and stroke in the total population have been declining slightly. However, death rates from cancer have increased for the total population and increased by 7% for all elderly persons between 1970 and 1977 (National Center for Health Statistics, 1979).

The continuing decline in mortality rates and the current low fertility level strongly suggest that the aged will continue to constitute a significant percentage of the population in the future.

The Elderly in the Year 2000

Although this section focuses on the number and proportion of elderly in the year 2000, it is important to remember that this exercise is not as futuristic as it may appear. In terms of numbers of elderly, we can be fairly confident in our statements because—barring any dramatic increase in deaths—the future aged of the year 2000 are already alive today. Projections of the elderly population at the beginning of the 21st century involve estimates of mortality, which is the most stable demographic process (Barclay, 1958).

In contrast, however, forecasting the proportion of elderly persons in the year 2000 is made difficult by the fact that projections of the total population must be considered, including birth rate, which is much less stable than the mortality rate; hence, such projections are less reliable (Barclay, 1958). This is not to suggest that the figures presented in this chapter are part of a methodological game, but rather that, as with any projection, accuracy depends on the validity of the underlying assumptions. Here, assumptions underlying the projections will be specified where possible so that the reader can appreciate what Sheppard and Rix (1977) call "the risky game of population projections."

Just as the aging of America continued to increase during the 1970s, it is expected to do so during the last two decades of this century. Assuming the current fertility level (1.7 children per woman), the elderly will account for about 13% of the total population by the year 2000. Table 6–3 shows this projected growth of the elderly that will be reflected in the median age, which, under the current level of fertility, would increase by about 7 years to 37.3 years in the year 2000. An increase in fertility rates to replacement level (2.1 children per woman) would, however, cause the population to age at a slower rate and would reduce the median age to 35.5 years.

Longer life expectancy for women is expected to continue in the near future. It is projected that the average life expectancy for both sexes in the year 2000 will be 74.1 years. For men, the life expectancy value for 2000 is 70.0 years, as compared with 78.3 years for women (Bureau of the Census, 1979).

The dramatic growth of the older population often overshadows the unprecedented changes occurring within that population. It is forecasted that the age group that will grow most rapidly will be the group 85 years and older. During the next two decades, the number of people 65 years and over is expected to increase by about 28%. This compares to the increase for the oldest age group (85 and over), projected to be approximately 64%,

TABLE 6–3.—POPULATION PROJECTION FOR THE UNITED STATES FOR 65 YEARS AND OLDER: 1985–2000*

PROJECTIONS	65 YEARS AND OLDER (millions)	PERCENT OF TOTAL POPULATION 65 YEARS AND OLDER	MEDIAN AGE OF TOTAL POPULATION
Series I			
1985	27,305	11.4	30.7
1990	29,824	11.7	31.4
1995	31,401	11.7	32.1
2000	31,822	11.3	32.5
Series II			
1985	27,305	11.7	31.5
1990	29,824	12.2	32.8
1995	31,401	12.4	34.2
2000	31,822	12.2	35.5
Series III			
1985	27,305	11.9	32.0
1990	29,824	12.6	33.7
1995	31,401	13.0	35.5
2000	31,822	12.9	37.3

*Projections as of July 1, 1976.

Source: U.S. Department of Commerce, Bureau of the Census. *Current Population Reports*, series P-25, no. 704, table H pp. 10–11. U.S. Government Printing Office, 1977. Levels of complete cohort fertility assumed are: Series I, 2.7 children per woman; Series II, 2.1 children per woman; Series III, 1.7 children per woman. Assumed level of net immigration (immigration minus emigration) is 400,000 per year.

while the elderly 75 and over are expected to increase by 53% "Of the 7 million increase in the size of the older population likely to occur between 1980 and 2000 almost three fourths of it (5 million) will be concentrated in the group 75 years of age and over" (Soldo, 1980). This differential growth within the older population continues the trend of the 1970s, which will result in some 44% of the elderly population being 75 years of age or older in the year 2000.

The divergence between white and black life expectancy at birth is expected to continue in the decades ahead (see Table 5–4). The declining ratio of men to women for the black population is expected to continue through the year 2000. The current ratio is projected to drop from approximately 70.7 men to 67.8 men per 100 women in the year 2000 (Bureau of the Census, 1978). "The Census Bureau projects 3 million blacks 65 and over for the year 2000 which, if borne out, would increase the older black population by 46% in the next two decades, 21 percentage points more than the older white population over that time span" (Soldo, 1980). Similar growth is also projected by the Census Bureau for elderly of Spanish origin.

One aspect of the aging population that is abundantly evident to those who provide services to the elderly is the massive proportional deficit of men to women when age increases. The higher mortality rates for men 65 and over as reflected in a diminished increase in the older male population is illustrated by Table 6–4. This higher mortality rate for men has had a significant impact on the composition of the male and female population over 65. It is projected that by the year 2000 there will be 66 men for every 100 women. In every successive age category the decrease in the number of men per 100 women becomes more striking.

The divergence between the number of elderly women and men is very evident among the group 85 years and older, where in the year 2000 it is projected that there will be 39 males for every 100 females.

TABLE 6–4.—PROJECTED PERCENTAGE INCREASE OF THE POPULATION 65 YEARS OLD AND OVER, BY AGE AND SEX: 1976–2000

SEX AND PERIOD	65 AND OVER	65–74	75–84	85 AND OVER
Male				
1976–2000	36	24	55	69
Female				
1976–2000	41	22	58	101

Source: U.S. Department of Commerce, Bureau of the Census. *Current Population Reports,* series P-23, no. 78, p. 10. U.S. Government Printing Office, 1979.

Health Care—Present Trends and Future Needs

Projections suggest that our society can reasonably anticipate that the elderly will continue to grow in numbers and, by the year 2000, based on current fertility levels, will constitute about 13% of the population. More specifically, we have noted that the greatest growth is occurring in the segment of the aged population that is 75 years or older. In the initial decades subsequent to the 21st century the aged population is expected to experience even greater growth so that, by the year 2030, the elderly, depending on fertility rates, will represent 13% to 21% of the population (Bureau of the Census, 1977).

The growing number of elderly, especially the old-old, is substantially altering the age structure of our society and putting increasing demands on our health care system. The Bureau of the Census projects that by 2050 female life expectancy will be 81 years and male life expectancy will have increased to about 72 years. Thus, the future society will be composed of an even greater percentage of old-old, who characteristically are the most vulnerable to physiologic decrements and who may find themselves with inadequate resources to meet related needs.

The growth in the numbers of aged in the next 20 years will affect our health care system in several fundamental ways. While age itself does not cause death, the aged as a group have higher incidences of chronic illness and often must cope with multiple chronic illnesses. "Eighty-five percent of the elderly suffer from at least one chronic condition, and 42% of those over age 65 are limited in activity because of chronic conditions" (Kane et al., 1980). Because their health problems are often chronic, the elderly require the services of the health care system on a much more frequent and long-term basis. This is mirrored in the fact that the noninstitutionalized elderly averaged 6.3 physician visits per year in 1978, compared to 4.6 visits for those under 65 years (Health Interview Survey, 1978). In addition, those 65 and older in 1978 averaged 11 short-stay hospital days compared to those under 65, who averaged almost half that number—5.8 days (Health Interview Survey, 1978).

Although mortality from the three leading causes of death among the aged—cardiovascular disease, malignant neoplasms, and cerebrovascular disease—is being reduced, these afflictions probably will not be eradicated by the dawn of the 21st century. It is, of course, difficult to accurately predict the health care status and utilization rates of the elderly in the year 2000. However, it appears that future generations of elderly will benefit from changing habits in physical exercise and diet, higher levels of education, and reduction of childhood diseases. In addition to being better educated and more mobile, they will be healthier longer, but there is "no evidence to suggest that they will be less incapacitated in the final phase preceding their death" (Tobin, 1978).

Because of the alterations occurring in the age structure of our society and the inherent implications of these changes, it is critical to plan health care services that can adequately meet the needs of this population. To plan for the health care needs of the elderly in the year 2000, a number of issues must be addressed. These issues include, but are not limited to, the assumptions that underlie our current health care model, the social support network available to the elderly, the cost of health care, the types of care available, and the training of the professionals and paraprofessionals who provide the care.

Recognizing the incidence of chronic illness among the elderly and the increasing numbers of old-old should make us keenly aware of the need to change the assumptions that underlie our current health care system. The major elements of the present system are based on the acute care model, which does not adequately serve older adults who are often beset with chronic health problems. One problem that must be addressed is the lack of personnel trained in gerontology and geriatric medicine. This inadequacy in trained personnel was reflected in testimony before the House Select Committee on Aging in 1978. It was reported that less than one half of our medical schools offer courses in geriatrics, and only three schools offer a specialization in this area (Subcommittee on Health and Long-term Care, 1978). Further, in 1971, only 27 out of 512 nursing schools had programs or courses in geriatrics (Subcommittee on Health and Long-term Care, 1978). These discouraging statistics point out some fundamental problems in providing services to the aged. First, there is a pervasive attitude that growing old means growing progressively sicker. We have come to accept poor health as a condition of advancing years. Second, many service providers dislike treating the aged because of the cultural view that old age is an unavoidable misfortune (Mutschler, 1971).

In the future, as suggested by Rice (1981), the supply of physicians will be more than adequate. With current educational trends, however, it is reasonable to ask if physicians will be adequately trained in geriatric medicine. Given that 23% of each health care dollar goes directly for professional services of physicians and other health care providers, and the unavoidable fact that the number of aged will increase significantly in the future, the importance of personnel adequately trained in geriatrics cannot be emphasized enough.

The changing structure of the family will significantly affect the health needs of the aged. The kinship network is rapidly altering because of scientific and technological advances that are changing the way we live and relate to one another. The impact of these changes is reflected in the decline of single elderly 75 and over who are living with relatives (45% in 1950; 25% in 1977). Because women outlive men, a higher proportion of single aged are women. In 1977, nearly 70% of women over 75 were widows, compared to 24% of the men in the same age category. A major trend in living arrangements "has been a decline in the overall number of multigenerational households reflecting the greater tendency of female widows to live by themselves and the equal tendency of males to remain married or remarry and maintain themselves as heads of their own households" (Mindel, 1979). Increased geographic mobility will continue to separate the aged and their families. The number of aged residing with families other than a spouse is declining (Kane et al., 1980); thus, the aged will increasingly look toward community services to help meet their health care needs.

A further question that urgently needs our consideration is the adequacy of health services for the elderly in the 21st century, and the cost of these services. Less than 5% of the population over 65 lives in nursing homes; however, the proportion rises significantly when age increases. By age 85 and over, almost 22% are living in nursing homes. Based on current occupancy rates, and assuming average length of stay does not change, 3 million beds will be needed shortly after the turn of the century—an increase of approximately 1.6 million beds from the current level of 1.4 million (Rice, 1981).

Future need for short-stay hospital beds is a more complex issue. Factors that interact to determine supply and demand include utilization rates, length of stay, admission policy, and national guidelines for health planning that call for four hospital beds per 1,000 persons. Given these factors, the suggestion by Rice (1981) to constantly monitor the situation to assure an adequate supply of hospital beds in the future seems reasonable.

In addition to the need for more nursing home and hospital beds in the 21st century is the need to change the current configuration of health care services to better serve the elderly in the year 2000. Tobin (1975) has identified three important types of service delivery to the aged. The first is the community-based organization that integrates a range of services under one setting and is designed to delay or prevent premature institutionalization. These services, individualized to meet the particular needs of the client, consist of both social and health services. Second is a smaller (20–50 beds), free-standing, community-based facility that provides custodial care services. This decentralized facility is architecturally designed to assure maximum mobility and social interaction of the residents and is linked with other medical facilities, as well as the social service system, to ensure a continuum of care. Finally, Tobin identifies a third form of social health service—the hospice—as an area of probable growth in the future. This care center helps terminally ill patients and their families through the dying process by controlling pain and by maintaining maximum social supports.

Many people currently working in the field of aging criticize the multitude of services offered today for their lack of integration. A continuum of services is needed to meet the various health needs of the older person throughout the aging process. Thus, such services as geriatric day care, home health care, homemaker services, and hospice care, must be more closely coordinated with those of the hospital, the long-term care facility, and the community in order to achieve adequate, efficiently delivered health care for the aged in the future.

Currently, about 29% of the health care dollar is spent on those over age 65. Medical expenses for the aged are approximately three times those for people under 65. The cost of health care has been steadily escalating and has become a major economic concern. The changing age distribution of the population is significantly affecting health services for the elderly, whose portion of total health care costs is greater than that of any other age group. In 1977, the per capita health care expenditure for the elderly was $1,745.17, or 3.4 times the per capita expenditure of $514.25 for those under 65 (National Center for Health Statistics, 1980).

In 1978, health care expenditures totaled $192 billion; and by the year 2000 it is projected that, with current rates of inflation, approximately one trillion dollars will be spent. Therefore, society faces critical choices in resource allocation. Should society invest huge amounts of money to eradicate death-causing disease and to extend life, or should funds be channeled into the development of well-integrated community health services?

In deciding on the allocation of resources to meet these needs, Tobin (1975) has argued that "our society will not allocate sufficient funds for therapeutic institutional care for the very-old, saying among other things, that it is very costly to hire personnel for the unpleasant task of caring for the chronically-ill aged." Thus it is clear that the decision on allocation of health care resources is one of the fundamental choices determining the future direction of health care and the ability of the health care system to meet the evolving needs of the elderly in the year 2000.

Conclusion

Since the future certainly begins in the present, projections about the aged in the year 2000 can be made with relative confidence because the people who will be 65 in the year 2000 are alive today. An educated guess about the scenario for the next 20 years suggests that continued medical advances will reduce mortality rates and, given current birth rates, that a significantly larger and more diverse elderly population will exist by the year 2000. The diversity of the elderly can be characterized by perhaps three groups: (1) old-old, (2) minorities, and (3) women. These three characteristics may be labeled what O'Neill (1981) refers to as "drivers of change," and they will certainly shape the future of the elderly population and our society.

In order to ensure that the future needs of the elderly can be met, fundamental changes must be made in our health care system and in the training of the people who work in that system. However, it is important to keep in mind the point made by the Commission on the Year 2000: "A complex society is not changed by a flick of the wrist" (Bell, 1967). To paraphrase the noted futurist Daniel Bell, the United States in the year 2000 will be more *like* the United States in the year 1982 than *different*. From the current political, business, and social trends, one can assume that the basic framework of our health care system will remain to the beginning of the 21st century without any dramatic changes.

This scenario does not negate the fact that the future is of the utmost importance and that it will be shaped by the "drivers of change" mentioned earlier. Technological innovation is rapidly changing "future expectations" into "present memories," and no one knows how life-extending research will transform the basic structures of society. What we can be certain about is that the beginning of the 21st century is less than 20 years away and "the future is an absolute reflection of the present" (Peterson et al., 1976). Past treatment of social issues in the United States suggests that adequate planning for the health care needs of the elderly in the year 2000 will not occur in earnest until the future is the present.

This educated guess about the next 20 years should not be an excuse to lull ourselves into a state of complacency because to do so is at our *own* peril.

REFERENCES

Barclay G.W.: *Techniques of Population Analysis*. New York, John Wiley & Sons, 1958.

Bell D. (ed.): *Toward The Year 2000: Work in Progress*. Boston, Beacon Press, 1967.

Brotman H.B.: The aging society. *Aging* January/February:2–5, 1981.

Clark R.L., Spengler J.J.: *The Economics of Individual and Population Aging*. Cambridge, Cambridge University Press, 1980.

Clark R., Spengler J.: Population aging in the twenty-first century. *Aging* January/February:6–13, 1978.

Conniff R.: Living longer. *NEXT* May/June:38,40–45, 1981.

Cunningham R.M.: The bed you shrink may be your own. *Hospitals* 52:105–107, 1978.

Golant S.M.: Residential concentrations of the future elderly. *Gerontologist* 15:16–23, 1975.

Gordon T.J. (ed.): The year 2050: Reflections of a futurist, in *The Lamp*. Exxon Corporation, Spring, 1981, pp. 26–31.

Herbers J.: Sharp rise of elderly population in 70's portends future increases. *New York Times* May 24, pp. 1,14, 1981.
Hickey T.: *Health and Aging*. Belmont, Calif., Brooks/Cole Publishing, 1980.
Kane R., Solomon D., Beck J., et al.: *Geriatrics in the United States: Manpower Projections and Training Considerations,* Rand Publication Series. Santa Monica, Calif., Rand Corporation, 1980.
Mindel C.H.: Multigenerational family households: Recent trends and implications for the future. *Gerontologist* 16:456–463, 1979.
Mutschler P.: Factors affecting choice of and perservation in social work with the aged. *Gerontologist* 11:231–241, 1971.
Neugarten B.L.: The future and the young-old. *Gerontologist* 15:32–37, 1975.
O'Neill G.K.: *2081: A Hopeful View of the Human Future*. New York, Simon & Schuster, 1981.
Palmore E.B.: The future status of the aged. *Gerontologist* 16:297–302, 1976.
Palmore E.B.: Potential demographic contributions to gerontology. *Gerontologist* 13:236–242, 1973.
Peterson D., Powell C., Robertson L.: Aging in America, toward the year 2000. *Gerontologist* 16:264–269, 1976.
Rice D.P.: The aging of America: Economic woes may dim the elderly's golden years. *The Review* March/April:3, 15, 17–18, 22, 24, 26, 28, 30, 32–33, 1981.
Sheppard H.L., Rix S.E.: *The Graying of Working America*. New York, Macmillan Publishing Co., 1977.
Soldo B.J.: America's elderly in the 1980's. *Popul. Bull.* 35(4):9, 1980.
Taggert P.: The elderly population expansion. *Life Care Directors Digest* 4(1):n.p., 1980.
Tobin S.: The future elderly: Needs and services. *Aging* January/February:22–26, 1978.
Tobin S.: Social and health services for the future aged. *Gerontologist* 15:32–37, 1975.
Toffler A.: *The Third Wave*. New York, William Morrow & Co., 1980.
U.S. Congress, House of Representatives. Special Committee on Aging: *The Graying of Nations: Implications*. 95th Congress, 1st sess. U.S. Government Printing Office, 1977.
U.S. Congress, House of Representatives. Subcommittee on Federal, State and Community Services: *Aging in the World of Tommorrow (Part I),* Comm. pub. no. 95–108, 95th Congress, 1st sess. U.S. Government Printing Office, 1977.
U.S. Congress, House of Representatives. Subcommittee on Health and Long-Term Care: *Future of Health Care and the Elderly (Geriatric Medicine),* Comm. pub. no. 95–151, 95th Congress, 2d sess. U.S. Government Printing Office, 1978.
U.S. Congress, House of Representatives. Subcommittee on Human Services: *Life Extension and Tomorrow's Elderly,* Comm. pub. no. 95–127, 95th Congress, 2d sess. U.S. Government Printing Office, 1978.
U.S. Congress, House of Representatives. Select Committee on Aging: *Future Directions for an Aging Policy—A Human Services Model: A Report by the Subcommittee on Human Services*. U.S. Government Printing Office, 1980.
U.S. Department of Commerce, Bureau of the Census: *Current Population Reports,* Series P-25, no. 601. *Projections of the Population of the United States: 1975 to 2050*. U.S. Government Printing Office, 1975.
U.S. Department of Commerce, Bureau of the Census: *Current Population Reports,* Series P-25, no. 704. *Projections of the Population of the United States: 1977 to 2050*. U.S. Government Printing Office, 1977.

U.S. Department of Commerce, Bureau of the Census: *Current Population Reports,* Series P-23, no. 59. *Demographic Aspects of Aging and the Older Population in the United States,* by Siegel J. U.S. Government Printing Office, 1978.

U.S. Department of Commerce, Bureau of the Census: *Current Population Reports,* Series P-20, no. 338. *Marital Status and Living Arrangements.* U.S. Government Printing Office, 1978.

U.S. Department of Commerce, Bureau of the Census: *Current Population Reports,* Series P-23, no. 78. *Prospective Trends in the Size and Structure of the Elderly Population, Impact of Mortality Trends, and Some Implications,* by Siegel J. U.S. Government Printing Office, 1979.

U.S. Department of Commerce, Bureau of the Census: *Current Population Reports,* Series P-20, no. 361. *Persons of Spanish Origin in the United States: March, 1980 (Advance Report).* U.S. Government Printing Office, 1981.

U.S. Department of Commerce, Bureau of the Census: *Supplementary Reports,* PC80–S1–1. *Age, Sex, Race, and Spanish Origin of the Population by Regions, Divisions, and States: 1980.* U.S. Government Printing Office, 1981.

U.S. Department of Health, Education, and Welfare. Public Health Service: *National Center for Health Statistics.* Vital and Heath Statistics. *Current Estimates from the Health Interview Survey: United States—1978, no. 130.* U.S. Government Printing Office, 1979.

U.S. Department of Health, Education, and Welfare. Public Health Service: *National Center for Health Statistics.* Vital and Health Statistics. *Health United States 1979.* U.S. Government Printing Office, 1980.

Wiseman R.F.: *Spatial Aspects of Aging.* Washington, D.C., Association of American Geographers, 1978.

PART II

Medical Science

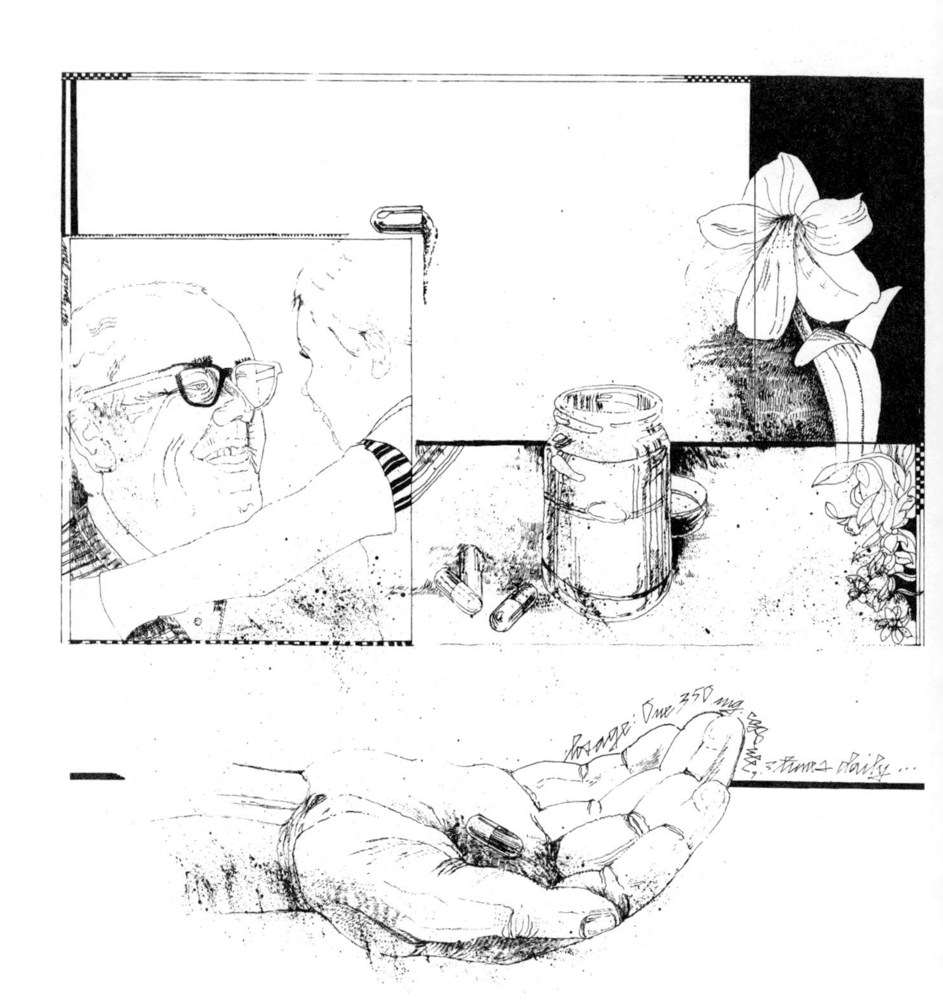
Dosage: One 350 mg. capsule, 3 times daily ...

7

MEDICAL HEALTH PROBLEMS AND HEALTH CARE ISSUES

Seymour Eisenberg, M.D.

MAXIMUM LIFE span for humans is approximately 110 years; this has not changed for thousands of years and is probably an immutable, genetically determined biologic limit. On the other hand, mean life span, or life expectancy, has increased from 46 years in 1900 to about 73–74 years in 1978. This increase has resulted almost completely from prevention of premature deaths in persons under 50; life expectancy in the over-60 population has not changed significantly in the past 80 years. It has been suggested (Fries, 1980) that a life expectancy of 85 may be attained by 2020 and that this may be the best achievable span.

Everyone engaged in the care of the elderly must be aware of these facts—not to encourage an attitude of hopelessness but to point out the finite limits of what one might hope to achieve. Every vigorous aged person who becomes ill must be treated as though he or she is advantaged genetically and is destined to reach an age near maximum life span. Patients with debilitating disorders may have sustained obviously irreparable injury and under these circumstances one may have to modify goals and alter expectations.

The aging process is characterized by progressively decreasing organ reserve. In the young, organ performance can increase as much as tenfold; or, expressed another way, for ordinary activity and circumstances organs may need to function at only a fraction of their total capacity. The elderly, on the other hand, have no such safety factor, no functional reserve; most organs are functioning at or near capacity during ordinary activities. When subjected to stress, the aged experience this inadequacy and it contributes to an overall difficulty in handling threatening stressful situations or illness.

Although there are cumulative disabilities that result from advancing years, old age is not an illness or an affliction. The majority (70%) of elderly people are quite satisfied with the state of their health. Moreover, inclusion of the 65–75 age group, the young elderly, in these considerations of the medical illnesses of the geriatric population will reveal a great number of active, vigorous people who may admit to some decline in function and some minor health problems but, in the main, require little attention. They would, and should, object to being considered outside the medical mainstream. It is true that certain diseases are almost completely limited to the elderly and that during these later years chronic disorders, often multiple, appear. Moreover, many common diseases are encountered with clinical manifestations that differ remarkably from those found in younger patients.

It is essential that people who work with the elderly be aware of the specific diseases associated with aging as well as the common complaints and problems of the aged. It is important not to mistake illness for aging changes and to consider any symptoms, particularly new ones, meaningful until proved otherwise. Thus, this chapter will include the important features of common illnesses likely to be encountered, signs of deterioration or complications of the basic problems, adverse reactions to treatment, and danger signals requiring more sophisticated attention.

Illnesses of the Elderly

These are disorders occurring almost exclusively in elderly persons.

Senile Dementia

Apprehension about this problem is foremost in the minds of aging persons and their relatives. True dementia of the Alzheimer type—or organic brain syndrome—must be distinguished from reversible causes of dementia, such as depression or simple forgetfulness. Senile dementia is associated with recognizable changes in the brain and carries with it a bleak prognosis. These people are unaware of themselves as well as their family, place, or time. They are unable to care for themselves and usually require institutional care. The diagnosis should be made by a physician who is particularly competent in this area, since reversible disorders may masquerade as true dementia, leading to consignment of the patient to inappropriate and intolerable surroundings.

Complications

There is slow deterioration with time, the average life span being five years from onset. These individuals often aspirate and may develop dehydration if not carefully observed. A frequent cause of death is infection, such as bronchopneumonia.

Danger Signals

The sudden onset of coma or fever in a demented subject requires that professional judgment be rendered on the nature of the problem, the treatment that should be instituted, and how vigorous that treatment should be. Such decisions should not be left to a nonprofessional. Afflicted patients are apt to develop pneumonia, urinary tract infections, skin infections, and other problems that might be obscured by their inability to communicate their symptoms adequately.

Hypothermia

For reasons not fully understood, aging is associated with a decreased capability of adapting to temperature changes; the elderly are particularly vulnerable to cold. This is not an infrequent cause of death, and great care must be taken to protect the elderly in circumstances of extreme cold. The care is usually appropriate except where the aged are isolated and neglected. When ambient temperatures are only moderately low and the danger appears minimal, precautions may not be adequate. Much of this is a central nervous system effect but it may involve lessened activity of the thyroid, decrease in heat-retention properties of the skin, decrease in shiver response, and so on.

The complaints indicating this problem are not specific. The alert aged may complain of being cold, but the syndrome may be apparent only by a decrease in responsiveness, by apathy, and ultimately by coma. The patient is cold to the touch and his temperature may be below 90 F. This constitutes an emergency and the patient should be transferred to a major hospital where body core temperature can be monitored and restored. Prior to this time, warming blankets should be used. The best guidelines for the health care provider are being aware of the problem and taking proper preventive action.

Diabetic Hyperosmolar Coma

This is one of many major complications of diabetes mellitus that is almost exclusively confined to the elderly. Adult onset diabetes mellitus is an extremely common problem in elderly patients, particularly women. Most do not require insulin but are managed satisfactorily with oral drugs and diet. The hyperosmolar state is an infrequent but alarming complication. The main symptom of the problem is an inordinate rise in blood sugar—which is often only modestly elevated in elderly subjects. Their usual 200–350 mg/100 ml blood sugar levels rise to the 750–2,000 mg/100 ml range. At this level, the glucose becomes a major determinant of osmolality, meaning that it draws water from cells; when this occurs in the brain, the result is stupor and then coma. There is little, if any, tendency to develop diabetic ketoacidosis, the better known and most dreaded complication of juvenile diabetes. The hyperosmolar state may be precipitated by an underlying serious medical disorder such as an acute myocardial infarction or "heart attack." There is significant mortality associated with this problem even with prompt and seemingly effective therapy.

Other complications of the elderly diabetic might be considered at this point, although these are not strictly limited to the elderly patient.

Foot ulcers, infection, and gangrene are examples of the many catastrophic problems that may develop in the feet of diabetic patients. These are mainly the result of severe interference with blood supply to the feet caused by obliterative arterial disease (atherosclerosis). Foot care must be impeccable; the slightest cut, the most trivial infection requires active treatment. Careful observation of the feet, care of the skin and nails, and avoidance of heat are some of the precautions. If feasible, active participation by a podiatrist in this phase of patient care will practically eliminate this type of problem. Of particular danger is the seemingly innocuous application of heat; these patients frequently have underlying peripheral neuritis that diminishes their pain/temperature perception and makes them susceptible to burns.

Complications of diabetes with which supervisory personnel should be acquainted include hypoglycemic (low blood sugar) reactions to insulin or drugs used to treat this disorder. These are extremely dangerous incidents and require modification of the treatment program. A hypoglycemic event can vary in severity from nervousness and apprehension to loss of consciousness to coma. The administration of glucose, perhaps as sweetened orange juice, may be life-saving. Other problems include a higher frequency of urinary tract infections, tuberculosis, heart attacks, peripheral neuritis, and fainting on assuming erect posture.

Temporal Arteritis and Polymyalgia Rheumatica

These are distinct syndromes; however, they frequently occur together, and the diagnosis of one suggests the likelihood of a patient developing the other. Temporal arteritis is a giant cell inflammatory disorder of the temporal and other arteries. There is pain and tenderness in one or both temple areas, and the diagnosis may be established by biopsy. A dreaded complication of this disorder is involvement of the major artery supplying the retina, which not infrequently results in sudden loss of vision on the affected side.

Polymyalgia rheumatica is a painful disorder of the shoulders and occasionally the hips in elderly patients. The major complaint is pain and stiffness that is much worse at night and that can be so incapacitating that movement is quite difficult. A particular feature of the illness is an extremely fast sedimentation rate, a commonly performed and usually nonspecific measure of the rate at which red blood cells sediment in an appropriate tube. A specific feature of the illness is a highly gratifying and dramatic response to adrenal cortical steroids. Once initiated, treatment is continued, not only to ameliorate the symptoms but to guard against an increased possibility of visual loss if there is concomitant temporal arteritis.

Osteoporosis

This is a disorder that is not limited to the elderly but occurs in this population group with sufficient frequency to qualify as an age-associated disease. The underlying problem is demineralization of bone, and it is this loss of density and basic bone strength that doubtless leads to the fractured hips, wrists, and vertebrae that plague the elderly. The disorder is of uncertain etiology but it is closely coupled with the menopause and other hormonal disturbances, with inactivity, inadequate calcium intake, and certain other disorders. There are no specific symptoms of the disorder, although some patients may complain of vague discomfort. The mineral loss is detected readily by radiographic examination.

There is some controversy about the reversibility of these changes once they have occurred, but progression of the disorder can certainly be halted. High-calcium diets and estrogens have been employed with questionable success. Once the diagnosis is apparent, increased precautions must be taken to guard against trauma. Loss of height with progressive aging is a result of reduced thickness, and sometimes collapse, of the vertebrae.

Patients with advanced demineralization are extremely fragile. It is imperative that health care deliverers (HCDs) realize that they must be assisted and moved gingerly, that a minor fall—even stepping into a depression—can result in severe fractures and complete disability and debility. This is a primary problem of the elderly; it has been estimated that there are 200,000 hip fractures per year in this country and some 100,000 wrist fractures (Marx, 1980). The problem is compounded by the fact that persons with these fragile, vulnerable bones are actually asymptomatic; the presence of severe demineralization is first seen in a pathologic fracture—one precipitated by no trauma or trivial trauma. Moreover, healing is poor. Pins and prostheses may not remain securely in place; there are many life-threatening complications during treatment of the hip fracture; and it can be a tragic setback in the general state of health, activity, and independence of these patients.

Osteoporosis is a major problem for the elderly. Much work is being done to develop effective treatment and, more important, preventive programs.

Osteoarthritis (Degenerative Arthritis)

This problem is almost universal among the aged, although the spectrum of severity is wide—for example, all have x-ray changes, some have minimal discomfort, and others may have severe, incapacitating disease. The problem primarily involves the cartilage and is a wearing, thinning process due to attrition. Weight-bearing joints, such as the knees and hips, are most prominently involved. Ultimately the digits and other joints of the upper extremities become involved, compromising fine movements of the fingers. There is *always* spurring of the spinal vertebrae, but, again, the degree of discomfort varies considerably.

Often, patients merely accept their discomfort as "growing old," which is a mistake for them and for professionals as well. Aspirin and other anti-inflammatory agents are quite beneficial. Intermittent local injection of steroids into more severely affected joints may be necessary—and affords a great deal of relief.

There are no notable complications or precautions. The patient should *not* be too active on weight-bearing joints as this can exacerbate the problem. If the patient is obese, weight loss should be encouraged. Heat applications and physiotherapy may afford some relief under certain circumstances. Finally, when the disease is sufficiently incapacitating and crippling, surgical joint replacement may be extremely beneficial.

Prostatic Hypertrophy

Simple benign overgrowth of the prostate and, in particular, of the segment through which the urethra courses can lead to gradual obliteration of the outflow tract from the bladder. It occurs in the majority of men but the severity of the problem varies. There is little implication of malignancy, but if the obstruction remains for any length of time, there is damage to the bladder, infection is frequent, and ultimately there is kidney damage. Often the patient appears with acute obstruction requiring emergency drainage procedures.

The usual symptoms are frequent urination with hesitancy, dribbling, and difficulty in starting the stream. The patient must awaken frequently to pass small volumes of urine.

The only way of coping with this problem definitively is by surgery. Drainage procedures, as with a Foley catheter, are merely temporary and, further, their chronic use inevitably results in infection. It is imperative, therefore, that surgery be undertaken whenever possible. This can be accomplished today through advances in surgical and anesthetic techniques for patients once considered prohibitively high risks. The most common procedure is one in which the obstructing tissue is reamed out by an instrument inserted through the penile urethra. If the gland is excessively large or cancer is suspected, complete, and more formidable, removal of the prostate may be required.

In patients who, for one reason or another, are unable to undergo surgery, use of a Foley catheter becomes mandatory. Proper care of this drainage system poses a challenge to all personnel involved in patient care. Proper attachment of the catheter to the drainage tube and then to the drainage bag is essential. Breaks in continuity of the system lead to infection, and intermittent careful irrigation may be required to ensure proper flow. Even under the best of circumstances infection is likely; but proper care and exercise of the most stringent aseptic precautions will perhaps minimize the problem.

Common Diseases in the Elderly

The following are disorders that are not encountered solely in the elderly but are certainly more common in this age group and are responsible for much of their disability.

Malignant Tumors

There are several tumors that occur much more frequently in the elderly than in younger people. The possibility of cure in most of these cases depends on early detection, and it is incumbent on those in close contact with these people to have some knowledge of their symptoms in order to see that adequate medical evaluation is obtained.

Carcinoma of the Colon

This is a common and potentially curable tumor in the elderly. In parts of the colon, it manifests as only an insidiously developing anemia; tests for blood in the stools are usually positive. In more terminal parts of the colon and in the rectum, bright red blood on the stools, abdominal pain, and changes in bowel habit may be present. Anemia may be overlooked if one sees a patient daily, but a relative who sees the individual only intermittently may remark that he or she appears pale and weak, whereupon it becomes evident to everyone. Sudden onset of constipation or the appearance of blood in the stool requires medical investigation and should not be ascribed to diet, hemorrhoids, or simply to advancing years. It cannot be emphasized too strongly that the alert nurse or paraprofessional may be the initiator of events that lead to cure.

Management is surgical, with resection of the involved bowel and examination for evidence of spread. This tumor tends to be slow-growing in the elderly, and even if complete cure is not achieved, the course may be quite slow. There are no satisfactory chemotherapeutic agents or combination of agents for carcinoma of the colon.

COMPLICATIONS—Problems, other than recognizing the danger signals of a primary tumor, would be symptoms indicating spread to other tissues and organs. The liver is frequently involved, and jaundice and abdominal pain would be danger signals of impending deterioration. Recurrence of bleeding, abdominal pain with distention, and severe constipation might be similarly interpreted—and would require medical attention.

Carcinoma of the Stomach

This is no longer a particularly common tumor. Unfortunately, when the tumor becomes symptomatic, it is often too late to effect a surgical cure. The primary symptoms are loss of appetite, a feeling of fullness or pain in the upper abdomen, vomiting blood, and evidence of blood in the stools (tarry stools or positive test). The diagnosis may be strongly suspected in contrast (barium) x-ray examination of the stomach and can be confirmed by endoscopy. Treatment is surgical and, although the outlook is bleak, the lesion is considered curable until proved otherwise.

Danger signals following operation would be general deterioration, weight loss, loss of appetite, symptoms of obstruction, and evidence of spread of the tumor. It often spreads to bone; severe bone pain is, therefore, an ominous development.

Carcinoma of the Prostate

This is not an uncommon problem in the aged. Unfortunately, management is rather unsatisfactory once the tumor spreads; it usually spreads to bone and looms as a distinct possibility when an elderly man complains of severe and unrelenting pain about the pelvis and lower back. Occasionally the tumor may lead to obstruction of urine flow, which might be fortunate if it calls attention to the presence of a problem before the tumor spreads. Otherwise, it is detected on rectal examination as a hard mass in the usually firm, smooth prostate gland.

Treatment includes radical removal of the gland surgically when the tumor is confined to the prostate. Once it has spread, removal of the testes and administration of estrogens may be beneficial. Radiation therapy is of some value.

COMPLICATIONS.—Bone pain and anemia are the principal problems. The tumor may spread to the lungs and to distant sites but this is not common.

Carcinoma of the Esophagus

This is perhaps more a disorder of the young elderly (60–65). The primary symptom is difficulty in swallowing that becomes progressively worse. It should always be taken seriously and usually indicates the presence of significant disease. This tumor is difficult to manage. When it is located in the most distant part of the esophagus, it may be treated surgically. However, the overall results are gloomy. X-ray is not curative but *may* provide some symptomatic relief.

Multiple Myeloma

A tumor of bone or bone marrow, this complicated disorder is characterized by production of abnormal amounts of protein by the cells responsible for the disorder. It may present in several ways but the the outstanding symptoms are bone pain and anemia. There is usually severe osteoporosis—demineralization of bone. Kidney failure is frequent, as is spontaneous or pathologic fracture of the vertebrae.

This is a slowly progressive disorder, the course of which can often be partially altered. There are no particular complications of which health care deliverers should be aware. Bone pain may be helped by radiation therapy and the weakness of severe anemia may necessitate transfusions. Bleeding can be a problem, but this is uncommon. Dehydration must be carefully avoided since this can hasten kidney failure. Where bone demineralization is particularly prominent one should exercise extra precautions to avoid trauma.

Chronic Lymphatic Leukemia

This is ordinarily a very slowly progressive disorder, indications being extreme enlargement of the spleen, visibly enlarged lymph nodes, and an exceedingly high white blood cell count. If the patient is not particularly anemic and has no symptoms, treatment may be delayed. Occasionally, transformation to a more acute, malignant form of the disease occurs, whereupon extremely sophisticated management becomes necessary.

One should be aware that the disorder is present and that change in the character of the disease may occur. Bleeding and infection can become problems. Occasionally the lymph nodes and spleen are of sufficient size to warrant treatment because of mechanical disturbances and for cosmetic reasons.

Myxedema

The cause of this disorder is inadequate function of the thyroid gland. It can develop as a primary disease of the thyroid or may be associated with other glandular disturbances. This disorder is characterized by fatigability, intolerance for cold, coarsening of the skin and hair, hoarseness, and slowing of thought processes that can masquerade as dementia. The significance of this disease is that it is completely reversible by taking either the hormone or an extract of thyroid by mouth.

Complications are not common once the disorder is recognized and treatment is instituted. If untreated, this disorder can be lethal. When treated, there is some danger, particularly in the elderly, of making heart disease more symptomatic. Therefore, the development of chest pain would require immediate medical assessment.

Heart Disease

Considering the various types of heart disease under one category, this is by far the commonest cause of death and disability in the elderly. It is important that the student or professional gerontologist understand in some depth the various ways that heart disease can affect the elderly and how these may be distinguished rather than being subsumed under the general terms heart trouble, heart attacks, and so on.

Congestive Heart Failure

An extremely common disorder in the elderly, this basic problem is inadequate function of the heart muscle due to a variety of causes—hypertension, coronary artery disease, and perhaps, according to some, age itself. Manifestations are shortness of breath and swelling of the feet and ankles. There are other causes of both these symptoms, but the possibility of heart disease must be considered when these appear. The elderly elderly (> 85) may not be as aware that they are having difficulty breathing, so that simple observation of rapid respirations (> 20 per minute) or of difficulty in lying flat might alert one to the possibility of this problem. Symptoms may develop acutely, particularly shortness of breath; in this instance, medical attention is urgently needed since fatal fluid overload in the lungs may occur.

The mainstays of treatment are digitalis, diuretics (agents to promote salt and water excretion), and a salt-restricted diet. With this program, significant improvement usually occurs. Treatment, however, is not curative and recurrences are frequent, particularly when patients deviate from their medication and diet.

Complications.—These patients are particularly vulnerable to infection; pneumonia is not infrequent. Moreover, infection often aggravates the underlying heart disease, leading to acute recurrences of the basic congestive state. Influenza is particularly dangerous in these patients; they should receive an appropriate vaccine, and amantadine (a new antiviral agent) therapy might be considered if they do develop true influenza. Complications include development of phlebitis or clots in the leg veins that are apt to become dislodged with fatal or potentially fatal consequences. They immediately traverse the venous system and the heart, and lodge in the lungs. This constitutes a major problem in these people and may require drugs to prevent blood clotting. The occurrence of this problem of a clot lodging in the lung may be subtle, with only worsening of congestive failure; or it may be dramatic, with acute shortness of breath, chest pain, and the coughing up of blood—an obvious life-threatening situation.

Complications of treatment.—Elderly people are particularly prone to digitalis overdosage; this occurs primarily because they have a decrease in muscle mass and diminished kidney function. Therefore, the drug is distributed in a smaller space and is excreted more slowly. Manifestations of digitalis overdosage are loss of appetite, yellow vision or other visual disturbances (spots, halos, etc.), irregularities of the heartbeat, and, ultimately, delirium. Medical evaluation is imperative at this point.

Diuretics cause certain problems. The blood potassium is frequently lowered, which can cause weakness and heart irregularities. Many physicians will attempt to avoid this by prescribing supplemental potassium when treatment is initiated. The blood level should be determined occasionally as either low or high levels may develop, and both are hazardous.

These patients should be weighed daily and the results carefully recorded. One of the better ways to perceive that the patient is lapsing back into congestive heart failure is by detecting a sudden gain in weight. This should prompt consultation with the patient's physician since it probably represents fluid accumulation.

Coronary Artery Disease

By no means limited to the elderly, this disorder is a common cause of disability and death in older persons. The problem in this disease results from blockage in the coronary arteries, the heart's own blood supply, by a fatty substance that deposits as a result of genetic predisposition, high blood cholesterol, hypertension, smoking, and perhaps sedentary lifestyle. The chief symptom of this disorder is chest pain, which may indicate a temporary inadequacy of blood flow to the heart or a severe and protracted deficit of blood supply leading to the death of varying amounts of heart muscle. The first is characteristic of angina pectoris, while the latter is a brief description of a myocardial infarction or heart attack. Angina pectoris is a clinical syndrome characterized by chest pain on exertion that is relieved by rest or by nitroglycerin tablets placed under the tongue. A heart attack or myocardial infarction, associated with protracted pain, sweating, and nausea and vomiting, requires immediate hospitalization.

Unfortunately, elderly subjects do not always experience pain with their attacks—of either type. One is therefore deprived of the usual clue that a serious problem exists. A sudden deterioration in well-being with weakness, shortness of breath, and perhaps fainting should alert one to the possibility that an infarction may have occurred.

COMPLICATIONS.—Following myocardial infarction, patients are liable to develop various problems. If the damage is extensive they may complain of weakness and fatigability; if severe and incapacitating, it may indicate an extremely poor prognosis. These patients frequently develop congestive heart failure, as previously described, and they are prone to develop irregularities in cardiac rhythm, some of which have lethal implications. Lastly, they are prone to further attacks and to sudden death.

COMPLICATIONS OF TREATMENT.—Patients should always carry nitroglycerin tablets; with time, these tend to lose their potency and should be replaced with fresh ones. Many patients are placed on long-acting nitrates and propranolol, an agent that acts primarily by slowing the heart rate, which may occasionally become too slow, requiring a decreased dosage. Other types of agents frequently prescribed are those given to prevent heart irregularities. There are many side effects of agents given to control heart rhythm that are too numerous to detail. These agents have many imperfections, and what works for one patient may not work for another.

Heart Block

This category includes several disorders that are characterized by sudden slowing of the heart rate which may be associated with loss of consciousness. There is an impulse-conducting system in the heart that is similar to an electric circuit. It may be broken at any point, from the primary initiating focus (sinus node) to the outermost reaches of the heart muscle. Fainting attacks in the elderly must not be ascribed simply to "old age"; it is imperative that the precise cause be sought. If it is one of the conduction disturbances described here, a cardiac pacemaker may be lifesaving since the break in the circuit can be bypassed.

COMPLICATIONS.—Cardiac pacemakers are very sophisticated devices that may develop flaws in their mechanism; moreover, the power source has a limited life span, like any battery, so careful follow-up is mandatory. Any recurrence of symptoms, such as dizzy spells or fainting, requires immediate assessment. There are now ways to monitor the performance of these devices by ordinary telephone, and it is a distinct advantage for patients to be followed in this manner where possible.

Aneurysms

These are balloon-like dilatations of arteries. They may occur almost anywhere, but the major problems are with aneurysms of the aorta—the major artery leaving the heart—in the chest or abdomen. These cause few symptoms until they are quite large or begin to leak. In the chest, they usually show up as an unexpected finding on x-ray. In the abdomen, there is a large pulsating mass that may be perceived by the patient but is usually first noted by a physician. This can cause pain, which usually indicates recent enlargement and impending disaster.

Treatment for this life-threatening problem is surgery; and if the aneurysms are enlarging or are above a certain size, it should be done immediately. If a patient who has a known aneurysm develops discomfort or states that it is getting larger, immediate medical attention is mandatory.

COMPLICATIONS.—Once the surgery has been performed and the aneurysm successfully removed, it is essential that the patient be observed for cold feet, sudden pain in one or both legs, discoloration of the legs, and so on. These symptoms require immediate assessment by the patient's physician.

Peripheral Vascular Disease

This disorder is the result of deposits in major arteries (usually those of the lower extremities) of the same material that is present in the coronary arteries of people who have heart attacks. Gradual narrowing of the arteries occurs to the point where the blood supply becomes inadequate. At first the symptoms may be mild, consisting mostly of pain in the calves when walking that is relieved by rest. Later, pain becomes more severe and occurs during rest, particularly at night; a feeling of numbness and coldness in one or both feet is noted. It may involve only a toe or may include the entire leg. Ultimately, there is death of tissue due to inadequate blood supply, resulting in gangrene that leads to eventual loss of part or all of the extremity.

This is a major problem in elderly patients. Complaints of pain or odd sensations in the feet or legs should arouse suspicion that it could be this disease. The patient may have no complaints, yet one observes that a toe or foot is blue and cool to the touch. Any problem of this nature requires medical attention. It is particularly common in patients with diabetes, as previously discussed. These people require extremely careful foot care with particularly close observation of minor cuts, abrasions, or infections. Applying heat may be dangerous since the blood supply—because of narrowing of the arteries—cannot be increased to meet the augmented demands imposed by the heat.

Hypertension and Strokes

These problems are presented together because it has become clear in recent years that control of hypertension drastically reduces the incidence of strokes. At the same time, the health care provider should understand that there are other causes of strokes and also that hypertension can cause problems other than strokes.

Hypertension

Blood pressure tends to rise with advancing age, and this has led to some confusion about what is normal for an elderly patient and what the goals of treatment should be. By and large, more severe hypertension (higher levels of blood pressure) is encountered in younger persons (<60). On the other hand, effects on target organs that suffer most from sustained increased blood pressure for years occur in the preelderly and young elderly. These include heart failure and coronary artery disease, kidney failure, and strokes.

It is imperative that hypertension in the elderly be treated, although just how aggressively is a subject of some debate. Some would argue that lowering the pressure *too much* endangers organs and can lead to strokes. Although this may be true for sudden decreases in blood pressure, appropriate gradual control of blood pressure unquestionably reduces the incidence of strokes and probably of heart failure (*J.A.M.A.*, 1979). Moreover, diastolic pressure should probably be reduced below 90 (Tobian, 1982). There is some evidence that systolic hypertension alone is associated with complications, so this too should be treated.

COMPLICATIONS.—The complications of hypertensive disease itself have been noted: strokes, congestive heart failure, coronary artery disease, and kidney failure. Strokes will be presented in more detail below; congestive heart failure has been discussed. Manifestations of kidney failure are subtle and beyond the scope of this presentation; they consist mostly of changes in blood chemistry that culminate in what is termed "uremia"—a piling up in the body of waste products usually excreted by the kidney.

Complications of treatment are important for the health care provider. One complication is failure to comply with or inadequacy of the prescribed program. Therefore, blood pressure should be monitored so that unacceptable and dangerous increases in pressure can be dealt with promptly. Other complications include a tendency to sudden decreases in blood pressure on standing, often causing dizziness or fainting. This should be brought to the attention of the patient's physician. Other problems resulting from treatment might include weakness due to low blood potassium levels, worsening chest pain, worsening heart failure, and, rarely, swelling of the feet and ankles.

Strokes

A stroke is also known as a cerebrovascular accident (CVA). There are several types and several causes but the net effect is destruction of some part of the brain where cells lack the capacity to reproduce themselves so that loss is irreversible. One type, the cerebral hemorrhage, is almost always seen in severe hypertensives and is a dramatic, often lethal event. A cerebral thrombosis, the most common type in elderly people, occurs when a clot forms in one of the arteries to a portion of the brain. The commonest location is an artery that affects pathways to an entire side of the body and face, resulting in partial or complete paralysis of half the entire body. Speech may be completely and irrevocably lost if the dominant side is affected. The stroke may be preceded by transient episodes from which there is complete recovery; it is important that these incidents be brought to the attention of a physician since specific measures might be instituted to prevent a final paralyzing event.

COMPLICATIONS.—These complications are what might occur in anyone forced into a position of complete dependence and invalidism. If patients are moved too infrequently, bed sores develop. They have difficulty with secretions so that aspiration and/or bronchopneumonia are frequent. If they are not properly cared for, a water deficit or malnutrition may occur. If aphasic (unable to speak), they cannot communicate their needs. It is always difficult to tell just how much improvement can be expected. Physical therapy should be continued until no further improvement is evident. There is no doubt that a stroke almost literally destroys apparently healthy, vigorous people. It is a bitter pill for the patient, relatives, and friends. Health care providers must be aware of all this because he or she may be at an interpersonal contact point and can do much to provide guarded optimism and encouragement to all concerned. In some patients there is little return of function and the outlook for a life of any quality is grim. On the other hand, improvement to the point of almost negligible incapacity is possible. If the patient is depressed and does not cooperate, there are definite limits to what can be accomplished.

Depression, Suicide, and Alcoholism

Health care providers *must* be completely aware of the psychological problems associated with aging. These run the gamut from minor depression to alcoholism to severe depression and suicide. For many people, the golden years are gray; they perceive themselves to be neglected and abandoned, their opinions are no longer sought or heeded, and their lives as useful members of society seem to be at an end. Many simply retreat and brood, often with the "aid" of alcohol; the frequency of serious drinking in this age group is considerable. The suicide rate in the elderly is inordinately high; people over 65 constitute 10% to 12% of the population, but are responsible for 25% of the suicides (*J.A.M.A.*, 1979). The rate probably would be even greater if all methods of self-destruction were taken into account: refusal to eat, self-neglect, automobile "accidents," overmedication, refusal to take medication, and other subtle actions.

It is imperative that this particular aspect of patient care be properly emphasized so that every effort is made to prevent needless tragedy. These people require support and, occasionally, professional psychiatric help. If depression is severe, antidepressant medications are often needed. Sedatives or tranquilizers have little place in treatment of the elderly unless they are agitated and difficult to manage.

COMPLICATIONS.—This type of problem has complications that one might anticipate. Among the more prominent are increasingly antisocial behavior, withdrawal, and personality disintegration. A change in personality may frequently occur soon after a stressful illness or a fall; irrational and agitated patients who are being treated with potent psychoactive drugs may develop a complication—tardive dyskinesia—that is similar to acutely acquired parkinsonism, with facial grimacing and chewing movements of the mouth and tongue. This requires immediate evaluation by a physician.

Danger signals for health care providers to be aware of are sudden changes in mood and personality and a tendency for a previously friendly person to become morose, withdrawn, and suspicious. Previous participation in various activities may cease, and a loss of interest in friends, relatives, and events may occur. Appetite will be noted to decline and weight loss soon becomes evident.

Bronchopneumonia

This is the type of pneumonia likely to occur in debilitated and elderly patients. It is caused by any number of bacteria and is frequently a complication of other disorders, such as heart failure, stroke, or surgery. Patients who are immobile and unable to turn are particularly likely to develop this type of pneumonia—especially when they have difficulty swallowing and have problems with aspiration of their own secretions and food. Prompt recognition and administration of antibiotics have altered the outcome of this previously terminal illness.

COMPLICATIONS.—Provided the patient survives the illness, there are no immediate complications. The pneumonia usually clears completely but occasionally there are problems that persist. Convalescence may be somewhat protracted, depending on the physical state of the patient before the illness. Seemingly minor respiratory infections during this period are a cause for concern and close observation lest the pneumonia recur.

Common Symptoms of the Elderly and Their Significance

The symptoms are discussed in sufficient depth to provide general guidelines to health care providers but are not intended to substitute for assessment by a physician. When symptoms persist, and particularly if they worsen, the best judgment is always to have the patient seen by a doctor. It is far better to err on the side of obtaining a needless evaluation than to jeopardize a patient's well-being by well-intentioned but inappropriate judgments of medical need.

Forgetfulness

This seems to be one of the most common complaints of the elderly. Every "slip of the mind" that was dismissed casually when younger now becomes a cause for concern. Is "senility" far behind?

There actually exists a tendency toward forgetfulness when aging. This does not imply imminent deterioration of mental function. Many people complain specifically of problems in remembering names, which is merely a source of embarrassment. There may be some difficulty in learning new material, whereas remote memory remains intact.

This entire area of intellectual function and the question of mental deterioration can be tested objectively. Most people with simple forgetfulness display little impairment, if any. People with true dementia are disoriented about time, place, and/or person. They are unable to perform simple mathematical problems and have little ability to comprehend or interpret proverbs. The vast majority of people who survive to the ninth or tenth decade retain their mental faculties. The gradual loss of nerve cells and decrease in brain weight have been interpreted as evidence of inexorable deterioration—which is a false association. Most (63%) of the elderly elderly who are institutionalized have some degree of dementia. On the other hand, the vast majority in this age group are not institutionalized and are *not* demented.

Weakness and Fatigability

These symptoms are not limited to the elderly but are perhaps more prominent in this age group. There is a loss of muscle mass with advancing years, and it is as yet unclear whether this can be prevented by increased activity and exercise. On the other hand, it is abundantly clear that inactivity causes loss of function that, once gone, may be irretrievable. It is therefore imperative that all elderly persons who are not physically limited participate in an active exercise program, one designed to maintain muscle mass as well as endurance.

The symptoms do not reflect only muscle function. They could be due to anemia, decreased thyroid function, decreased adrenal gland function, low serum potassium, congestive heart failure, a disturbance in heart rhythm, and, possibly, an underlying neurosis. The sudden onset of weakness in a previously vigorous person certainly requires assessment by a physician.

Diminishing Vision or Blindness

The elderly have two particular eye problems: cataracts and macular degeneration (an aging change of uncertain causation in the most crucial portion of the retina). Persons with cataracts may complain of halos and diminished vision with particular difficulty seeing or reading in bright light. Cataracts are being treated surgically with increasing success, and the use of the implanted lens has increased the effectiveness of the procedure. It is essential that elderly people whose visual disturbances become distressingly prominent be evaluated by an ophthalmologist. The condition of the underlying retina may not become apparent until the cataract is removed, so guarantees of improvement must be avoided. Other disorders of the eye that might affect vision are degeneration of the optic nerve or retina, usually associated with generalized disorders such as diabetes and hypertension (particularly untreated and severe), and with certain medications that can increase intraocular pressure or cause dilatation of the pupil. Sudden onset of blindness may indicate a clot in the central artery of the retina, perhaps associated with temporal arteritis (discussed at some length in the section on specific diseases of the elderly).

Deafness

There is a gradual loss of hearing with age, particularly in certain sound frequencies. The entire mechanism of sound perception is a complicated physiologic process and there is no precise, singular defect in the elderly. It varies from cerumen or wax in the external ear to degeneration of the nerve. The most common problem is an aging change in the inner ear or perhaps a vascular disturbance. Studies of audiograms in individuals over a period of years reveal a gradual loss of hearing in particular ranges of the sound spectrum.

It is particularly important that this sensory loss be recognized as early as possible in order to exclude curable, reversible disorders. Additionally, for those people where no specific medical intervention can be undertaken to reverse a problem, a hearing aid should be obtained. Its use requires considerable dexterity and proper regulation is not simple. If the hearing aid does not result in significant improvement, one has to urge lipreading instruction, loud buzzers instead of doorbells, amplification equipment for the telephone and television, and similar ploys to circumvent the problem.

It has been observed that older people tolerate loss of sight better than they do loss of hearing. Partially deaf people frequently undergo significant personality changes. They suspect that people consider them unintelligent because they cannot respond appropriately to comments or questions. They begin to feel somewhat paranoid, overlooked, dismissed, and avoided. Their voices become louder and more strident, and there is clearly a personality change; they become garrulous, grumpy, unhappy, and paranoid—especially if they were not particularly pleasant before. They require much understanding, explanation, and help. This entire problem can be ameliorated in a major way by health care deliverers who understand the difficulties the patient is experiencing, particularly the effects on personality.

Loss of Appetite

It is clear that older people experience a decrease in appetite with advancing years. There is a progressive loss in the number of taste buds on the tongue, and this is considered by many to be a major causative factor. There could be others: a decrease in sensitivity of a central nervous system appetite center or centers, problems with teeth or dentures, problems with swallowing, and a change in metabolic demand. People become less active as they age and their caloric requirements would be expected to lessen. In addition, there is a significant loss in lean body mass, and one could argue that this decreases the need for food, although some might say that it is the decrease in caloric intake that results in the weight loss. Lastly, many of these subjects have chronic illnesses that in themselves could blunt the appetite or require taking medications that tend to induce nausea and distaste for food. It will be recalled that digitalis overdosage is frequent in the elderly, and the *first* symptom of intoxication with this agent is loss of appetite.

The elderly may have other problems that affect nutrition adversely. Many have dental problems and some are edentulous and do not have proper prostheses (false teeth). Others have problems initiating the swallowing mechanism, stemming from lack of coordination of the actions that propel a bolus of food into the esophagus. After they aspirate several times they become fearful of asphyxiation and will swallow only the simplest foods. At times, they are observed to chew a bolus for protracted periods and finally expectorate it in disgust. Finally, some elderly persons have difficulty in swallowing that is due to motor paralysis or incoordination of the muscles in the esophagus. Food tends to become lodged in the esophagus—in the chest—under this circumstance.

These problems require careful management. Many patients are on bland, tasteless diets prescribed by their physician. He might be apprised of their problems with eating and be willing to compromise their dietary program in the interest of increased palatability and improved nutrition. Many elderly patients like ice cream because it is soft, tasty, and easy to manage. An imaginative dietitian can do wonders in dealing with this problem. Patients can be assisted to overcome their apprehension and shown that they can manage food if the texture is appropriate.

One final circumstance requires comment. Some elderly elderly patients may suddenly refuse all food. This becomes a major ethical problem since it may be their way of passively ending their lives. Whether one intubates them, cajoles them, and so on is a matter of judgment and family wishes. It may at times be a transient depression, and if the patient is somehow supported for a brief period, oral feeding may again be possible. There are no strict guidelines. If the patient steadfastly refuses food and water despite a period of assisted alimentation (feeding), it is likely that prolonged support of this sort is probably doomed to failure.

Dizziness

Many older people complain of spells of giddiness, light-headedness, feelings of detachment from their surroundings, amnesia, or a feeling that everything is spinning about them. Among these various ways of presenting with what appear to be variations on a single theme might lurk symptoms of severe disease. One has to be cautious in attempting to cope with this seemingly innocuous problem and not accept the subject's resigned, "I guess I'm just getting old," explanation. For true loss of consciousness or true amnesia, evaluation by a physician is essential. If there is actual spinning of the room, evaluation in some depth is also indicated. The problem is that the elderly do have diminished circulation of blood to the brain. A transient, acute further decline of blood flow classically has more specific symptoms, such as paralysis or unilateral blindness of short duration; a more modest decrease in blood flow, as might occur with standing, can cause only vague "giddiness."

The health care deliverer may be assuming too much responsibility by attempting to evaluate the need for medical attention—particularly if the symptoms are new, are increasing in frequency and/or severity, and are the cause of mounting concern to the patient. If the symptoms have been evaluated in the past and there has been little change in the character or tempo of the complaint, it is likely that further investigation would yield little information. On the other hand, any substantial change requires thoughtful, cautious assessment.

Shortness of Breath

Shortness of breath on exertion, even with minimal exercise, is a common complaint of the elderly. The symptom must be distinguished from fatigue as their causes tend to be different. Aging is associated with a decline in heart function and changes in stiffness and elasticity of the lungs. This combination of functional change in two critical organs leads to a sharply limited reserve so that, although there is no air hunger at rest, modest activity exceeds the capacity of the heart and lungs to meet increased oxygen needs. If this symptom remains unchanged, there is little cause for alarm. Development of shortness of breath at rest, and in particular at night, casts a new and more ominous light on the problem. It is also more likely to be a reflection of significant disease if it is associated with swelling of the feet and ankles.

Gait and Balance Disturbances

It requires little training to observe that the elderly develop an uncertain, hesitant gait that culminates in a type of locomotion that can best be termed a "shuffle." Coordination of the nervous and muscular systems that produces a forceful, confident stride is evidently lost, and the precise nature of the defects may not always be clear. There is loss of muscle mass and strength, as has been noted. The myriad pathways and connections in the brain and nervous system are complicated and sophisticated; the elderly probably suffer several breaks in this network and their precise locations are not always apparent, even to experts. One problem, of course, is lack of confidence and fear of falling; this can be helped with walking aids, physiotherapy, and encouragement. The shuffle most resembles the classic gait with short steps of a person with parkinsonism, and it may indeed be distantly related to this disease.

Elderly people who have this problem are apt to avoid activity and remain in the relative safety of their bed or chair. This will ultimately aggravate the situation since the muscles will further lose their strength and tone. They should be encourgaed to walk, perhaps with assistance initially. Our goal should be for everyone to walk "ramrod straight" with a firm, unhesitating step. This may not always be possible but it is eminently conceivable that gait deterioration can be largely or partially prevented.

Insomnia

This is a common complaint to which the elderly often tend to ascribe their declining vigor, at least in part. There are abundant theories on why sleep patterns change, including the likely fact that less sleep is needed and the probable fact that naps during the day diminish the need for nocturnal sleep. There is a great deal of investigation into the physiology of sleep and abnormal sleep patterns. Prinz (1977) has shown that older men sleep less soundly, have 90% less stage 4 or deep sleep and 27% less rapid eye movement sleep, and experience twice as much wakefulness at night compared to a control group of normal young men. The problem is not an easy one to manage satisfactorily. Sedatives are certainly to be avoided and there probably is no such thing as a "minor" tranquilizer in an elderly subject. Some evidence shows that calcium provided by milk or yogurt exerts a beneficial effect on sleep. Occasionally, a small amount of wine is helpful. It is hoped that with increased knowledge of sleep mechanisms, new agents will emerge that will be more satisfactory than those currently available.

Constipation

The elderly, at least in this country, seem to have the fixed idea that proper bowel elimination is mandatory if good health is to be enjoyed. This attitude is unfortunate in that it leads to needless taking of cathartics (laxatives) and enemas. These, in turn, tend to decrease bowel tone, a sort of deconditioning process. Ultimately, there develops almost complete loss of bowel function and dependence on the very agents that caused the problem. Much of the obsession with bowel activity stems from folklore and advertising. The simple fact is that a daily bowel movement is not essential and there are no adverse effects on health from irregularity of bowel movements. Many of the current elderly have already been victimized by their laxative habits, and it is naive to think that one can rapidly reverse this attitude or the resultant decrease in bowel tone. The current fad for bran and other fiber products may do much to alter the habits of a new generation of elderly. It is perhaps judicious to use mild cathartics occasionally in our current older population to prevent fecal impaction, particularly when there is a history of this problem. Bulk laxatives are preferred; stool softeners may be worthwhile if there is a problem with consistency of the stool. Agents that act by stimulating the bowel should rarely be used.

Aches and Pains

Many people have vague aches and pains that are of little consequence. Most of these do *not* imply serious underlying disease and, in the main, are best ignored if self-limited. The elderly seem to have more complaints of this nature; some actually become hypochondriacal in their later years—people who had never complained previously. Little is gained by adopting a patronizing attitude, nor is it advisable to say, "Well, you *are* getting older and what did you expect?" All symptoms have potential significance and it is a mistake not to hear patients out—even if the complaints seem tedious and repetitious. Reasonable explanations of symptoms (slight osteoarthritis or changes in muscle and muscle attachments with age) are usually helpful. One should be alert to changes in the frequency and severity of discomfort. A patient who develops intractable, severe low back pain instead of his previous bothersome discomfort is likely to be experiencing more than just a flare-up of his arthritis. Medical assessment is in order.

Feelings of Uselessness and Abandonment

This section devoted to common complaints in the elderly may seem an inappropriate place to discuss the psychology of aging since the problem may or may not be verbalized; when it is, it is apt to be in a resigned, forlorn "what's the use" manner. There is no question that this is one of the more important aspects of dealing with and caring for the elderly. Almost always there is a serious psychological problem when individuals suffer loss of power and position, loss of credibility, and decrease in income; there is the almost universal perception that the world is rushing by and there is no visible role for the elderly. People react in different ways to this diminishing role. Those who previously wielded little authority or influence and exerted little presence perhaps feel it the least; those who occupied positions of authority, whose opinions were sought and respected, have considerable difficulty in coping. For many it is a bitter pill to swallow and some come to terms with it very slowly. This is particularly true when their severance from the scene of their power is not clean and incisive, and they are permitted an honorary but superficial and superfluous limping role. The new regime simply cannot "do it properly" and things "never are as they were in the good old days." There may be few complaints and most suffer what they perceive to be their "fallen image" in quiet and with some degree of despair. It is not universally thus, but is very common. If the baton is passed to a son or daughter or close relative, it may be more painless, but not necessarily so.

These problems tend to be more prominent in the period immediately following retirement or "promotion to chairman of the board." With time, a new set of interests is developed along with more self-appreciation of the "grand old man or woman" role. Those who adjust the best do not continue to dwell on the past but instead look to the future and new horizons.

It is imperative that persons in contact with the elderly be aware of these psychological frailties. Proper support and proper appreciation for what they were and what they might become will help them over this hurdle and into a new and promising phase of their lives. Positive attitudes about the future should be substituted for preoccupation with past glories. It is not always a simple task.

REFERENCES

Five-year findings of the hypertension detection and follow-up program. *J.A.M.A.* 242:2562–2571, 1979.

Fries J.F.: Aging, natural death, and the compression of morbidity. *N. Engl. J. Med.* 303:130–135, 1980.

Marx J.L.: Osteoporosis: New help for thinning bones. *Science* 207:628–630, 1980.

Prinz P.N.: Sleep patterns in the healthy and aged: Relationship with intellectual function. *J. Gerontol.* 32:179–186, 1977.

Tobian L.: Personal communication, 1982.

8

SUBSTANCE ABUSE

Leonard Naeger, Ph.D.

ELDERLY PATIENTS present unique drug utilization problems for health professionals charged with their care. A systematic discussion of these problems must begin with fundamental definitions of drug misuse and abuse. Next, those physiologic changes that inevitably accompany aging, and that alter drug response, demand attention. Then, the drugs used most frequently among elderly patients can be considered: nonprescription products, nonscheduled prescription drugs, and scheduled prescription drugs.*

Understanding drug response problems in any patient, regardless of age, depends initially on distinguishing among three terms. The first of these, *drug use,* refers to a patient taking a drug specifically and exclusively according to the physician's directions. A patient who "uses" a drug complies strictly with the prescribed regimen.

Involuntary deviation from the physician's orders is commonly referred to as *drug misuse*. Examples of misuse include unnecessary or unauthorized refills of prescriptions that lead to overuse of substances intended only for temporary or acute conditions. Drugs may also be misused when necessary refills are omitted, leading to premature termination of therapeutic programs. The problems in either case most frequently arise from one of several causes. Physicians may simply neglect to inform their patients in detail about the program of drug therapy. Or a patient's misunderstanding of a physician's written or verbal orders may result in deviation from a prescribed regimen. Finally, patients may be physically deterred from full compliance with planned drug therapy. For example, the dosage form may be unpalatable, or the application of the drug product may be physically inconvenient, difficult, or painful. These latter causes of misuse may be of special concern for elderly patients.

Willful deviation from the prescribed regimen is termed *drug abuse*. Most commonly, substances that induce euphoria or relieve discomfort are

---

*It has been determined that scheduled drugs have especially dangerous addictive potential. They are classified "scheduled" according to this potential by the FDA and their dissemination is strictly controlled by law.

abused (e.g., minor tranquilizers and analgesics). Drug misuse and, more commonly, drug abuse can lead to acute dependence (addiction). Dependence may be either psychological or physiologic; some substances produce both. Physiologic dependence has by far the most serious consequences. Therefore, the relative benefits of agents known to produce such dependence must be weighed carefully against their addictive potential. Above all, it must be remembered that, while some drugs are more likely to produce dependence than others, all drugs can produce some degree of psychological dependence and are thus subject to abuse.

Drug response, including the variables of use, misuse, and abuse, is complicated among elderly patients by significant physiologic changes that accompany aging. Such changes affect the absorption, metabolism, and excretion of any substance—including drugs.

Alteration of absorption may change drug response substantially. However, the exact direction or magnitude of the changes is extremely difficult to predict. Gastrointestinal acid secretion and motility change with age. In the digestive tract, drugs will generally remain more stable because they are less subject to chemical and mechanical degradation. For this reason, the amount of drug absorbed should be increased in elderly patients. However, as blood flow to all organs, including the digestive tract, decreases with age, so does overall absorptive capacity. Thus, in most elderly patients, factors that both enhance and depress drug absorption are at work; they may even cancel each other in some cases.

Once drugs have been absorbed into the circulation, they are distributed throughout the body, taken up by specific tissues, and metabolized. All materials absorbed after digestion travel via the portal circulation for processing in the liver. This first step in distribution is called *first pass metabolism;* it is of particular concern among elderly patients because of physiologic changes that affect the liver. As with gastrointestinal absorption, changes in liver function may enhance and/or depress drug action.

On the one hand, elderly people experience a 20% to 60% decrease in blood flow to the liver. So, the same factor that limits the absorption of drugs from the digestive tract limits their transport to the liver. On the other hand, liver capacity itself decreases with age. Since it is one of the jobs of the liver to remove certain substances from the circulation, many drugs are much less effectively metabolized by this organ among aged patients. This is particularly true of such fat-soluble drugs as hypnotics and minor tranquilizers (e.g., Librium and Valium). Such drugs may have an exaggerated effect in the elderly because of less efficient liver processing.

Blood leaving the liver distributes absorbed substances, including drugs, throughout the body for metabolism by various tissues. Many drugs, specifically those soluble only in oil or fat solvents, do not dissolve in the blood. Instead, they may "ride" to their sites of action as tiny suspended particles—in a "free" state—or bound to a protein in the blood plasma. There are a limited number of such "protein seats" available in the blood, and many different undissolved substances may compete for rides. Significantly, *only* the *unbound* or *free* drugs are active. Since the plasma protein concentration decreases as liver function is reduced, a smaller proportion of any drug in the circulation of an elderly patient will be transported in the bound or inactive state. Therefore, a given concentration of a drug will generally exert greater pharmacologic activity in an elderly patient, because more of it is in the free or active form.

In addition to a decrease in plasma protein concentration, several other factors relating to circulation combine to affect drug response. As we age, we tend to experience a decline of lean muscle mass and a relative increase of fatty tissue. Blood perfuses or flows less efficiently through fatty tissue than through lean muscle. Thus, among the elderly, blood flow is concentrated in a more limited area. This concentration of blood flow is further enhanced by the general decline in vascular (blood vessel) volume that accompanies aging. Finally, certain vascular conditions such as sclerosis narrow the blood vessels, thus causing even greater restriction in circulation. While this general diminution of circulatory capacity may inhibit the distribution of some drugs to sites of action, it also concentrates greater amounts of all drugs in the free or active form in limited areas. Overall, circulatory changes among elderly patients probably increase the pharmacologic activity of most drugs.

Many substances in the blood pass ultimately into the kidneys for excretion. It is estimated that renal (kidney) capacity decreases approximately 1% per year beyond the age of 40. Many water-soluble substances normally excreted by the kidneys may remain in the circulation in elderly patients. Potent water-soluble drugs such as the cardiac glycoside digoxin (Lanoxin) may thus retain their activity for extended periods of time.

Nonprescription Products

General physiologic changes affecting drug response in elderly patients have an impact on all specific questions pertaining to drug misuse and abuse. The first class of drugs with abuse potential are the over-the-counter (OTC) preparations. Such products may be purchased without a prescription. The OTC products most commonly taken by older patients will be discussed in the following order: (1) analgesics, (2) laxatives, (3) cough and cold preparations, (4) antacids, (5) vitamins, and (6) ethanol.

Over-the-counter analgesics are used quite heavily by elderly patients to relieve pain and to reduce inflammation in conditions such as arthritis. Aspirin and acetaminophen are two of the most common nonprescription analgesics. Both drugs relieve fever and pain, but only aspirin reduces inflammation as well. Aspirin may irritate the gastrointestinal tract, but the degree of irritation may be reduced if the aspirin is taken with a large glassful of water or after meals. Aspirin should be avoided in certain situations, particularly for various conditions common among older patients: aspirin allergy, gout, ulcers, and conditions treated by oral anticoagulants (e.g., Coumadin). Although it is less common today, aspirin has been combined with phenacetin and caffeine. Two of these APC tablets (e.g., Empirin Compound) are generally taken three times a day. Such a regimen, followed for extended periods, may lead to renal damage or exaggerate an already deteriorating kidney condition. Aspirin or APC tablets may be replaced in many of these conditions by acetaminophen, which is generally less irritating to the digestive tract that either aspirin or APC.

OTC laxative preparations are frequently misused or abused by the elderly. Decreased energy requirements lead to diminished food intake, and hence diminished excretory function among the aged. Yet the presumption persists that a daily bowel movement is "normal," resulting in excessive reliance on artificial stimulants or softeners. Misuse or abuse of laxatives may generate a variety of obvious problems among geriatric patients.

Mineral oil laxatives taken over an extended period may lead to paraffinoma, a waxy buildup on the wall of the colon. More seriously, these oil-based products may prevent absorption of any oil-soluble substance from the gastrointestinal tract. Not only may the oil-soluble vitamins—A, D, E, and K—dissolve and thus remain unabsorbed, but also any oil-soluble drugs may be eliminated without achieving their therapeutic effect. Any laxative taken for prolonged periods may lead to a loss of intrinsic bowel tone and motility. Furthermore, dependence on laxatives can lead to diarrhea and the corresponding risks of dehydration, depletion of vital ion potassium, and acidosis through excessive loss of basic ions.

Several nonprescription preparations for symptoms of the common cold are frequently used by the elderly, who occasionally misuse and abuse these drugs. In addition to the analgesics discussed earlier, these comprise the antitussives, expectorants, bronchodilators, decongestants, and antihistamines.

"Chest colds" are frequently accompanied by coughs. It is commonly assumed that they should be routinely suppressed by antitussive agents such as dextromethorphan or codeine. Codeine may depress respiration and should be used with caution in patients with respiratory difficulties. While it is reasonable to treat dry, hacking coughs (smoker's cough) and those that disrupt sleep with antitussives, not all coughs should be suppressed. "Productive" coughs that clear excessive mucus secretion from the respiratory tract ought to be encouraged. Occasionally, patients will attempt to suppress the cough, yet encourage mucus clearance by taking a combination antitussive and expectorant that contains either guaifenesin or potassium iodide (e.g., Robitussin DM). This practice, however, is largely ineffective. The viscosity of expelled fluid depends ultimately on the patient's general state of hydration rather than on the contents of the expectorant, and the cough itself is necessary for efficient expulsion of the excess mucus.

OTC bronchodilating agents such as ephedrine are frequently used to provide relief from chest congestion characteristic of the common cold. However, bronchodilators also stimulate the heart. They often complicate conditions such as angina and cardiac arrhythmias. Since older adults frequently suffer heart difficulties, they should either avoid bronchodilator therapy altogether or use it only with extreme care under a physician's supervision.

Because colds frequently stimulate nasal congestion, nonprescription decongestants and antihistamines are popular sources of relief. However, both kinds of preparations cause side effects that are potentially dangerous, to elderly patients in particular. Congestion itself results from excessive dilation of vessels in the nasal mucosa. Decongestants (e.g., Neo-synephrine) constrict nasal arterioles to provide temporary relief. However, they also constrict blood vessels in other parts of the body, causing a potentially dangerous elevation in blood pressure. Patients suffering from hypertension should avoid systemic decongestants or use them only with extreme care. The excess secretions that accompany nasal congestion are often treated with antihistamines (e.g., Chlor-trimeton). They should be used with great care since they can cause excessive dryness of both the nose and the mouth; inhibition of tear formation may lead to eye irritation as well. Antihistamines may also complicate glaucoma by reducing the effectiveness of drugs used to treat that condition.

In general, elderly patients seeking relief from symptoms of the common cold should check with a physician before using even nonprescription medications. Such consultation is crucial in patients with cardiovascular abnormalities.

OTC antacid preparations are among the most frequently used nonprescription products. They are drugs that react with hydrochloric acid in the stomach and small intestine to produce a more alkaline milieu. Antacids are especially popular among elderly patients with ulcers and other gastrointestinal complaints. These preparations come in compounds that utilize four separate ions: calcium, aluminum, magnesium, and sodium. Excessive ingestion of each variety presents potential dangers of a particular kind.

Calcium carbonate is an inexpensive agent that is easily incorporated into various dosage forms (e.g., Tums tablets, Chooz gum, Bisodol powder). Although it is an effective neutralizing agent, it has been associated with acid rebound (renewed acid secretion at a level similar to that experienced prior to neutralization). In addition, doses of calcium carbonate in excess of 20 gm per day may cause systemic hypercalcemia.

Aluminum hydroxide (e.g., Amphogel) is a neutralizing agent that may also be used therapeutically to remove excessive concentrations of phosphate from the body. Misuse of the antacid can cause a variety of problems. As it interacts with dietary phosphate, it may prevent the nutrient's absorption and, in excessive amounts, aluminum hydroxide can lead to demineralization of bone. It has significant constipating ability. It can, through interaction, prevent the absorption of various drugs (e.g., tetracycline), and prolonged use of the agent may produce symptoms of systemic aluminum toxicity in patients with renal impairment.

Magnesium hydroxide (e.g., Milk of Magnesia) and other magnesium salts have excellent neutralizing capacity, but cause increases in peristaltic activity that may lead to diarrhea. Since this side effect is countered by the activity of aluminum salts, many commercial antacids contain mixtures of the two salts that are designed to prevent alterations of normal peristaltic activity (e.g., Di-Gel, Maalox). As with aluminum salts, prolonged use of magnesium compounds may induce toxicity in patients with renal impairment.

Sodium bicarbonate (e.g., Alka-Seltzer) is a systemic antacid because it is absorbed in amounts sufficient to cause alkalinization of the plasma and urine. Thus, it may cause acid rebound and alter the urinary excretion rate of a variety of other drugs. While its use has been declining over the past two or three decades, it is still preferred by large numbers of elderly patients.

OTC Vitamins

One significant problem with OTC vitamin therapy among elderly patients has already been touched on, namely, the threat to absorption of fat-soluble vitamins (A, D, E, K) posed by misuse of mineral oil laxatives. The other problem of note is associated with the relatively recent popularity of ingesting high doses of vitamin C as a nostrum for the common cold. While its effectiveness against the cold remains speculative, vitamin C definitely acidifies the urine. This lowering of urinary pH will cause increased excretion of alkaline drugs (e.g., antiarrhythmic) and increased renal reabsorption, hence retention, of acidic drugs (e.g., aspirin).

Ethanol

While conventional cultural attitudes may make the definition at first seem curious, ethanol ought to be considered an OTC drug. Alcohol is a general depressant of body function. It complicates therapy involving other depressant agents by increasing the depth of depression experienced by patients. Ethanol enhances the absorption and delays the metabolism of tranquilizers and hypnotics (e.g., Librium, Valium); thus it exaggerates their sedative effect. In addition, it augments the hypotensive effect of antihypertensive agents. Most problems involving ethanol result from misuse through excessive ingestion of the drug.

Nonscheduled Prescription Products

Nonscheduled prescription products constitute the second class of drugs with potential for misuse and abuse among elderly patients. Like OTC products, many of these agents are used to treat chronic conditions and so are subject to heavy use. However, a substantial number are used for more acute problems than those addressed by nonprescription products. They are generally more potent than OTC preparations and they require a physician's direct order for their use. The classes of drugs that most frequently present response problems among elderly patients are: (1) analgesics, (2) antibiotics, (3) antihypertensives, (4) cardiac medications, (5) drugs for diabetes, (6) eye medications, (7) antidepressants, (8) major tranquilizers, and (9) male and female hormones.

Analgesics

When OTC analgesics prove inadequate in alleviating discomfort, more potent nonnarcotics (thus unscheduled) are frequently prescribed. Because such agents have more potency milligram for milligram than OTC preparations, fewer need to be taken. The most important of these have been classified as nonsteroidal, anti-inflammatory drugs (NSAID). Many of these drugs, including Motrin, Naflon, and Naprosyn, are used to treat chronic inflammatory conditions such as arthritis and occasionally other types of minor pain. Actually, these agents have analgesic, anti-inflammatory and antipyretic (fever-reducing) activity comparable to aspirin. Their advantage for the elderly lies in the reduced levels of gastrointestinal irritation they cause.

Antibiotics

Many antibiotics that are ingested orally can facilitate an intestinal fungal infection, since they eradicate bacteria that normally keep the fungus in check. However, the antibiotics themselves are not frequently toxic to patients. Drugs such as sulfonamides, penicillin, ampicillin, cephalosporins, and erythromycin produce few side effects. Tetracycline may cause diarrhea and permit fungal infections in the oral cavity and in vaginal tissue. Chloramphenicol may produce anemia, and aminoglycosides are toxic to the kidney and cause potential hearing deficits, but these latter drugs are prescribed only with careful supervision. Nevertheless, in spite of the generally mild side effects, antibiotic therapy presents among the most difficult of drug response problems. These problems are centered on patient compliance; quite often, medication is discontinued before the prescribed period of time has elapsed. Patients may well experience symptomatic relief quite early in the therapeutic program, and may then stop taking the drug. This is especially true if the regimen is somehow uncomfortable or inconvenient. Unfortunately, such casual compliance can easily lead to bacterial resistance. Lethal organisms that do not respond to normal antibiotic therapy can develop easily. Thus, the importance of consuming the entire amount of antibacterial medication exactly as prescribed cannot be overemphasized.

The necessity for strict and complete compliance with the prescribed regimen applies to all antibiotic therapy. In addition, two particular conditions for which antibiotics are prescribed deserve special mention because of their frequency among elderly patients. The first of these, the upper respiratory infection, is generally caused by a virus rather than by bacteria. Thus, such infections are not susceptible to antibiotic therapy. Prescription of antibiotics, "just to be sure," may lead to substantial drug misuse in such cases. Respiratory infections that do originate with bacteria usually respond to penicillin or a similar agent. Regardless of their origin, however, respiratory infections may be complicated by drugs that depress respiration generally. Among these, propranolol (Inderal) and nadolol (Corgard) are agents to counter angina and cardiac arrhythmia which are often prescribed for elderly patients.

The second condition common among geriatric patients is the urinary tract infection, including cystitis. Anatomically, women are more susceptible to urinary tract infections than men. However, elderly men present a special case, since an enlarged prostate often interferes with complete emptying of the bladder. Such instances may easily lead to urinary tract infection. Uncomplicated infections respond to sulfonamide therapy. However, resistance is not uncommon, and more potent drugs or combinations of drugs, some with potentially serious side effects, must be used. Naturally, with a longer treatment program and more drugs involved in the regimen, the ideal of full compliance becomes increasingly important, even as it becomes more difficult to realize.

Antihypertensive Agents

High blood pressure readings are recorded in many people over the age of 60. While various drugs are used to treat this condition, diuretics are most frequently prescribed for the milder forms of hypertension. Of these, the thiazide diuretics (e.g., Diuril, Oretic, Esidrex, Enduron, Renese) are often encountered. They cause loss of sodium and water and help relieve swelling due to accumulation of fluid. Diuretics can increase plasma uric acid concentrations, often precipitating gout attacks. They also reduce plasma potassium concentrations, a circumstance that increases the activity of the digitalis glycosides (e.g., Digoxin). In individuals whose potassium levels are not adequately maintained, long-term diuretic therapy can produce symptoms similar to those suffered by patients with diabetes mellitus. Levels of this vital ion may be increased by dietary (fruits, juices, and green leafy vegetables) or synthetic supplement. Diuretics usually produce their activity for several hours; thus they should be taken in the morning to avoid the inconvenience of nocturnal urination.

Acute hypertension requires more potent antihypertensive agents (e.g., Dibenzyline, Minipress, Catapres). While these drugs are generally effective, the precise quantitative results are difficult to predict. They may, for example, cause a sudden and excessive drop in blood pressure. This is especially likely in patients who are also taking tranquilizers and antidepressants. In addition, if use of these agents is suddenly discontinued, a rebound hypertensive crisis may ensue. Overall, drugs used to treat acute hypertension may be accompanied by drowsiness and dizziness. A result of orthostatic or postural hypotension (a drug-induced exaggeration of the slight dizziness that normally accompanies a rapid shift from sitting or lying to standing), this latter side effect is of special concern among the elderly, whose generally more brittle bones may easily fracture in a fall.

Cardiac Medications

Because of relatively greater incidence of heart problems among older patients, cardiac medications are of special importance. These agents fall into four broad categories: anticoagulants, antianginal agents, antiarrhythmic agents, and drugs used to treat congestive heart failure.

After a heart attack, anticoagulants are often used to prevent development of fatal blood clots. When the danger is acute, clotting may be prevented by intravenous administration of heparin, a natural product that interacts only infrequently with other drugs. However, heparin may prompt bleeding, particularly in elderly women. Heparin is inappropriate for chronic anticoagulant therapy, since it is not absorbed when administered orally. Instead, patients may be given drugs that inhibit platelet aggregation, the initial stage of clot formation, (e.g., aspirin, Persantin). More intense anticoagulant therapy will require warfarin (Coumadin), an orally administered drug. Patients taking warfarin must have their blood monitored regularly for bleeding tendencies. In addition, the drug interacts with many classes of agents, particularly analgesics, tranquilizers, and antibiotics.

Angina pectoris is a condition characterized by intense chest pain and shortness of breath. Patients generally experience attacks during exercise, although these may also occur during rest. Nitroglycerin tablets are used to control the acute phase of the attack. They are placed beneath the tongue to ensure rapid action. However, they must not be taken too frequently during an attack; they can cause excessive peripheral vasodilation, which can in turn cause a more rapid heart beat that may intensify the attack. Nitroglycerin tablets are relatively unstable and should be kept tightly capped in the original bottle. Old tablets should be discarded and replaced periodically with fresh tablets. The incidence of angina attacks may be reduced by the prophylactic use of such drugs as propranolol (Inderal). However, these agents may depress respiration, thus complicating an asthmatic condition. They should be used with extreme care by the elderly, many of whom experience respiratory difficulties.

Certain agents have been found effective in restoring regular rhythmicity to an irregularly beating heart. These antiarrhythmic agents are frequently lifesaving. Arrhythmias associated with heart attacks are prevented by intravenous administration of drugs such as lidocaine. Once normal rhythm has been restored, various oral medications will help prevent the return of abnormalities. While their therapeutic actions are similar, their side effects vary. Patients taking quinidine may experience tinnitus (ringing in the ears), procainamide (Pronestyl) may prompt skin eruptions, and disopyramide (Norpace) may cause dry mouth.

Congestive heart failure is an insidious condition whose gradual onset is prompted by a progressively weakening heart muscle. To compensate for the decreased capacity attending this weakness, the heart increases its rate. The cardiac glycoside, digitalis, increases the strength of each individual contraction, thus allowing the heart to slow. However, digitalis is a potentially dangerous drug because of its numerous interactions with other agents. For example, either a decrease in potassium concentration (a result of diuretic therapy) or an increase in calcium level (a result of antacid ingestion) will effectively increase digitalis activity. Unfortunately, fatigue and lethargy, the symptoms of digitalis toxicity, are exactly those that characterize congestive heart failure. Thus, patients frequently compound the toxicity by taking more digitalis. As a rule of thumb, digitalis is not administered to patients whose heart is beating at fewer than 60 beats per minute. A physician's advice should always be sought if a question arises.

Diabetes Mellitus

Patients who suffer from diabetes mellitus produce urine with an abnormally high sugar content. The condition is caused by plasma levels of the hormone insulin that are insufficient to utilize glucose. Since the sugar cannot supply energy to the body's cells, it is lost in the urine. As this disease becomes increasingly frequent and acute with age, it becomes more and more important to reestablish adequate plasma insulin levels. This can be accomplished either by injecting insulin or by giving drugs that release the body's natural insulin from its site of synthesis in the pancreas; the choice of treatment depends on the cause of the insulin deficiency.

The first of these insulin deficiencies is known as insulin-dependent diabetes mellitus (IDDM) or brittle juvenile diabetes. In this condition (not limited to the young), the pancreas loses its ability to synthesize the hormone. Since insulin is decomposed by the enzymes and acids in the stomach, it cannot be administered orally and must be injected. Various insulin preparations are available in two strengths, 40 units/ml and 100 units/ml. Because compliance is perhaps the major consideration in successful insulin therapy, the 100-unit dosage form is preferable because it can be more conveniently measured. For example, a prescription for 43 units simply requires drawing up 0.43 ml in the syringe; in each instance, the number of units prescribed equals the equivalent decimal fraction of a milliliter of the 100 unit/ml preparation. Insulin preparations vary according to onset and duration of action; however, all must be refrigerated to prevent degradation.

The second condition, non-insulin-dependent diabetes mellitus (NIDDM), develops later in life and has come to be known as mature onset diabetes mellitus. More common among women than men, it appears frequently in persons who are obese, over 50, and have relatives who are also diabetic. In this state, the pancreas produces sufficient insulin, but the hormone is not secreted in sufficient quantities to control blood sugar. Drugs such as Orinase, Dymelor, Tolinase, and Diabinese can help many patients, but these agents interact frequently with other drugs and may produce exaggerated side effects. Frequently, non-insulin-dependent diabetes mellitus will resolve itself if sufferers reduce their weight significantly toward an ideal level.

Drugs Used in the Eye

Several drugs are used to diagnose and treat eye disorders in the elderly. The eye's pupil acts as a gate regulating the amount of light allowed to strike the sensitive portion at the back of the eye—the retina. A physician will dilate the pupil to examine the retina for symptoms or complications associated with hypertension, glaucoma, or diabetes mellitus. Most frequently atropine, but sometimes homatropine or epinephrine, may be used to open the pupil. Patients should be accompanied to the physician's office for an eye examination, because the drugs that dilate the pupil may compromise vision for several hours, making it difficult to read, drive, or carry out any activity that requires focusing on specific objects.

When pressure within the eye increases, small blood vessels that supply oxygen to the peripheral cells of the retina are compressed. Decreased blood flow may result in cellular death, and thus loss of light sensitivity in that portion of the eye. Loss of vision develops insidiously at the external fringes of the visual field, frequently going unnoticed by the patient. Ultimately blindness results from this condition known as glaucoma. Glaucoma is treated by reducing the pressure in two ways: reducing the rate of fluid formation or draining excess fluid directly. Acetazolamide (Diamox) reduces fluid formation when administered orally, and agents such as pilocarpine or echothiophate (Phospholine Iodide) accelerate the escape of fluid from the interior of the eye when applied topically. Strict compliance with the prescribed regimen is particularly important to ensure the effectiveness of the latter drugs. A common side effect of antihistamines, for example, that is exaggerated by age is suppression of tear formation. Some of the topical preparations therefore contain carboxymethylcellulose (CMC), a lubricant that ensures the eye's comfort during therapy.

Antidepressants

Two major categories of drugs are prescribed in treating depression. The first of these antidepressants, the monoamine oxidase (MAO) inhibitors (e.g., Parnate, Nardil, Eutonyl, Marplan), can be involved in serious drug and food interactions. Patients taking these agents should avoid alcohol, caffeine, and some dairy products—some of which can, in combination with the drug, prompt a fatal hypertensive crisis. Because of their potential for serious interactions with other substances, the MAO inhibitors are reserved for use exclusively in resistant cases.

The second class of antidepressant, the tricyclics (e.g., Elavil, Tofranil, Norpramin), are less toxic than the MAO inhibitors; still, they can produce side effects such as cardiac complications, drowsiness, dry mouth, and hypotension. Like the antibiotics, tricyclic antidepressants present substantial compliance problems. Because these agents exert their therapeutic effect only after a period of two to four weeks, patients frequently stop taking them because of the irritating side effects. They must understand the necessity for pursuing the regimen, perhaps for several months to a year, to prevent relapse. A new group of antidepressants, the tetracyclics (e.g., Ludiomil), has been reported to have a more rapid onset of action with fewer toxicities than the tricyclics. The newer agents are, however, more expensive than the more commonly prescribed antidepressants.

Major Tranquilizers

The major tranquilizers are commonly known as the phenothiazines and include such agents as Thorazine, Mellaril, Compazine, and Stelazine. They are most often prescribed for long-term use by patients with exaggerated mental problems. Major tranquilizers may produce a variety of side effects including drowsiness, hypotension, dry mouth, and constipation. Stool softeners such as Colace can alleviate the gastrointestinal complications, and chewing gum or dissolving hard candy may help relieve dryness in the mouth. Some patients on long-term therapy have developed "tremors" or Parkinson-like symptoms. These generally subside if dosages are adjusted downward, and drugs such as Cogentin and Artane can help reduce the severity of these symptoms.

Male and Female Hormones

Because of their side effects, male hormones are infrequently used therapeutically. The practice of treating tumors in female organs with testosterone or methyl testosterone is rapidly falling into disfavor. However, female hormones or estrogens are commonly used to relieve a variety of postmenopausal symptoms. Such estrogenic agents as Premarin and diethylstilbestrol (DES) can help prevent hot flashes, vaginal irritation, and headaches. They may also be useful in helping prevent calcium loss from bones, which is a particular problem in women over the age of 40. Some practitioners have suggested that estrogen may be useful in preventing atherosclerosis. In early menopausal therapy, estrogen can be supplied by birth control pill regimens that are 21 days long, followed by a 7-day period for withdrawal bleeding. This break in therapy also helps prevent pain in the breasts. Estrogen therapy has been associated with an increased risk of cancer. While the estrogenic agents do not themselves cause the tumors, they do fuel their abnormally rapid growth. Frequent checkups are essential to monitor for neoplastic growth, and these hormonal agents should be avoided altogether by women who have symptoms of heart failure or migraine headaches.

Scheduled Prescription Products

Scheduled prescription products make up the third class of drugs with abuse potential among elderly patients. Many of the agents in this category are used to treat psychological disorders over long periods of time. Their psychoactive characteristics, combined with their frequently serious liability of causing physical addiction, require that great care be exercised in their use. A brief definition of scheduling will precede discussion of specific drugs in this class. Then, the agents themselves will be considered in the following order: (1) narcotic analgesics, (2) minor tranquilizers, and (3) hypnotic agents.

Scheduling

Scheduling is a means of assigning uniform classification to certain drugs according to their potential for addiction. Schedule I agents are illegal for general use. Heroin is the best known of such drugs. Drugs placed on Schedule II may not be prescribed by telephone, except in emergencies, and prescriptions for them may not be refilled. Schedule III and Schedule IV agents may be prescribed by telephone and prescriptions may be refilled up to five times or for six months, whichever occurs first. Finally, Schedule V drugs include certain OTC medications for which the purchaser must sign. While a remarkable degree of uniformity exists among the various scheduling authorities, some agents appear on different schedules in a few states. The precise schedule designation for any particular drug should therefore be verified locally.

Narcotic Analgesics

A number of narcotic substances are used to treat the symptoms of pain. As their potency increases, so does the addiction liability. Morphine, codeine, and meperidine (Demerol) are highly addictive physiologically. Drugs such as Darvon and Talwin are less addictive, but potential for abuse is quite high because their use is so widespread. They are frequently used in combination with aspirin and acetaminophen.

Narcotics may depress respiration, decrease blood pressure, and cause constipation. Occasionally they are prescribed to help control diarrhea or to suppress the cough reflex.

Minor Tranquilizers

Minor tranquilizers are among the most frequently abused medications. Most of them (e.g., Valium, Librium, Serax, Tranxene) are very similar in chemical structure and pharmacologic activity. They are indicated for treatment of acute, temporary disturbances that are not deep-seated illnesses. Minor tranquilizers have been used as nighttime sedatives, muscle relaxants, and in therapy for alcoholism. They should be used only as necessary and constant use should be discouraged. Special care must be taken to limit drinking with these agents, since alcohol increases blood levels by suppressing their metabolism and enhancing their absorption.

A single dose of the minor tranquilizers may yield effects for up to 24 hours. They may produce exaggerated effects in elderly patients; thus a downward dosage adjustment is often required. If the drug is administered just prior to bedtime, many side effects can be minimized or may wear off completely by the time the patient awakes in the morning. Some physicians will instruct patients to take the drug four times daily, especially when the patient benefits psychologically from the act of ingesting the medication.

Hypnotic Agents

Many drugs used to help patients fall asleep have particularly widespread use among the elderly. During the past several years, the more toxic hypnotics, especially the barbiturates (e.g., Seconal, Nembutal, Tuinal) and the central nervous system depressants (e.g., Doriden, Quaalude, Noludar, Placidyl), have been discontinued in favor of safer agents such as chloral hydrate and particularly Dalmane and Restoril. The latter are similar in structure to the minor tranquilizers and are much safer than the older agents.

Before a patient is given a nighttime hypnotic, one should make sure that the drug is actually needed. Some patients will be able to fall asleep on their own if they are discouraged from taking late afternoon or early evening naps. Restricting the use of caffeine-containing beverages (coffee, tea, colas) during evening hours may also allow the patient to sleep more easily. In some situations, institutionalized patients are given hypnotics because the night shift is "short on help," and they do not want to contend with "bothersome" disturbances.

Summary

It remains, in summary, to repeat briefly the cautions mentioned elsewhere. All medications are capable of misuse or abuse. People responsible for the care of elderly patients must exercise special care, since those under their supervision are more likely both to be taking a variety of medications and to have problems in safely accommodating normal adult dosage levels.

BIBLIOGRAPHY

Adams G. (ed.): The use of drugs in geriatric medicine, in *Essentials of Geriatric Medicine*. New York, Oxford University Press, 1977.

Asperheim M.K.: *Pharmacology: An Introductory Text,* ed. 5. Philadelphia, W.B. Saunders Co., 1981.

Atkinson I.: An investigation into the ability of elderly patients continuing to take prescribed drugs after discharge from hospital and recommendations concerning improving the situation. *Gerontology* 24(3):225–234, 1978.

Barnes C.: Alcohol use among older persons. *J. Am. Geriatr. Soc.* 27:244, 1972.

Caransos G.J., Stewart R.B., Cluff L.E.: Drug-induced illness leading to hospitalization. *J.A.M.A.* 228:713–717, 1974.

Chapron D., Lawson I.: Drug prescribing and care of the elderly, in Reichel W. (ed.): *Topics in Long Term Care*. Baltimore, Williams & Wilkins Co., 1981.

Cooper J.W.: Drug therapy in the elderly. *Am. Pharm.* NS18(7):25–31, 1978.

Davis R.H.: *Drugs and the Elderly*. Los Angeles, University of Southern California Press, 1975.

Davison W.: Neurological and mental disturbances due to drugs. *Age Ageing* 7:119–126, 1978.

Drug problems of the elderly: The show goes on. *Am. Pharm.* NS20(9):9–10, 1981.

Gabriel M., Gagnon J.P., Bryan C.K.: Improving patient compliance through the use of a daily drug reminder chart. *Am. J. Public Health* 67:968, 1977.

Geriatric Drug Interactions. East Hanover, N.J., Sandoz Pharmaceuticals, 1979.

Gerson C.K.: Pharmaceutical service in home health care. *Am. Pharm.* 20(8):50–51, 1980.

Goth A.: *Medical Pharmacology,* ed. 9. St. Louis, C.V. Mosby Co., 1978.

Gotz B., Gotz V.: Drugs and the elderly. *Am. J. Nurs.* 78(8):1347–1351, 1978.

Green B.: The politics of psychoactive drug use in old age. *Gerontologist* 18(6):525–529, 1978.

Howard J.B.: Nursing home medication costs. *J. Am. Geriatr. Soc.* 26(5):228–230, 1978.

Karock M.: Drugs and the elderly. *Can. Med. Assoc. J.* 118(10):132–136, 1978.

Katzoff J.: A pharmacist in a home health agency. *Am. Pharm.* 20(8):52–54, 1980.

Keeping Track of Your Medicines (Publication no. 78–705b). U.S. Department of Health, Education and Welfare, Public Health Service. Rockville, Md., National Institute on Drug Abuse, 1978.

Krupka L.R., Vener A.M.: Hazards of drug use among the elderly. *Gerontologist* 19(1):90–95, 1979.

Lamy P.P., Vestal R.: Drug prescribing for the elderly, in Reichel W. (ed.): *Topics in Long Term Care*. Baltimore, Williams & Wilkins Co., 1981.

Lamy P.P.: The food/drug connection in elderly patients. *Am. Pharm.* 18(7):30–31, 1978.

Lamy P.P., Kitler M.E.: Drugs and the geriatric patient. *J. Am. Geriatr. Soc.* 1:23–33, 1971.

Monitoring Drug Therapy in the Long-Term Care Facility. Washington, D.C., American Pharmaceutical Association, 1978.

More Than Dispensing. Washington, D.C., American Pharmaceutical Association, 1980.

Perspectives on Geriatric Medicine (Publication no. NIH81–1924). U.S. Department of Health and Human Services. U.S. Government Printing Office, 1979.

Pharmaceutical Services in the Long Term Care Facility. Washington, D.C., American Health Care Association, 1975.

Pharmacy and the Elderly: An Assessment of Pharmacy Education Based on the Needs of the Elderly and Recommendations for Increasing Geriatric Aspects of Pharmacy Curricula (Publication no. 80–37). U.S. Department of Health, Education and Welfare-HRA. Washington, D.C., Center for Human Services, 1979.

Physicians' Desk Reference, ed. 34. Oradell, N.J., Medical Economics Company, 1980.

Poe W.D., Holloway D.A.: *Drugs and the Aged*. New York, McGraw-Hill Book Co., 1980.

Roe D.A.: Drugs, diet and nutrition. *Am. Pharm*. 18(10):62–64, 1978.

Saving Money with Generic Medicines: Can You? U.S. Department of Health, Education and Welfare, Public Health Service. Rockville, Md., National Institute on Drug Abuse, 1979.

Segal J.L., et al.: Drug utilization and prescribing patterns in a skilled nursing facility: The need for a rational approach to therapeutics. *J. Am. Geriatr. Soc*. 27:117–122, 1979.

Smith C.: Use of drugs in the aged. *Johns Hopkins Med. J*. 145(2):61–64, 1979.

Stanaszek W.F.: The hospital pharmacist and the geriatric patient: Drug therapy considerations. *Hospital Formulary Management* 2:18–24, 1974.

U.S. Department of Health, Education and Welfare, Food and Drug Administration: *Drug Bulletin* Feb./Mar., 2:2, 1979.

Using Your Medicines Wisely: A Guide for the Elderly (Publication no. 78–705a). U.S. Department of Health, Education and Welfare, Public Health and Human Services. Rockville, Md., National Institute on Drug Abuse, 1978.

Vancura E.J.: Guard against unpredictable drug responses in the aging. *Geriatrics* 34(4):63–65, 1979.

Ventnor A.M., et al.: Drug usage and health characteristics. *J. Am. Geriatr. Soc*. 27(2)83–89, 1979.

Vestal R.E.: Drug use in the elderly: A review of problems and special considerations. *Drugs* 16:358–382, 1978.

Ward M., Blatman M.: Drug therapy in the elderly. *Am. Fam. Physician* 19(2):143–152, 1979.

9

SENSORY CHANGES IN AGING

Carol J. Dye, Ph.D.

AS IN OTHER physiologic systems, the senses decline in function with the aging of the organism. The extent and pattern of the decline for each of the senses vary considerably. Some sensory functions show a gradual, consistent decrease over time. Such is the case with narrowing of pupil size in the eye. Other functions may show changes fairly rapidly at first and then the rate at which further changes occur slows down. An example is farsightedness in vision that develops with age. Other patterns of change may be identified. There is also variability in the time of the life span when sensory changes begin. For example, much of the decline in the eye begins in the 40s and 50s. However, changes in the sense of taste seem to occur somewhat later—in the 60s and 70s. The practitioner dealing with older adults needs to be aware of these patterns and times of onset, not only to accommodate the environment to these individuals but also to identify pathologic deviation from normal aging.

Determining what is normal and what is pathologic in sensory decline is complicated by the amount of variation found within the aged population. In the data presented in this chapter, the mean values for the performance of groups of older adults will be presented and compared to the mean performance of younger groups of persons. Comparisions of the means of these various age groups typically reflect a steady decline in functioning in each of the senses over the life span. What these means fail to show is that there tends to be much greater variability in the performance of the older group. The young group may earn scores between 15 and 20, whereas the older group may earn scores between 7 and 20. A very important point to be made about this greater variability is that we must be especially careful not to stereotype our approach to older people. While some are showing many of the disabilities of age, others are still functioning at a relatively unimpaired level. For all older individuals, we need to check whether they can hear before we start shouting, and whether they can read regular print assisted by their glasses before we give them large-print material, or assume in other ways that their senses are deficient. In the following review of the sensory changes with age, these issues will recur.

Changes in Vision

There are a number of areas in which age affects vision. Some of these are related to changes in muscle tone; others are due to changes in the rapidity with which photochemical processes occur; and still others are due to accumulative processes within the eyes. Perhaps the two most noticeable changes are in acuity and in the ability to focus on objects at close distances (Duane, 1931; Friedenwald, 1952; Hofstetter, 1954).

Visual acuity is the ability to see objects at far distances. It is generally considered that the standard for the normal individual is the ability to see certain fixed objects distinctly at 40 feet. As a person ages, however, this same object can be seen distinctly only 20 feet away with the better eye. The ratios are expressed as 20/40, with the distance a normally sighted person can distinguish the object represented by the second figure, and the adjusted distance by the first figure. Defective visual acuity (less than 20/40) is present at the rate of about 22 per 100 persons in the 12- to 14-year age group. This increases only slightly up to age 45 years. From that age on, however, there is a steady and dramatic increase in the number of persons with defective vision.

In the 75- to 79-year age group, only 15 per 100 persons have 20/20 vision, even with correction. As can be seen, changes in visual acuity are not likely to be noticed by the individual until the 40s and 50s; but by 70 years, poor vision is the rule for the average person. These data are the result of examination in clinic settings under conditions of average lighting. In real life situations, the amount of light on an object greatly influences visual acuity. If the lighting is dim, acuity is greatly decreased. On the other hand, if the level of illumination is above average, acuity is increased. Another factor affecting acuity is the amount of contrast between object and background. Contrast sensitivity declines with age (Weiss, 1959). Subtle differences in shadings or colors will reduce acuity, whereas greater differences improve it. Acuity in old age, then, can often be improved if levels of illumination are increased and if the contrast between object and background is optimal.

The loss of ability to focus at close distances due to loss of elasticity of the lens of the eye is actually a change that begins early in childhood. It is so gradual during adolescence and early maturity that it is generally not noticed by the individual. During the 40s and early 50s, the rate of change accelerates (Bruckner, 1967) so that individuals become aware of greater farsightedness. For example, they notice that they cannot read comfortably while holding material at the same distance from their eyes as they had previously. There is a standard statement people make at this time—that if the person is to continue reading he will "have to get either longer arms or glasses." From the 40s up to the early 50s, the rate of decline in this ability becomes more gradual. The same considerations of illumination and contrast mentioned above apply to visual accommodation at close distances.

For the previously normal sighted individual, aging changes in acuity and accommodation mean that there is a restriction of the range of vision since both distant and close vision are affected. Generally, glasses for reading, at first, and then bifocals correct these deficits. There is a need to increase the amount of correction as the individual continues to age. As the data on visual acuity indicate, in advanced old age the person may not be able to see very well even with glasses.

Another change that occurs in visual ability with age is in adaptation to dark, that is, rapidity with which the individual adapts to changes in levels of illumination, as when going from a lighted to a darkened room. Two aspects of this visual adjustment are important to aging. One is the rate at which the adaptation occurs and the other is the level reached when the adjustment is completed. Some data seem to indicate that both rate and final level achieved are affected by age (McFarland et al., 1960; Domey et al., 1960). That the final level of accommodation is affected by age is shown in the correlation of .90 of these two variables (McFarland, 1955). The reason for a slowing in the rate of adaptation is that there is a slowing of the photochemical processes in the eye. The reason for the decline in final level of accommodation is the increased opacity of the lens in old age that prevents some of the available light from entering the eye.

Of course, the same problems experienced in adapting to the dark will occur when the individual moves from a darkened environment to an illuminated one. Problems in adaptation will occur in places where there are spots of light, such as on a highway at night. The problem of adaptation to changes in levels of illumination will be evident for the older adult in such situations as entering a darkened movie house, awakening at night and turning on a bedside light, or walking down a darkened street punctuated by occasional streetlights.

There are other problems related to adaptation to levels of illumination by the aging eye. One has to do with visual glare. As indicated above, the lens clouds as the eye ages. This not only causes less light to enter the eye, but also causes a scattering or diffusion of the light. Epithelial cells that have been loosened and scattered on the anterior portion of the eye, plus material accumulated in the vitreous, also contribute to this scattering of the light rays entering the eye. The result is that visual images become increasingly blurred. Additionally, the scattering of light rays makes glare much more visually disruptive in the older adult, since intensive stimulation randomly affects many parts of the retina. If this happens while the person is driving on a rainy highway at night, the temporary disorientation may have serious consequences. Another common source of glare is that occurring at night from light-colored enameled or tiled walls in bathrooms. It has been noted that the elderly seem to prefer more dimly lit, darker-surfaced rooms (Botwinick, 1978). This may be because of the problems they experience with glare.

Clouding of the lens in the aged eye may eventuate in cataracts. It is not certain whether this relatively complete clouding of the lens with serious impairment in vision is a pathologic process or a manifestation of aging that occurs sooner in some persons than in others. The incidence of cataracts in the elderly is not great, however, though the rate increases with age. For example, in a Duke University study, 9%, 18%, and 36% of persons in their 60s, 70s, and 80s, respectively, were found to have cataracts (Fozard et al., 1977). If cataracts are diagnosed, the clouded lens can be removed surgically. This is an easily performed procedure today, resulting in vastly improved vision. Of course, contact lenses or eyeglasses must be worn to replace the lens that has been removed.

In addition to greater clarity in vision, removal of the clouded lens from the eye results in other visual changes. A positive result is that the individual is less prone to the effects of glare. Objects appear about one-third larger than they did previously; the individual becomes more farsighted than he was before; and with more light entering the eye, normal levels of lighting may appear much brighter. Removal of the lens in cataract surgery may not make for completely clear vision, however. The cornea of the eye changes shape and flattens with age, and irregularities in images may occur as a result of these distortions (Fozard et al., 1977). This is called astigmatism and may also be corrected by specially ground lenses for the eye.

Another normal aging change in vision resulting in reduced illumination to the eye is a decrease in the size of the pupil over the life span. There is a correlation of approximately −.55 with age and pupil size (Feinberg and Podolac, 1965). A decrease in pupil size is one of the changes that is gradual over the life span, beginning at about 20 years of age. Not only does the size of the pupil decrease, but it also reacts less effectively and more slowly to changes in the level of illumination, and eventually may not react at all. By age 85, only one third of the people have pupils that respond to light (DHEW, no date). Overall, the lenticular and pupillary changes and the accumulation of opacities in the vitreous result in a linear decrease in light reaching the retina after age 20 (Weale, 1965). It can be easily understood from these data that increasing levels of environmental illumination for the aged are a necessity.

The lens not only clouds in old age but it also yellows, causing the filtering of shorter wavelengths of light—the blues and violets. Consequently, color perception is not as accurate. Gilbert (1957) showed that ability to discriminate colors gradually declines after 20 years of age. This decline accelerates and becomes most noticeable in the 70s and beyond (Dalderup and Fredericks, 1969). While the blue part of the spectrum is affected most, there is an overall decline for the entire continuum. Not all the problems of color perception are due to yellowed lenses. While removal of the lens during cataract surgery improves color vision, colors do not become as distinct as they were in younger years. As a practical demonstration of changes in color perception in old age, take a piece of yellow acetate and place it over various colored objects. Note how the yellow objects become almost indistinguishable, the blue ones become green, and the red ones remain red but lose their vividness. This change in color perception is important for the older adult in situations where he needs to discriminate colors in order to determine behavior. Matching the colors in clothes, following color codes in an institutional environment, and taking pills denoted by color are some of the activities affected.

One other point needs to be mentioned about age changes in the eye. As the individual ages, the elevator muscles that allow an upward gaze atrophy from disuse. The average upward gaze is 40, 33, 26, and 16 degrees, respectively, groups 5–14, 35–44, 55–64, and 75–94 years of age, respectively (Chamberlain, 1970). Consequently, the older person must raise his or her head when an upward glance is necessary. As a result, some older adults who are bent over or who have arthritis that interferes with normal neck movement may not see street or door signs placed above head level.

The overall result of changes in the aging eye is that the elderly will likely require eyeglasses to read or see for distance, take more time to accommodate to changes in level of illumination, and generally require greater levels of illumination. Visual changes that occur with age may force the older adult to restrict activity. He may cease driving at night because of problems experienced with dark adaptation and glare. Walking activities may be restricted both indoors and outdoors because of increasing uncertainty in depth perception and blurring of vision. To the outside observer, the older adult may appear to be uncertain and cautious. Much can be done within the environment to optimize functioning in old age. Providing diffuse and adequate levels of illumination in all areas of the living environment is an important requirement. Diffuse, even lighting reduces the need for continual visual adaptation and the need to distinguish objects in shadows. Adequate lighting will increase acuity. Soft finishes and appropriate colors should be chosen for walls to reduce glare. Bright colors that contrast sharply with background colors should be used to outline doorways, thresholds, steps, and stairways. While these environmental supports would greatly help older people, they are obviously safety features for all ages.

Changes in Hearing

In 1969, the Department of Health, Education and Welfare estimated that there were approximately 236,000 legally deaf individuals in the United States. This number did not include approximately 6 million individuals who had bilateral hearing loss of sufficient magnitude to be a significant handicap in everyday functioning and another 2.5 million with unilateral hearing impairment (DHEW, 1969). These data are important for the gerontologist since hearing difficulties are relatively infrequent among the young. Within the 45–54 age group, 19% show some beginning difficulty in hearing. By the time these individuals reach 75 to 79 years of age, about 75% have impairments (DHEW, 1975). As with the eye, there are changes in the anatomical structure and the mechanical and neurologic functions of the auditory apparatus. One structural change is a lengthening of the pinna of the ear. The significance of this for functioning has not been established, but it certainly contributes to the identification of aging in the individual. Another structural change is the degeneration of hair cells, directly affecting the ability to sense incoming sounds. Additionally, there is greater chance of accumulating wax and fluid in the middle ear, further contributing to loss of sound perception (Corso, 1977).

The basic presbycusic change in function is that high-pitched sounds become inaudible and hearing becomes increasingly restricted to low-frequency sounds. The normal ear picks up sounds in a range of 20 to 20,000 vibrations per second (Hz), although to hear sounds at the extreme ends of this continuum, the loudness of those tones must be increased. Changes in hearing ability become apparent in the 50s and affect perception of sounds above 1000 Hz. This is the sound approximately two octaves above middle C (Botwinick, 1978). As hearing loss progresses with age, more of the lower-frequency sounds become inaudible.

Hearing loss above 1000 Hz is significant since this is approximately in the middle of the speech frequency range. Most of the consonants that are spoken range between 1000 Hz and 3000 Hz. The voiceless consonants (s, f, p, t, k, ch, sh, st) are the highest-frequency consonants at 3000 Hz. Vowel sounds fall below 300 Hz in adults and children (Grey and Weise, 1959) so that they should still be heard in old age, but consonants are the letters by which spoken words are recognized. If these become unintelligible with age, then speech, the chief means of interpersonal communication, will be affected and restricted significantly. Feldman and Reger (1967) found that after 50 years of age understanding of speech became increasingly affected by losses in hearing, until age 80, when there was a 25% loss of understanding.

Not only does auditory threshold decline with age, but the ability to discriminate between two pitches also declines; and, not unexpectedly, the greatest problem in pitch discrimination is in the ranges where hearing loss is greatest. The amount of difference between two sounds necessary to discriminate them increases as a linear function of age up to 55 years. After that time, the increase in difference between the two pitches is dramatic, especially for the higher frequencies (Corso, 1977).

Some hearing loss documented as occurring with age may, in fact, be due to the wear and tear of a noise-polluted environment (Kryter, 1970; Lebo and Reddell, 1972). It is known that older populations existing in environments with lower noise levels show a smaller percentage of hearing impaired adults (Rosen et al., 1962; Rosen et al., 1964; Bergman, 1966). Also, it is suggested that the often noted difference in hearing impairment between men and women in old age is due to exposure of the male ear to industrial and other noises. It is not clear at this point how much loss documented as accompanying aging is due to this type of stress. Functionally, the hearing loss that occurs in high noise environments appears the same as that with aging. However, Corso has proposed that the differences between the two are physiologically quite distinct (1976). More study is needed in this area, with obvious implications for environmental noise control (Lebo and Reddell, 1972).

One of the problems in assessing auditory thresholds of the elderly is their noted cautiousness in responding to auditory signals. Investigators interested in auditory thresholds of older adults (Rees and Botwinick, 1971; Craik, 1969) note that they are more cautious in reporting having heard a signal. Attentiveness to and ability to focus on the task are also important response variables that may affect the results of assessments of sensory thresholds. It is well known that older adults have more difficulty in focusing on and maintaining attention on a task. The likely effect of these response variables is an overestimation of the amount of hearing loss within the older population.

A solution to the loss of higher frequencies and pitch discrimination problems of presbycusis is to increase the volume of incoming signals. One way to do that is to use a hearing aid, which amplifies sound and, therefore, does assist hearing to some extent. There is a drawback to hearing aids, however, in that they amplify all sounds. Random sounds not normally perceived by the individual, such as an airplane flying overhead or an object dropping on the floor, will be amplified as well as significant sounds and can prove distracting. A tape recorder does the same thing; it demonstrates practically what the older adult experiences when wearing a hearing aid. It is possible, thus, that adjustment to a hearing aid could be difficult and frustrating. The inconvenience of it, plus the image that a hearing aid designates the individual as being old, may discourage a person from using one.

It has already been stated that speech perception is likely to be affected by changes that occur in the ear during aging. Central nervous system (CNS) factors also affect speech perception (Calearo and Lazzaroni, 1957; Jerger, 1971). As with other bodily functions, the CNS slows in the rate with which it processes incoming signals. Compared to younger persons, the aged take longer to process each signal. If sounds are separated sufficiently in time to allow for this, the older adult will be able to process the signals adequately. If, however, signals come too rapidly, some will be missed. Take as an example this request made of the older adult: "Please come into my office so that I may talk to you about your diabetes." Slowed CNS processing of this auditory message may cause the older adult to miss every third syllable so that he hears only: "Please come ____ to my ____ ice so ____ I may ____ to you a ____ your diabetes." As can be seen, the slowing of CNS processes, together with the loss of consonants in high frequencies, could result in the loss of much communication. The solution to the problem of CNS slowing is to reduce the amount of auditory information given to an older adult per unit of time. Instead of *increasing the volume, slowing the rate* of speech is likely to have greater benefit for communication.

Since hearing is related to speech, it would be expected that auditory loss in old age would affect speech also. If so, it is at present unclear how this takes place. It has been noted by many people, however, that as a person becomes more hard of hearing, he seems to speak louder. Researchers have found that the frequency range of the older voice is smaller, and there is a decrease in vocal intensity and a decline in voice quality (Luchsinger and Arnold, 1965). How these vocal changes are affected by changes in hearing and how the vocal apparatus ages are yet to be determined.

Changes in Taste

Data in the sensory area of taste perception over the life span are sparse and at times contradictory, due mainly to the greater difficulty of doing research in this area. As in other systems, there are anatomical and neurologic changes in taste that occur with age. These changes affect the ability of the older adult to make discriminations in tastes and to enjoy eating.

Unquestionably, as in other parts of the body, the nerves of the gustatory system atrophy with age. In addition, there is a change in number and in distribution of taste buds (Arey, Tremain, and Monzingo, 1935; Mochizuki, 1939). The child has taste buds not only on the upper part of the tongue but also on the lips, tonsils, uvula, and underside of the tongue (Moncrieff, 1951). Some of these sensors survive through maturity but others atrophy early in life. Then, at about 60 years of age, there appears to be accelerated atrophy of the taste buds and a loss of papillae. In childhood, the individual has an average of 248 functioning taste buds per papilla; by the time he reaches 74 to 85 years, there are only about 88. In addition, one half of those still functioning are stunted. Consequently, there is about an 80% loss in taste buds over the life span (DHEW, no date).

The data on taste perception show this loss in sensory apparatus. Taste thresholds for the four basic substances—sweet, sour, salty, and bitter—increase with age; that is, it takes more concentrated solutions to have an effect. Studies in this area consistently reflect this fact, although the extent of increase of threshold over age varies (Richter and Campbell, 1940; Bourliere, Cendron, and Rapaport, 1958; Byrd and Gertman, 1959; Cooper, Bilash, and Zubek, 1959; Langan and Yearick, 1976). Some of the variation may be due to experimental procedures used in the study, the group sampled, or the substance studied. Few studies have assessed all basic substances in the same population, but this was done in the Cooper, Bilash, and Zubek (1959) study. These investigators found that there was very little change in any threshold until after the late 50s. Then, bitter showed the greatest increase in threshold, while sour increased the least and at a later point in the life span than the other substances. There is some indication that the extent of increase in threshold may be declining over recent years, and the point at which it begins may be occurring later in the life span. Dye and Koziatek (1981) compared their results of threshold testing of sucrose in younger and older adults to previous studies and they noted improvement in sensitivity of the older adults over the past four decades. Possibly this indicates that more recent cohorts of elderly are more youthful and in better physical condition.

Taste sensitivity is modified by a number of other variables that may complicate and accentuate the taste problem for any older adult. Long-time habits of food consumption will modify food preferences in later life. In a study of Indian laborers who ate large quantities of the sour tamarind fruit, Moskowitz (1975) documented a noticeable increase in preference for sour tastes, although preferences for different tastes matched baselines from other populations. It seems that strong food preferences could be evident over a lifetime, having important implications for diet, adequate nutrition, and weight control in later years. Some documentation of this by Garcia, Battese, and Brewer (1975), in a study of dietary patterns over the life span, showed a cohort effect but no influence of age on consumption patterns.

Lifetime habits affect taste perception in another way, too. Some habits such as smoking and alcoholism seem to diminish taste sensitivity. An older adult who has smoked or consumed large quantities of alcohol over his lifetime would likely experience even less enjoyment from food. Disease states also influence taste sensitivity—sometimes increasing it and at other times decreasing it (Henkin, 1967).

Threshold testing with basic tastes in solution is only one way to assess taste sensitivity. An important question is whether the elderly are able to discriminate among food substances as well as younger persons can. Recent research by Schiffman (1977) showed that food samples processed to control for differences in texture were also discriminated and identified less well by older adults. So it seems that no matter what the form of food, the older adult is likely to gain less of a taste sensation from what he masticates. Often the older adult may complain that things do not taste the same as they once did. The data on loss of taste buds and perception of basic tastes and food substances explain, at least in part, the basis for this complaint. Lacking here is research that explores possible changes in the hedonic aspects of food and taste over the life span. Perceived pleasantness of food substances is the motivator for eating. While clinically it is noted that the elderly complain of experiencing less enjoyment from eating, there are no data on this important variable. Since eating is an important basic pleasure in life, decreased acuity in this sensation may contribute to negative moods in the elderly.

Changes in Smell

Taste and smell are usually discussed together since they are related experientially. Taste is greatly dependent on smell. Note, for example, that things do not taste as good when one has a cold that clogs the nose. Masking odors of foods decreases enjoyment. Much of the enjoyment of food comes from the pleasant smells arising from cooking it and serving it. If there is a decline in olfaction with age, this may also affect age in relation to taste.

Data regarding the effect of aging on smell are even sparser than those for taste, perhaps also because of the special problems that must be overcome to conduct studies in this area. Some early studies of aging of the olfactory apparatus and nerve fibers showed neural loss and structural atrophy over the life span (Smith, 1935, 1942; Mesolella, 1934). However, these early results did not determine whether the conditions were due to normal aging or to disease processes. It may have been that factors concomitant with aging, such as poor health, produced the apparent age relationships. For example, a study of olfactory perception of diesel exhaust fumes indicated that older persons found the fumes less objectionable (Springer and

Dietzmann, 1977). At first, this would seem to show less sensitivity in the elderly. However, the older adults tested also rated themselves as in poor health. When their ratings were compared to others of various ages who also considered themselves in poor health, the perceptions were similar. Health status, not age, seemed to affect ratings of the fumes.

Other recent data indicate that sensitivity to smell may not decline in normal older adults. In a study by Engen (1977), the ability to identify a smoky odor showed such variability in both a young (20–22 years) and an older (60–74 years) group that it would have been difficult to sort the individuals into their respective age groups based on their perception scores. Still other data (Kimbrell and Furchgott, 1963) seem to show differential age decline in olfactory sensitivity for different odors. This coincides with the findings for the basic substances in taste.

As can be seen, this area has yet to be explored. Extrapolating from the age findings for the other senses, it would seem unusual indeed if the sense of smell did not show some decline based on anatomical and neurologic changes. It also seems that the notion of wide individual variability, as described at the beginning of this chapter, is particularly relevant in this area, with concomitant variables such as health status having an important influence in determining those individual differences.

Pain

Pain is a sensation with a great psychological component to its perception. This psychological component is made up of sociocultural (Chapman, 1944; Schluderman and Zubek, 1962), cognitive, motivational (Melzack and Casey, 1968), and suggestion (Melzack, 1973) factors. Therefore, at any age, actual sensation pain thresholds that are free of contamination by these other factors are difficult to determine.

Early studies in this area indicated that there were no age-related changes in pain sensitivity (Hardy et al., 1943; Birren, Schapiro, and Miller, 1950; Wilder, 1940; Sherman, 1943). While these results were found in the laboratory, clinically it has been noted that older adults are able to tolerate more pain than younger ones without as much discomfort. This same finding has been noted by dentists and health care professionals. Elderly people seem able to experience serious illness without the agony felt by younger persons, and to undergo minor surgery or dental work without the need for anesthesia often necessary at younger ages. Two possibilities arise to explain these clinical findings. One is based on the psychological component of pain perception. Since the present group of older adults were born at a time when pain-reducing medications were not so readily available, they may have had to learn to handle higher levels of pain without complaining than younger persons do in today's world. The second possibility is that since it is known that neurons in all parts of the body die with age, pain sensations may no longer be as reliable or intense.

Clark and Mehl (1971) separated decision variables from sensory thresholds in a signal detection study of pain perception. They found that older persons adopted a higher criterion of pain than younger people. The older subjects seemed to need more evidence before they reported pain, whereas the younger subjects reported pain much more readily. Whether this is a situation like that noted in audiological testing with older adults, indicating greater cautiousness, or whether it is a cohort effect is not known from the results of the study. In reference to actual sensation of pain, Clark and Mehl (1971) found that older women were less sensitive to similar intensities of stimulation than were the younger and older men and younger women. The only problem with this study is that the "old" subjects included were between the ages of 30 and 67 and were not within the age range typically considered old. Yet the results are interesting since they separate criteria and sensation factors in perception.

A possible loss of sensation to pain at older ages appears to have implications for health care, since it might be easier to have older adults in physical therapy, and so on, and to engage them in more strenuous activities. On the other hand, older adults have more somatic complaints than younger persons. Whether these complaints are actually pain-related or just general discomfort has not been determined; also, whether these complaints come from populations with distinct characteristics, such as poor health status, has to be determined. Whatever the case, reduction in sensitivity to pain in old age may be the one area in which loss of sensory processes results in a positive effect.

Other Special Senses

There are a number of other areas in which people receive sensations from the body that enable them to survive in the environment. These include sensations from the skin and the viscera, kinesthetic perceptions, and temperature sensitivity. Maintaining function in these areas allows the individual to acknowledge (*a*) the touch of objects or people; (*b*) body position, in order to avoid falls; and (*c*) the warmth or coldness of an object or environment so as to react protectively and to dress appropriately. Generally, data pertaining to these senses indicate that age brings a decline in them but, as with the other senses, it is far from clear whether the decline is due to age itself or to diseases and injuries concomitant with age (Kenshalo, 1977). Much of the research does not report on concomitant variables that may affect sensation in the populations studied, so it is not known which variables besides age might determine loss of sensitivity. It is known, however, that not all older adults show declines in these areas. For example, in a study of vibratory sensitivity, Skre (1972) reported that only 5% of his population showed impairment in this sense in the upper extremities, while 40% showed impairment in the lower extremities of the body. Consequently, there is a great deal of variability in the manner in which age affects these special sensitivities.

A basic question, then, is whether possible loss of sensitivity occurs because of slowing of peripheral nerve conduction, loss of neurons with age, or CNS processing factors. It is well known that neural loss occurs with age (Brody and Vijayashanker, 1977). Consequently, it should be expected that sensitivity would be reduced for that reason alone. There is no agreement, however, on whether there is a concomitant slowing in neural conduction with age. Wayner and Emmers (1958) were unable to show a slowing of peripheral nerve responses in rats. Weiss (1965), in exploring speed of response in humans, concluded that the slowed response time was due to CNS processes and not to peripheral nerve conduction. While neural processes may account for some of the decline in sensitivity of the special senses with aging, they may not be the only processes that cause a decline. Again, aging of body structures may also determine declines in sensitivity. An example of this is the change in structure of the skin that affects cutaneous sensations. As can be seen, age changes in the special senses is another area requiring much more research. Questions remain on the effect of disease and injury in producing an aging effect in sensory data, underlying etiology of aging or other changes that occur over the life span, and the specific processes that produce a decline.

Conclusions

As the discussion shows, most sensory decline over the life span occurs from middle maturity onward. Though some age changes occur earlier, they are so gradual that they are generally not noticed by the individual. The effect of sensory loss in old age is for the individual to increasingly shut the world out from his experience, and he may feel diminished enjoyment from the environment. There are wide individual differences in this perception, however, depending on the extent of decline and on personality factors. Some older people dismiss these changes as petty annoyances; others continually lament them. Since the decline in functions starts at different times and occurs at different rates, it is likely there will be gradual adjustments to the changes as they set in. As one sense declines, another may be used to compensate for it. As sight diminishes, hearing may be relied on increasingly to gain necessary cues from the environment. Or if hearing is impaired, the individual can learn to supplement his understanding of speech through lipreading. If both these two very important senses decline, the chances are reduced that the individual can maintain independent living. This is likely to happen in only a very small percentage of the older population, probably far below 5%. Older adults who experience normal sensory decline learn to compensate. They take more time to perform tasks to be certain of their perceptions; they learn to use more than one sense to gain information in any situation; they restrict their activities to those environments in which they can feel secure; and they may learn to rely more on other people.

REFERENCES

Arey L.B., Tremain M.J., Monzingo F.L.: The numerical and topographical relation of taste buds to human circumvallate papillae throughout the lifespan. *Anat. Rec.* 64:9–25, 1935.

Bergman M.: Hearing in the Mabaans. *Arch. Otolaryngol.* 84:411–415, 1966.

Birren J.E., Schapiro H., Miller J.: The effect of salicylate upon pain sensitivity. *J. Pharmacol. Exp. Ther.* 100:67–71, 1950.

Botwinick J.: *Aging and Behavior,* ed. 2. New York, Springer Publishing Co., 1978.

Bourliere F., Cendron H., Rapaport A.: Modification avec l'âge des sénils gustatifs de perception et de reconnaissance aux saveurs salée et sucrée chez l'homme. *Gerontologia* 2:104–112, 1958.

Brody H., Vijayashanker N.: Anatomical changes in the nervous system, in Finch C.E., Hayflick L. (eds.): *Handbook of the Biology of Aging.* New York, Van Nostrand Reinhold, 1977.

Bruckner R.: Longitudinal research on the eye. *Gerontologia Clin.* 9:87–95, 1967.

Byrd B., Gertman S.: Taste sensitivity in aging persons. *Geriatrics* 14:381–384, 1959.

Calearo C., Lazzaroni A.: Speech intelligibility in relationship to the speech of the message. *Laryngoscope* 67:410–419, 1957.

Chamberlain W.: Restriction in upward gaze with advanced age. *Trans. Am. Ophthalmol. Soc.* 68:235–244, 1970.

Chapman W.: Measurement of pain sensitivity in normal control subjects and in psychoneurotic patients. *Psychosom. Med.* 6:252–255, 1944.

Clark W.C., Mehl L.: Thermal pain: A sensory decision theory analysis of the effect of age and sex on d′, various response criteria and 50% pain threshold. *J. Abnorm. Psychol.* 78:202–212, 1971.

Cooper R.M., Bilash L., Zubek J.P.: The effect of age on taste sensitivity. *J. Gerontol.* 14:56–58, 1959.

Corso J.: Auditory perception and communication, in Birren J.E., Schaie K.W. (eds.): *Handbook of the Psychology of Aging.* New York, Van Nostrand Reinhold, 1977.

Corso J.F.: Presbycusis as a complicating factor in evaluating noise-induced hearing loss, in Henderson D., Hamernick R.P., Dasanjh D.S., et al. (eds.): *Effects of Noise on Hearing.* New York, Raven Press, 1976.

Craik F.I.M.: Applications of signal detection theory to studies of aging, in Welford A.T. (ed.): *Interdisciplinary Topics in Gerontology*. New York, S. Karger, 1969.

Dalderup L.M., Fredericks M.L.C.: Colour sensitivity in old age. *J. Am. Geriatr. Soc.* 17:388–390, 1969.

Domey R.C., McFarland R.A., Chadwick E.: Dark adaptation as a function of age and time: II. A derivation. *J. Gerontol.* 15:267–279, 1960.

Duane A.: Accommodation. *Arch. Ophthalmol.* 5:1–14, 1931.

Dye C.J., Koziatek D.A.: Age and diabetes effects of threshold and hedonic perception of sucrose solutions. *J. Gerontol.* 36(3):310–315, 1981.

Engen T.: Taste and smell, in Birren J.E., Schaie K.W. (eds.): *Handbook of the Psychology of Aging*. New York, Van Nostrand Reinhold, 1977.

Feinberg R., Podolac E.: Latency of pupillary reflex to light and its relation to aging, in Welford A.T., Birren J.E. (eds.): *Behavior, Aging, and the Nervous System*. Springfield, Ill., Charles C Thomas, Publisher, 1965.

Feldman R.M., Reger S.N.: Relations among hearing, reaction time, and age. *J. Speech Hear. Res.* 10:479–495, 1967.

Fozard J.L., Wolf E., Bell B., et al.: Visual perception and communication, in Birren J.E., Schaie K.W. (eds.): *Handbook of the Psychology of Aging*. New York, Van Nostrand Reinhold, 1977.

Friedenwald J.S.: The eye, in Lansing A.I. (ed.): *Cowdrys Problems of Aging*, ed. 3. Baltimore, Williams & Wilkins Co., 1952.

Garcia P.A., Battese G.E., Brewer W.D.: Longitudinal study of age and cohort influences on dietary patterns. *J. Gerontol.* 30:349–356, 1975.

Gilbert J.G.: Age changes in color matching. *J. Gerontol.* 12:210–215, 1957.

Grey G.W., Weise C.N.: *Basis of Speech*. New York, Harper & Row, 1959.

Hardy J.D., Wolff H.G., Goodell H.: The pain threshold in man. *Am. J. Psychiatry* 99:744–751, 1943.

Henkin R.I.: Abnormalities of taste and olfaction in various disease states, in Kare M.R., Maller O. (eds.): *The Chemical Senses and Nutrition*. Baltimore, Johns Hopkins Press, 1967.

Hofstetter H.W.: Some interrelationships of age, refraction, and rate of refractive changes. *Am. J. Optom. & Arch. Am. Acad. Optom.* 31:161–169, 1954.

Jerger J.: Audiological findings in aging. Paper presented at meeting of the International Oto-Physiology Symposium. Ann Arbor, Mich., 1971.

Kenshalo D.R.: Age changes in touch, vibration, temperature kinestasis and pain sensitivity, in Birren J.E., Schaie K.W. (eds.): *Handbook of the Psychology of Aging*. New York, Van Nostrand Reinhold, 1977.

Kimbrell G.McA., Furchgott E.: The effect of aging on olfactory threshold. *J. Gerontol.* 18:364–365, 1963.

Kryter K.: *The Effects of Noise on Man*. New York, Academic Press, 1970.

Langan M.J., Yearick E.S.: The effects of improved oral hygiene in taste perception and nutrition of the elderly. *J. Gerontol.* 31:413–418, 1976.

Lebo C.P., Reddell R.C.: The presbycusis component in occupational hearing loss. *Laryngoscope* 82:1399–1409, 1972.

Luchsinger R., Arnold G.E.: *Voice-Speech-Language*. Belmont, Cal., Wadsworth Publishing Co., 1965.

McFarland R.A., Fisher M.B.: Alterations in dark adaptation as a function of age. *J. Gerontol.* 10:424–428, 1955.

McFarland R.A., Domey R.C., Warren A.B., et al.: Dark adaptation as a function of age: I. A statistical analysis. *J. Gerontol.* 15:149–154, 1960.

Melzack R.: *The Puzzle of Pain*. New York, Basic Books, 1973.

Melzack R.: *The Puzzle of Pain*. New York, Basic Books, 1973.
Melzack R., Casey K.L.: Sensory, motivational and central control determinants of pain, in Kenshalo D.R. (ed.): *The Skin Senses*. Springfield, Ill., Charles C Thomas, Publisher, 1968.
Mesolella V.: L'olfatto nelle diverse eta. *Arch. Italiano di Otologia Rinologia e Laringologia* 46:43–62, 1934.
Mochizuki Y.: Papilla foliata of Japanese. *Okajimas Folia Anat. Jpn.* 18:337–369, 1939.
Moncrieff R.W.: *The Chemical Senses*. London, Leonard Hill Ltd., 1951.
Moskowitz H.R.: Cross-cultural differences in simple taste preferences. *Science* 190:1217–1218, 1975.
Rees J., Botwinick J.: Detection and decision factors in auditory behavior of the elderly. *J. Gerontol.* 26:133–136, 1971.
Richter C.P., Campbell K.H.: Sucrose threshold of rats and humans. *Am. J. Physiol.* 128:291–297, 1940.
Rosen S., Bergman M., Plester D., et al.: Presbycusis study of a relatively noise-free population in the Sudan. *Ann. Otol.* 71:727–743, 1962.
Rosen S., Plester D., El-Mofty E., et al.: High frequency audiometry in presbycusis: A comparative study of the Mabaan tribe in the Sudan with urban populations. *Arch. Otol.* 79:18–32, 1964.
Schiffman S.: Food recognition by the elderly. *J. Gerontol.* 32:586–592, 1977.
Schluderman E., Zubek J.P.: Effect of age on pain sensitivity. *Percept. Mot. Skills* 14:295–301, 1962.
Sherman E.D.: Sensitivity to pain. *Can. Med. Assoc. J.* 48:437–441, 1943.
Skre H.: Neurological signs in a normal population. *Acta Neurol. Scand.* 48:575–606, 1972.
Smith C.S.: Age incidence of atrophy of olfactory nerves in man. *J. Comp. Neurol.* 77:589–595, 1942.
Smith C.: The change in volume of the olfactory and accessory olfactory bulbs of the albino rats during post-natal life. *J. Comp. Neurol.* 61:477–508, 1935.
Springer K.J., Dietzmann H.E.: Correlation studies of diesel exhaust odor measured by instrumental methods to human odor panel ratings. Paper presented at the Odor Conference at the Karolinska Institute, Stockholm, Sweden, 1977. In Engen T.: *Taste and Smell,* and in Birren J.E., Schaie K.W. (eds.): *Handbook of the Psychology of Aging*. New York, Van Nostrand Reinhold, 1977.
U.S. Department of Health, Education, and Welfare, Health Services Administration, National Center for Health Statistics: *Health United States,* 1975.
U.S Department of Health, Education, and Welfare: *Human Communication and Its Disorders*. Bethesda, Md., 1969.
U.S. Department of Health, Education, and Welfare: Working with older people: A guide to practice. *The Knowledge Base,* vol. 1. Rockville, Md., n.d.
Wayner J.I., Emmers R.: Spinal synaptic delay in young and aged rats. *Am. J. Physiol.* 194:403–405, 1958.
Weale R.A.: On the eye, in Welford A.J., Birren J.E. (eds.): *Aging, Behavior, and the Nervous System*. Springfield, Ill., Charles C Thomas, Publisher, 1965.
Weiss A.D.: The locus of reaction time change with set motivation and age. *J. Gerontol.* 20:60–64, 1965.
Weiss A.D.: Sensory function, in Birren J.E. (ed.): *Handbook of Aging and the Individual*. Chicago, University of Chicago Press, 1959.
Wilder R.M.: Sensitivity to pain. *Proceedings of Staff Meetings at Mayo Clinic.* 15:551–554, 1940.

10

MENTAL HEALTH AND AGING

Bert Hayslip, Jr, Ph.D.

ALL OF US, regardless of age or background, have our own ideas about what constitutes "abnormal" behavior; most of us feel we can identify the person who is experiencing a "problem." Furthermore, we assume that universal "signs" of problem behavior, that is, isolation, hostility, difficulty with relationships, diet and/or sleep disturbances, apathy or listlessness, and excessive worry, can apply with equal validity to everyone.

In addition to such standards (which we all, to greater or lesser degrees, internalize regarding psychological distress), we have ideas about what constitutes "appropriate" or "acceptable" behavior with advancing age. Thus, while we might tolerate rebellious or even irresponsible acts from an adolescent, such behavior would, at the very least, be frowned on in an adult. Unfortunately, due to myths and stereotypes about aging, deviations from the norm are not reinforced when they are observed in an older person. We all feel that there are appropriate ways for older people to act, whether the issue is retirement, institutionalization, grandparenthood, a marked change in health, or widowhood.

To the extent that older people behave in accordance with our expectations (i.e., "act their age"), we think well of them. In the event that these behavioral ground rules are broken, the older person is perceived as experiencing a problem; he may be labeled senile, or simply written off just because he is old. The real tragedy lies in the fact that many elderly themselves accept such age-related expectations, reinforcing both their views about themselves and our ideas about them (i.e., older people are isolated, sick, useless, sexless, unable and/or unwilling to learn and change, or senile).

This chapter explores current thinking about mental health and abnormal behavior in elderly persons. Our judgments about problem behaviors in the aged not only affect our personal relationships with older persons, but also influence the way we interact with them as professionals and how we ultimately shape our personal views about our own aging.

Defining Mental Health and Abnormal Behavior

As Ullmann and Krasner (1975) have noted, labeling an act abnormal has several consequences, the most important of which, from our perspective, implies that this act then becomes the concern of a psychologist, psychiatrist, or some other mental health professional. To label a given behavior as abnormal implies a kind of social control; an act is thus perceived as deviant (i.e., unlawful, inappropriate, disruptive, harmful, not understandable/predictable by usual standards). As the term "abnormal" suggests, such behavior is literally apart from the norm. Thus, society's expectations about how old people should behave, that is, what is expected at a given place or time for a given individual, set the standard. A *culturally relative* approach to abnormality then sets limits on what "good" behavior is in terms of what society in general and/or those in a given situation will tolerate.

Coleman (1976) alternatively rejects this approach in favor of one suggesting that abnormal or problematic behavior is *maladaptive;* it does not promote the well-being of the individual, and ultimately that of the group. Thus, any behavior (regardless of society's sanctions) that is counterproductive to the individual's growth and functioning, producing personal distress or group conflict, falls within this sphere.

These two perspectives represent the dominant approaches to defining abnormal behavior today. They both involve value judgments which, of course, are arbitrary, such as valuing human growth and survival and valuing socially acceptable behavior.

In addition to these approaches, a number of other more specific definitions of normal and abnormal have been proposed (Coleman, 1976; Ullmann and Krasner, 1975): (1) attempting to derive a formal definition of mental health (i.e., being able to adjust to and get along with others with a maximum of effectiveness and happiness); (2) having traits (i.e., realism, self-acceptance, competence) seen as crucial to normal behavior; (3) establishing specific criteria (personal distress, anxiety, guilt, conformity to norms) for abnormal behavior; and (4) proceeding from particular models of behavior (psychoanalytic, behavioral) to define abnormal behavior. Other definitions of abnormality frequently involve seeing someone for professional psychiatric treatment, or as specifically defined by psychiatric diagnosis, having a definable set of symptoms that lead to a label such as psychosis or mental illness. In this case it is assumed that some underlying disease state or causal agent (the medical model) is producing a set of symptoms in the patient that can be identified (a syndrome) and labeled and for which a specific treatment exists. Other yardsticks involve subjective definitions;

definitions by objective psychological tests; definitions of mental illness as the absence of mental health; statistical criteria, i.e., the person who is normal is like most other people (*and* normal to the same degree); and legal criteria, i.e., competence, commitment to an institution, and criminal responsibility for an act.

How have the criteria mentioned been used to define normal versus abnormal and maladaptive behavior in the aged?

Birren and Renner (1980) note that the concept of normality is difficult to apply since what is regarded as acceptable or deviant changes with time. Such a measure of normality encompasses (1) the statistical concept of the mean or average, (2) *perceived* statistical frequency related to value judgments, (3) socially acceptable behavior, and (4) biologically typical behaviors as a function of age. Concepts such as "maladjustment" (or, alternatively, good adjustment) are unacceptable in a universal sense because they are situational or age-specific in nature. From their perspective, Birren and Renner see mental health as made up of several components, organized hierarchically from somatic (physical), to affective/cognitive, to a philosophical/spiritual level. It is apparent that no one single definition or criterion will suffice. Furthermore, there is value in the argument that because abnormal and normal behavior can be learned and unlearned via the same principles (i.e., reinforcement, punishment), and because the same behavior may be, at different times and in different situations for different persons, *both* adaptive and maladaptive, the terms "abnormal" and "normal" or "mental illness" versus "mental health" are not clearly distinguishable; there are no sharp dichotomies. Thus, it may be appropriate to say that everyone displays aberrant behavior at one time or another.

Jahoda (1958) suggests six criteria for positive mental health: (1) positive self attitudes, (2) growth and self-actualization, (3) integration of the personality, (4) autonomy, (5) reality perception, and (6) mastery of environment. These are intended to represent maximum functioning. Birren and Renner (1979) note that these criteria lack precision and represent an agenda for defining mental health rather than a definition per se. In other words, the criteria perhaps define goals, but they tell us little about how to achieve positive mental health—especially for the elderly.

Birren and Renner (1979) further point out that applying these criteria to elderly persons presents some problems. For example, environmental mastery may be impossible, if not harmful, for those elderly who are in poor health, living on fixed incomes, isolated, or institutionalized. Positive mental health in such cases might be facilitated if the environmental demands were lessened. Similarly, autonomy and self-actualization may take on different forms for the older adult. Retirement, poor health, or widowhood may force the individual to give up previous activities; he may have to satisfy his needs for autonomy within a more restricted set of alternatives. Self-actualization may be redefined to focus on living in the present and reflected in how one's life was lived, rather than setting goals and making plans that are future-oriented. "In the one case there is the matter of preparing well for the race and in the other an evaluation of how well the race was won" (Birren and Renner, 1979). Thus, what constitutes positive mental health for the elderly person may not be identical to that for the adolescent. That mental health has typically been defined in terms of absence of mental illness suggests that we are just beginning to seriously describe this construct and to define various paths for attaining it across the life span.

Evidence of such a shift in perspective is the publication of the *Handbook of Mental Health and Aging* (Birren and Sloane, 1980) versus the pathology-oriented approach by Pfeiffer in "Psychopathology and Social Pathology" in the *Handbook of the Psychology of Aging* (Birren and Schaie, 1977).

From a pathology-oriented perspective, problems are also encountered when one attempts to apply conventional criteria to the aged. Using a single criterion of psychopathologic behavior with symptoms such as personal distress, discomfort to others, incompetence, or change from a previous state, misleading conclusions are frequently reached. "Personal distress could be a perfectly reasonable transient response to bereavement. Discomfort caused to others could be a reflection of the latter's hypersensitivity. Incompetence might result from the abnormal demands of a task. Change from a previous state might be for the better rather than for the worse" (Gurland, 1973). Also, Gurland goes on to discuss the inappropriateness of prevalence, etiology, maladaptation, or treatment as criteria for abnormal behavior in the aged. Using a prevalence approach, behaviors that are common to the elderly, such as depression, anxiety, paranoia, and hypochondriacal concerns, would ironically be considered "normal." Thus, the acceptance of such behaviors leads to paradoxical conclusions regarding abnormal behavior among the aged.

Etiologically, behaviors that are intrinsically caused are more likely to be called abnormal than those that are extrinsic in nature. Thus, behaviors presumably associated with brain cell changes are perceived as pathologic. Gurland (1973) notes that one's particular biases can lead to opposite conclusions, that is, the isolated elderly person could be seen as rejected by his community, withdrawn because of depression or paranoia, or disengaged in an adaptive sense. Particularly important is maladaptation as a criterion for pathology mentioned earlier. Behavior may be maladaptive for one purpose and quite adaptive for another; for example, obsessive-compulsive behaviors might help to structure one's time in an enforced retirement situation and schizoid detachment may help to protect one from the physical and psychosocial losses of later life. Depression may be adaptive in situations where prolonged isolation is the rule. Most interesting in this regard are the findings of Leiberman (1975), who found that traits such as neuroticism and hostility enhanced adaptation to forced relocation to a nursing home; such traits would be seen by many persons as highly undesirable in most interpersonal relationships. Finally, treatment may be a difficult standard to apply when it does not exist; for instance, lack of an appropriate treatment for depression would lead to somatic complaints, sleep disturbances, or constipation being viewed as "natural for old age." Many such complaints were seen as associated with depression after the development of antidepressant drugs.

Characteristics commonly associated with aging, such as cognitive impairment, depression, isolation, institutionalization, and diminished energy, may or may not be pathologic; and, as Gurland notes (1973), illustrate the difficulty in separating normal aging changes from those that are truly abnormal. Again, each of these "signs," despite their commonality, is difficult to apply in deciding who is abnormal. Cognitive impairment may not be universal (i.e., primary vs. secondary memory loss, encoding vs. retrieval deficit); self-reports frequently do not correspond with objective findings. Clinicians may not see patients with minimal levels of impairment (or patients whose losses are gradual), and thus are not as skilled in making discriminations at this end of the continuum.

In many cases depression is a difficult criterion since it is a common, predictable response to loss (of friends, family, job, skills) that normally accompanies old age; transient depression, moreover, is frequent among elderly persons. Isolation may result from role loss, a change in health, or loss of a spouse—all understandable outcomes of events over which there is little control. Isolation brought on by defensive, paranoid-like behavior that is delusionary is another matter, however. Institutionalization likewise fails as a criterion since it may be an inevitable consequence of the family's inability to care for a frail older member; many elderly are institutionalized when in fact they can function quite well on their own. Diminished energy may result from poor health and/or the side effects of drugs that may be prescribed for the older person. Lack of energy, in itself, does not suggest the older person is experiencing a psychological problem.

Since mental health professionals rarely see older persons (see Birren and Renner, 1980; Gatz, Smyer, and Lawton, 1980), labeling behaviors that may be distressful to them as abnormal relieves them of the responsibility to treat older adults as *persons;* they may instead view elderly disturbed persons as disturbed *because* they are old. Thus, much of the current thinking about mental health and mental illness serves to maintain the status quo, reinforcing the separateness of young and old and contributing to the neglect of genuine mental health problems that older adults may have. Too often, psychopathology is assessed (Schaie and Schaie, 1977), instead of the more positive, adaptive characteristics of behavior in the aged (Gurland, 1973). Thus, the terms "abnormal" or "psychopathology" are often administrative in nature. There are many (Coleman, 1976; Gurland, 1973) who feel such terms should be abandoned because of the negative "set" they create in the distinction between normal and abnormal, and because of the generally pessimistic orientation toward older adults created when such terms are used. One is left to deal with "mental health" as something left over after the "mental illness" is cleared up or treated.

It is not surprising that we have so much difficulty in defining mental health. One rarely goes to a counselor or a psychologist when he is untroubled! In addition, a pathology-oriented philosophy, frequently based on information about children, predisposes us to assume that *all* behavior that is distressing or unusual in the elderly *is* abnormal because of its biologic basis (i.e., brain cell changes producing dementia). It is quite logical to assume, then, that older persons cannot be treated therapeutically because the biologic processes underlying their behavior are irreversible. This "myth of untreatability" contributes to a general neglect of the problems older adults face (whether they be psychogenic or somatic in nature), resulting in a lack of mental health services (or poorly designed services) for older persons. Paradoxically, the consequent underutilization of available services (Birren and Renner, 1979, 1980; Gatz et al., 1980; Redick and Taube, 1980) for various reasons—cost, distrust, pride, inaccessibility, lack of knowledge, poorly trained staff (Kramer, Taube and Redick, 1973)—reinforces professional ignorance of and bias toward treating older persons. At the same time, it convinces staff that there are few needs or demands for such mental health services from the elderly! Retaining a pathology-oriented stance (including use of a classification system—DSM III) provides us with a "common language" for communicating with other mental health professionals, but it nevertheless works against the best interests of many older adults by deemphasizing mental health to the exclusion of mental illness and psychopathology.

Birren and Renner (1980) discuss the difficulty in both conceptualizing and assessing mental health in the elderly. Mental health, like aging, is a highly complex phenomenon, and in order to be accurately understood and measured it must be viewed from a variety of perspectives, each with many components. Birren and Renner (1980) suggest that in order to determine whether one is aging successfully or has positive mental health,

> one must have a grasp of the individual's goals in order to sense what it is he is trying to maximize internally and in relation to the environment. A low adjustment

or productivity may, in fact, be a high level maximization of potentials if one understands the individual's origins and available resources.

Such a view is all the more important in view of the tremendous heterogeneity found among older persons, relative to the young (Botwinick, 1978; Maddox and Douglas, 1974). A variety of factors bear on attaining mental health in later years, such as the importance of *maximizing* individual potential in relation to one's abilities, resources, and reference group demands (Birren and Renner, 1980). Implicit here are ideas of:

1. Competence (the ability to deal with environmental/interpersonal demands in a life-satisfying manner).
2. Awareness of one's needs (social, psychological, physical, spiritual).
3. The extent to which one is able to take advantage of new environmental opportunities and support.
4. Opportunity for, and personal desirability of, control over one's environment.
5. Willingness to abandon or change previous goals (or ways of meeting those goals).
6. External rewards or costs of a particular pattern of behavior (i.e., isolation from others, somatic distress, evoking feelings of belongingness and self-esteem in others).
7. Impact of events beyond one's control that affect oneself and others (e.g., widowhood, retirement, loss of independence, health).
8. Willingness to acknowledge older persons' feelings about death and dying.
9. The extent of family support and nature of family ties (Sussman, 1976).
10. Individual differences in the ability of both the elderly and their families to make decisions that imply change.
11. Discrepancy between intrapsychic versus socioadaptational levels of personality functioning and their relationship to life satisfaction in old age (Neugarten, 1977).

Birren and Renner (1980) consequently advocate an interactional approach to mental health in the later years, emphasizing the continuing dialectical (Riegel, 1976) nature of the relationship between what the older person thinks of (and expects from) himself, characteristics of the environment (and how these are perceived), and biologic status. The extent to which some older persons see old age in terms of freedom from interpersonal and sociocultural obligations while others see it as a "normless" period of life will determine which aspects of old age are internalized. Research by Brubaker and Powers (1976) suggests that prior self-concept mediates whether the positive or negative aspects of aging will be adopted. Not only are there wide individual differences in life satisfaction and morale among the elderly, but research by Harris and Associates (1975) suggest many important differences in how old age is viewed by the elderly versus the nonelderly general public. In most cases, elderly persons had more positive feelings about their lives and about being old than were attributed to them by younger persons. It is only when poor health, social isolation, low income, and inadequate housing are experienced simultaneously that older persons report low morale (Birren and Renner, 1980).

> Findings indicate that most individuals are able to adjust to changes in roles and expectations with age and to accommodate comfortably to the interactions between their needs and the opportunities of their environment. Indeed, for many older persons, growing older is accompanied by an increasing sense of personal mastery and social recognition from family and other reference groups. . . . While an optimistic point of view about the mental health of the older population in general is justified, there is every reason to be deeply concerned about the large numbers of older persons who are living lives in distress, for there are relatively more of them than in younger groups (Birren and Renner, 1980).

Thus, while we cannot be complacent about the unique problems some older persons experience, the forces that join to enable some to enjoy mental health and others to suffer from distress are complex and often have little to do with the aging process itself. Increased self-confidence, self-reliance, healthy attitudes about one's strengths and weaknesses, learning and maintaining effective coping skills, and an active stance toward the environment are prerequisites for good mental health in the elderly. Obviously, such assets benefit the young as well. Unrealistic expectations of self, narrowness of experience, emotional fragility, resistance to criticism, and a restrictive environment encourage development of unhealthy styles of coping in *both* the young and the old. As Birren and Renner (1980) note, the terms "mental health" and "self-actualization" might better be thought of as *competence* in view of the factors facilitating continued human growth and development *throughout* the life span.

While there are universal components of mental health at any age, several special considerations must be given when viewing this construct in the aged. Birren and Renner (1980) suggest five principles to promote a continued sense of growth in old age: (1) *life review* (Butler, 1963), including an evaluation of one's life, resolution of past conflicts, acceptance of life's successes and failures as one's own, and an integration of such (via introspection) to produce what Erikson (1959) has termed integrity, defined as a sense of completeness about the life cycle; (2) *reconciliation* of one's real life with the ideal; (3) *relevance* of a set of values; (4) *reverence* (self-esteem); and (5) *release* of stress, resulting from reconciliation. Birren and Renner (1980) suggest that the mentally healthy person of *any age* needs the ability to "respond to other individuals, to love, to be loved, and to cope with others in give-and-take relationships." Obviously, this requires a good sense of who one is and the courage to break off relationships that are destructive. As Birren and Renner note, "Such concepts may seem idealistic goals but they are not trivial, for unless we incorporate them into a philosophy not only for ourselves, but for those who have seen 65 years or more, is *real* progress in mental health possible?"

We need to (*a*) change our current decrement-oriented/pathologic attitudes about aging and the aged; (*b*) make mental health services as affordable, accessible, and acceptable for the aged as they are for the young; (*c*) supply enough adequately trained personnel to deal with disturbed elderly; and most important, (*d*) recognize that the factors contributing to positive mental health are complex, and while some universals exist, special requirements must be met to attain it in old age. Otherwise, the goals Birren and Renner have set for us will remain unfulfilled.

Mental Disorders in the Aged

We now turn from our discussion of mental health to a consideration of the major types of mental disorders occurring among the elderly. It must first be noted that several limitations exist that place qualifications on what we know about the dynamics and incidence of mental disorders in the aged.

Currently, major diagnostic categories are based on a revision of the system developed by the American Psychiatric Association, *Diagnostic and Statistical Manual of Mental Disorders,* ed. 3, 1980 *(DSM-III)*. Despite intended improvements (Gallagher, Thompson, and Levy, 1980) over previous versions of such a classificatory scheme, such changes remain to be assessed. Previous editions of *DSM* are known among clinicians (Davison and Neale, 1978) to be notoriously unreliable, based on symptomatology assumed to be characteristic of a given disorder. Since clinicians' contacts and experience with elderly clients is likely to be limited, problems in reliability may nevertheless occur with the new revision. *Any* typology (such as *DSM-III*) should be used with caution; it is simply a descriptive tool to aid the clinician in arriving at a diagnosis. Where inconsistencies arise, the clinician's own experience along with psychometric data should be used to improve validity. Moreover, such classificatory systems tell us little if anything about etiology. Thus, the data on mental disorders in the aged (previously based on *DSM-II*) should be seen as purely *descriptive* and should not be interpreted rigidly. This would avoid unnecessary and harmful "pigeonholing" or "labeling" of older persons, based on a set of symptoms (e.g., depression) that are often reported or interpreted differently by the aged relative to younger persons (Raskin and Jarvik, 1979). Generally, in order to reach a reliable "diagnosis," clients must be seen several times rather than just once.

Other major limitations to consider are: (1) techniques for gathering data on mental disorders may be flawed; and (2) the sample of persons from whom such information is gathered is likely to be misleading about the true incidence or dynamics of mental disorders in later life. Whether based on available case registers, general practices, field surveys, clinical interviews, or questionnaires, data collected are subject to error. Kay and Bergman (1980) and Gurland (1979) have discussed problems in case identification (reliability of psychiatric diagnosis, development of standardized interviews) that must be recognized in interpreting epidemiologic data on mental disorders. Given current elderly attitudes toward counseling (i.e., relating to distrust, inaccessibility, ignorance of services, pride, cost) and the negative attitudes clinicians hold toward treating the elderly (Butler and Lewis, 1977; Gatz et al., 1980; Kastenbaum, 1978), most available information about mental illness and aging must be seen as representing available case loads. These case loads are composed of elderly people who can afford treatment, are likely to be in better health, are more highly educated, and who often hold more positive attitudes toward treatment than their counterparts who do not show up at community mental health centers, private clinics, or hospitals, or who are treated within a nursing home setting.

The point is not that all data should be disregarded for these reasons, but that available data be interpreted with the above limitations in mind; rigid, hard and fast conclusions are premature, given the current state of research.

Psychopathology in the Elderly

Pfeiffer (1977) differentiates *intrapersonal* and *interpersonal* pathology in the aged. In either case, dysfunctional behavior results from the failure to adapt, in that issues related to loss, identity (life) review, and maintenance of activity to retain function are not dealt with satisfactorily (i.e., the individual's needs are not met, or are met at great expense to himself or others). Estimates of incidence of even mild psychological dysfunction are plagued by numerous problems (mentioned previously); however, Pfeiffer suggests that as many as 15% of all elderly suffer from some form of psychopathology. While frequency estimates vary by service locale (e.g., VA hospital vs. community mental health centers) and by type of disorder (e.g., organic brain syndrome vs. depression), others (Kay and Bergman, 1980;

Storandt, Siegler, and Elias, 1978) provide similar figures, whether data are based on actual cases receiving mental health services or are estimates made on the basis of previous epidemiologic studies.

Pfeiffer differentiates *functional* disorders (failures in adaptation occurring despite intact brain function) and *organic* disorders (failures in adaptation occurring because of impaired brain function). This distinction is important because it emphasizes the fact that each type of disorder demands both special diagnostic and assessment techniques and differing types of intervention. Both functional and organic disorders are considered intrapersonal, as contrasted with interpersonal disorders such as isolation, loneliness, family conflicts, or sexual disorders.

Organic brain syndromes (OBS) account for approximately half of all mental impairments among persons 65 years of age and older. Among persons who are institutionalized, its incidence increases; this is also true for those in each of the categories after age 65 (i.e., 65 to 75, 76 to 85). Their distinguishing characteristic is brain cell loss or dysfunction. Such losses are correlated with structural changes in the brain itself, such as decrease in brain weight, the presence of senile plaques (cholesterol-like deposits on brain cells), and the presence of neurofibrillary tangles (twisted nerve fibers). On examination, the brain has a characteristic appearance—it appears shrunken, a softening of tissue is present, gyri (convolutions) are smaller, and sulci (fissures) are wider.

Typically, terms such as "senile" or "dementia" are used when referring to elderly persons with OBS. Because such terms are frequently imprecise, misleading, and harmful, a careful description of symptoms is important to distinguish between forms of OBS that are reversible and those that are not.

Senility, despite its popularity among lay persons and the medical profession, tells us virtually nothing about the older person's actual condition or prognosis. Confusion, hostility, memory loss, and disorientation are often "explained" by "Well, what can you expect, you are old." Unfortunately, "old" frequently translates into "senile," which in turn often results in no effort at treatment. Senility is too often used as a "wastebasket" term when no identifiable cause can be found for the person's behavior. Its use is to describe age at onset; senility refers to the appearance of a disorder after the age of 65. Realistically, it has no redeeming scientific value as a diagnostic term; it frequently encourages a "give up" approach, making matters much worse for staff, family members, and elderly "victims" themselves. Treatment for those who are "senile" often consists of custodial care—in effect, no active treatment.

Another term frequently used to describe OBS is "dementia." In a general sense this is accurate in that we are describing a cluster of symptoms said to define cognitive loss (memory loss, disorientation, inability to learn new material or perform calculations, poor judgment). It can also be used to refer to an individual's level of functioning compared to someone with a similar educational background and social history. In some cases, it may refer to a person's status relative to what he had evidenced earlier (presumably when he was healthier and more capable). Another use of the term "dementia" is in reference to a specific group of diseases (Miller, 1977) with a variety of causes: Alzheimer's disease, Pick's disease, neurosyphilis, Huntington's chorea, Jakob-Creutzfeldt disease, normal pressure hydrocephalus, senile dementia, and arteriosclerotic dementia. The first six are referred to as presenile dementias, whereas senile dementia and arteriosclerotic dementia are senile dementias. In practice, among presenile dementias, all but Pick's disease and Alzheimer's disease are relatively rare (Eisdorfer and Cohen, 1978; Pfeiffer, 1977; Sloane, 1980). Senile dementia is generally considered to be more common than the cardiovascular variety among the senile dementias. There is disagreement on whether these and other forms of OBS can be reliably differentiated (Eisdorfer and Cohen, 1978; Pfeiffer, 1977; Raskin and Jarvik, 1979; Sloane, 1980); these types of dementia are often discernible after death and thus are confirmed only by histologic investigation. In no case does a diagnostic label show causal (etiologic) factors responsible for a given set of symptoms.

Pfeiffer (1977) notes that clinical manifestations of OBS vary little in the specific cause of brain cell death or impairment. They do vary greatly, however, in the extent of brain impairment, rapidity of onset, personality resources of the individual, and the quality of the surrounding environment. While symptoms such as anxiety, depression, hallucinations, delusions, hostility, withdrawal, and emotional lability *may* be associated with OBS, they do not guarantee its presence or absence. Several issues, according to Pfeiffer, are critical in accurate diagnosis and treatment of OBS:

1. Reversibility versus irreversibility of function.
2. Severity of organic impairment.
3. Acute onset versus chronic presence of organic impairment.
4. Diffuse versus localized extent of damage.
5. Progressive versus stable organic impairment.
6. Whether associated psychopathology is present.

As noted, there is a constellation of symptoms common to persons with forms of OBS: disorientation; impaired judgment; loss of memory (particularly for recent events); disturbed visual-motor coordination; confusion; and loss of ability to abstract, learn new material, or carry out tasks sequentially.

When onset is gradual and damage is localized, only highly intellectual functions are impaired. OBS is frequently preceded by a variety of emotional and behavioral changes, such as depression, apathy, withdrawal, and irritability. As the deficit becomes more long-standing, there are increases in disorientation as to time and place; forgetting of names, dates, telephone numbers; and memory loss. Eventually, memory for overlearned, highly meaningful, personal material deteriorates; behavior may become more impulsive and erratic; speech becomes garbled; motor control is lost; and the person may no longer realize where he is or be able to feed, dress, and otherwise care for himself. At this point, the person may not know his own name; this indicates the most severe organic loss and suggests the person is completely dependent on others for his care. Depending on rapidity of onset, the person may lapse into a coma or may develop infections and lose bowel control. At present, no known effective treatment exists for forms of OBS that are irreversible; the person eventually dies from the cumulative effects of physical ailments brought on by organic deterioration.

As pointed out, it is particularly important to distinguish between forms of OBS that are essentially irreversible (chronic) and those whose effects are reversible (acute), to avoid so-called false positives and false negatives. False positives refer to the tendency to diagnose elderly persons as organic, overlooking many symptoms that could otherwise be treated. Poor health, isolation, or depression often lead clinicians to give up on the elderly patient; he is diagnosed as organic (senile). False negatives imply that the person is not diagnosed as organic, and thus someone who may be suffering from an acute, reversible condition is denied treatment on the basis of his observable behavior. Acute disorders, if left untreated, frequently deteriorate into a condition that *is* irreversible. Irreversibility does not, however, imply untreatability. Patients with an accurate diagnosis of chronic OBS can be made more comfortable, depression and anxiety can be lessened, and family can be taught to care for the elderly person to ameliorate feelings of isolation and helplessness.

The major forms of irreversible dementia (where the severity of impairment can range from mild to severe, presence is chronic and diffuse in distribution throughout the brain) are senile dementia, arteriosclerotic dementia, Alzheimer's disease, Pick's disease, and Jakob-Creutzfeldt disease. Their principal clinical features have already been described. Severity of such manifestations relate to (1) amount of brain cell loss (the greater the loss, the more severe), (2) rapidity of loss (the more rapid, the more severe), (3) personality and intellectual resources (those with the most resources adapt to disease-related changes more effectively), and (4) the supportiveness of the environment (the more supportive, the fewer demands made on the individual). In general, rapid loss, poorly integrated personality resources (see previous discussion of mental health), poor social skills, and little education are factors that favor the development of associated psychopathology (depression, hostility, anxiety, withdrawal) in persons with irreversible dementia (OBS). Such symptoms are likely to be more prevalent in the early stages of the disorder. Alzheimer's disease and Pick's disease are early-onset variants of senile dementia, with Alzheimer's disease being rapidly progressive; in practice, they are virtually indistinguishable (Pfeiffer, 1977; Sloane, 1980). Pick's disease, however, is inherited, brain lesions are more localized, and personality changes are initially more severe (Eisdorfer and Cohen, 1978). Jakob-Creutzfeldt disease is also rapidly progressive, but it is viral in nature and may be transmitted under unusual circumstances. It is rare, however, as is Pick's disease.

Arteriosclerotic dementia involves a series of strokes, large and small. The extent of damage is localized and the course of the disorder is more variable, frequently leaving the personality undisturbed but with a great deal of emotional lability. Its onset is rapid, with considerable intellectual impairment that improves later. Memory loss is "patchy." Arteriosclerotic dementia is sometimes accompanied by epileptic seizures (in about 20% of all cases). As the effects of such strokes become cumulative, the disorder may resemble senile dementia. At this point, it can be identified by an analysis of cerebral blood flow. The restricted blood flow associated with arteriosclerosis (progressive hardening of cerebral blood vessel walls) and atherosclerosis (the narrowing and eventual closing of the vessel) cause impairment in this case. The disorder is frequently misdiagnosed as paranoia, due to accompanying delirium and hallucinations, and can be fatal. Despite its comparison with "hardening of the arteries," there is some debate (Marsden, 1978) about the causal nature of reduced cerebral blood flow in arteriosclerotic dementia, which accounts for approximately 10% to 20% of all dementias.

Huntington's chorea, normal pressure hydrocephalus, and neurosyphilis all produce dementia-like symptoms. Huntington's chorea is genetic in nature, but very rare (see Sloane, 1980, for a discussion). Neurosyphilis and normal pressure hydrocephalus are treatable (Sloane, 1980).

Acute (reversible) dementias present a diagnostic problem in that they frequently mimic symptoms of irreversible organicity, and if left untreated they may become chronic. Pfeiffer (1977) estimates that 10% to 20% of elderly persons with OBS have conditions that are in fact reversible. They may coexist (as may functional disorders) with irreversible organic brain syndromes in the same individual. Specific factors causing reversible OBS are many, for example, diabetes, hypoglycemia, hepatic or renal toxicity, vitamin deficiencies (especially B_{12}), viral infections (meningitis), hypertension, drug intoxication (e.g., sedatives, bromides, antidepressants, antipsychotics), malnutrition, metabolic imbalances resulting from inadequate fluid intake, congestive heart failure, intracranial tumors (normal pressure hydrocephalus), neurosyphilis (see above), acute alcohol intoxication, and pulmonary disease (emphysema). The key to differentiating acute and chronic OBS is a complete evaluation of the patient, that is, physical examination, clinical laboratory tests (to detect metabolic imbalances), radiologic studies (CAT scan), radioisotope analyses (brain scan, analysis of cerebral blood flow), a careful health history that includes an interview with the physician and family, and complete documentation of the drug regimen prescribed for the individual (Habot and Libow, 1980). Since anxiety, hallucinations, and delusions often accompany acute OBS, psychological testing is certainly appropriate. In addition, a complete cognitive evaluation should be performed, to include the assessment of memory impairment, orientation, language function, dyspraxic skills (ability to follow directions), use of numbers, and visual-spatial-constructional abilities. Preferably, such assessments should be repeated over a span of time, and will require the skills of many professionals (i.e., psychologists, internists, physicians, psychiatrists). A detailed examination of assessment procedures useful for differentiating acute and chronic OBS can be found in Eisdorfer and Cohen (1978), Sloane (1980), Pfeiffer (1977), Schaie and Schaie (1977), Miller (1980), Simon (1980), and Kahn and Miller (1978). Consistent with the above perspective on mental health and abnormal behavior, assessment of OBS is a multidisciplinary, complex task, beyond the skills of a single professional.

In addition to the separation of acute and chronic OBS, diagnostic confusion exists with respect to the differentiation of functional and organic dysfunction in the aged. The most common functional disorders (based on available data) in the aged are depression, paranoia, manic reactions, hypochondriasis, and schizophrenia. Also included in the nonorganic disorders are suicide, alcoholism, drug misuse, criminal behavior, adjustment reactions, transient anxiety states, and sleep disturbances. Pfeiffer (1977) views social isolation, loneliness, family conflicts, and sexual problems as "social pathologies." While this list is very diverse, all of the disorders cited share a common characteristic in that they can occur in the absence of impaired brain function.

Depression is perhaps the most widespread (Gurland, 1976) of the functional psychopathologies in the aged (see, however, Jarvik, 1976; Klerman, 1976). It varies in degree and severity, ranging from normal transient reactions to loss to paralyzing, prolonged depressions that are highly dysfunctional. While a great deal of literature exists regarding depression and aging (Raskin, 1979; Salzman and Shader, 1979; Stenback, 1980), most of it is based on clinical impression, rather than on empirical data, which makes it difficult to identify symptoms unique to depressed elderly, those characteristic of depression in general, and those unique to depressed versus nondepressed aged. Estimates vary by residence and sex, and depend on (*a*) whether psychiatric diagnosis or symptom pattern is used and (*b*) whether transient or chronic depressions are examined.

Apathy, withdrawal, loss of self-esteem, feelings of hopelessness and helplessness, suicidal thoughts, and a core of somatic complaints characterize depression in the aged. Typically, depression is a response to both psychosocial and physical losses, or to life changes over which the elderly person has little or no control (Seligman, 1975). Since elderly persons typically prefer to report somatic symptoms rather than psychogenic ones, particular concern must be paid to somatic complaints symptomatic of depression versus physical ailments that are genuinely illness-related and/or drug-induced. Thus, physical causes must first be eliminated before symptoms such as loss of appetite, fatigue, difficulty in sleeping, constipation, or weight loss are characterized as depressive in nature. Depression is sometimes accompanied by considerable tension, guilt, anxiety, paranoia, and agitation. Depression in the aged must be distinguished from depression preceding illness, "depressive equivalents," and "pseudodementia." "Depressive equivalents" refer to the individual's unconscious use of bodily symptoms to mimic depression. In this sense, depression results from anger turned inward that is displaced into physical complaints, and is thus related to hypochondriasis. It lacks the depressive mood characteristic of true functional depression; the person may explicitly deny feeling depressed, but chooses to present himself as such because it relieves him of the responsibility for his own hostile feelings. Depressive equivalents are in effect a call for help, but are difficult to treat in that symptoms serve a psychic function.

Pseudodementia is a condition with symptomatology that may mimic OBS. The person may appear confused, disoriented, exhibit memory loss, and so on. There is, however, no clear indication of organic impairment. In persons with depressive pseudodementia, affective (emotional) symptoms predominate relative to cognitive ones. Onset is acute, and memory loss in this case can be alleviated by cognitive training or antidepressant drugs.

Depression may also be superimposed on an existing organic condition, may be a function of drug toxicity (Salzman and Shader, 1979), or may exist as a response to cognitive losses in the early stages of true dementia (see Salzman and Shader, 1979; Stenback, 1980, for discussions of depression). Manic reactions are essentially mirror images of depression and may be treated with lithium carbonate (Pfeiffer, 1977).

Paranoid reactions in the aged are less serious than those in the young, and are most common (next to depression) in the aged. Paranoid ideation in the elderly is more down to earth, and is often an attempt to structure the environment in the face of change and/or sensory losses. Forgetfulness, hearing loss, isolation, or losses in taste discrimination often give rise to accusations of stealing, poisoning, rejection, and so on. For example, decreased sensitivity to foods might lead one to "accuse" his provider (family, staff member, live-in home aide) of poisoning him (particularly if some conflict was present). Correction of sensory deficits, administration of mild tranquilizers, and provision of support (e.g., memory aids) frequently lessen such accusations (see Pfeiffer, 1977; Post, 1980, for discussions).

Hypochondriasis is the next most common functional disorder in the aged. It suggests an intense preoccupation with one's bodily functions in the absence of physical pathology. Such persons are particularly resistant to psychological explanations for their "complaints," and must be evaluated at both the physical and psychological levels. They hold on to their symptoms and have made an unconscious choice to present themselves as physically ill despite the psychogenic (displaced aggression and hostility, guilt over unacceptable thoughts and actions) origin of their behavior (Gentry, 1978; Pfeiffer, 1977).

In a related vein, psychosomatic disorders (hyperventilation, ulcers, colon and urinary disturbances, constipation) can exist as part of a response to the loss of a significant other (spouse) in the aged. Physical health status is particularly important in determining such reactions, as is the quality of support in the environment.

Schizophrenia in the elderly is comparatively rare. It is characterized by a close-knit delusional system, late onset of hallucinations, and symptoms such as irritability, agitation, assaultiveness, memory loss, and disorientation of a progressively deteriorative nature (Raskin, 1979). It may accompany senile dementia or arteriosclerotic dementia. In many cases, however, elderly schizophrenics are most likely to be those residing in state hospitals or nursing homes who were diagnosed as such much earlier in life and have simply grown old in the institution. Often, their symptoms are the result of the isolation and depersonalization that accompanies years of custodial care.

Anxiety states in the aged may coexist with depression or OBS. They are typically transient in nature and often constitute a predominant reaction to physical loss, fear of dying alone or in pain (Peterson, 1980), impending surgery, or institutionalization. They are characterized by sleeplessness, obsessive eating, or loss of appetite. Older persons are prone to deny feeling anxious (Raskin, 1979). Such symptomatology is associated with what Pfeiffer (1977) terms "adjustment reactions," characterized by fear and panic, helplessness, tearfulness, tension, rapid heartbeat, sleeplessness, and shortness of breath. Support, ventilation of feelings, and mild tranquilizers (temporarily) constitute treatment for transient anxiety states in the aged.

Suicide is becoming a serious problem in the aged. While attempted suicide is usually a cry for help in the young, older persons (particularly white men) are serious when they attempt to take their own lives. They are less likely to use available suicide prevention services, so serious attention to *any* life-threatening cues is imperative with the potential elderly suicide, who is often depressed and socially isolated. Older persons almost always intend to die when they attempt suicide. Suicide may also take the form of indirect self-destructive behavior within institutions for many elderly (Hayslip, 1981; Miller, 1979; Stenback, 1980). While a variety of factors (e.g., impending retirement or institutionalization, illness, loss of spouse, loneliness) seem to precipitate suicide in the aged, the causal links are difficult to establish (Miller, 1979).

Alcoholism and drug abuse among the aged are becoming more widespread (Simon, 1980; Wood, 1978). Extensive research, however, is lacking; questions regarding motivation, chronicity, and the long-term consequences of such behavior remain to be investigated. In view of the many physical-psychosocial-economic stresses with which older persons have to cope, attention to such topics (as well as research) is likely to increase.

Pfeiffer (1977) refers to sexual difficulties, isolation, loneliness, and family conflicts as "social pathologies," because they are conditions frequently imposed on elderly persons as a function of forced retirement, institutionalization, death of friends and spouse, physical health problems, and discrimination in both the work world and housing. It may be stated that while these pathologies are not problems in and of themselves, they frequently *become* problems for the aged due to the myths surrounding elderly persons and the care they receive.

The trend toward institutionalization (as opposed to home-based care) for both the ill and the dying, preconceived notions about "role reversal" (where adult children sometimes impose on their elderly parents a child-like dependent role), myths and jokes about "dirty old men" and "sexless" older persons, and ideas about uselessness and a preference for others of one's own age (stemming from the notion of disengagement) all contribute to social pathology in the aged. Perhaps it would be better to say that such "problems" are cultural rather than individual in nature. Extensive discussions of such pathology are found in Kasl and Rosenfield (1980), Bengston and Treas (1980), Lowenthal and Robinson (1976), Sussman (1976), Comfort (1980), Corby and Solnick (1980), Peterson (1980). These specifically relate to how such factors contribute to the prevalence of mental health problems resulting from isolation, family conflict, lack of meaningful sexual relationships, and feelings of helplessness or devaluation in the aged. These social pathologies are particularly relevant to the previous discussions on an "adjustment" or "culturally relevant" approach to mental health and aging.

Assessing Mental Health and Psychopathology in the Aged

While a discussion of the development of specific scales for the measurement of mental health and psychopathology are beyond the scope of this chapter (Gallagher, Thompson, and Levy, 1980; Gurland, 1980; Lawton, Whelihan, and Belsky, 1980; Miller, 1980; Raskin and Jarvik, 1979; Sloane, 1980), some general comments on assessment are in order.

Regardless of what functions or presumed conditions are being measured, the assessment procedure must be comprehensive. That is, it must focus on as many dimensions of the person as possible, preferably from at least three perspectives: that of the elderly person, his family, and the physician. The quality of the surrounding environment must be assessed; a complete physical and neurologic examination should accompany any assessment, which should be conducted at least twice.

When specific scales are used, it is important that they be both reliable and valid with respect to the elderly; adequate (recent) norms must be used that apply to aged persons. Concern should be given to the conditions under which an assessment is done: physical surroundings should be conducive to the establishment of privacy, rapport, and trust; a clear explanation of the purpose of the assessment, as well as what will be done with the data collected, should be made to the person's satisfaction prior to the procedure. Physical handicaps, transient confusion or disorientation, sensory deficits, motivation for being assessed, response biases (carefulness, cautiousness, conformity), level of education, and familiarity with testing procedures are all personal variables that influence the quantity and quality of information gathered from elderly clients.

The physical characteristics of the test materials themselves affect testing: printing must be clear, with adequate contrast, on nonglare paper; instructions and formats for questions must be consistent and understandable; and lengthy, fatiguing procedures should be avoided. Test-specific anxiety, anxiety over having one's skills (which may be deficient) and physical and mental health assessed, pacing of the interview and testing, and spacing of anxiety-evoking questions are all critical considerations.

Personal qualities of the interviewer (Hilpert, Selzer, and Barton, 1975; Donnan and Mitchell, 1979), such as age and sex, as well as his adeptness in dealing with manipulative behavior, hostility, and defensiveness; his ability to speak clearly and distinctly; maintaining eye contact; touching; and perhaps most important, his treatment of the elderly person with respect, dignity, and concern, are of the utmost importance in conducting an assessment that preserves the aged person's sense of self-worth.

Concluding Comments on Mental Health and Aging

A comprehensive understanding of mental health in later years was stressed in this chapter. To further such an objective, the interested reader should be sensitive to issues pervading the development of gerontologic mental health as an emerging discipline. As with all young fields, divergent views compete on critical issues.

In the geropsychological literature, such issues relate to (1) views of aging that are age-specific versus approaches that are life-span developmental in nature (Baltes, Reese, and Lipsitt, 1980); (2) debates over how mental health services are to be organized (Cohen, 1980; Gatz, Smyer, and Lawton, 1980; NIMH, 1979c); (3) whether such services are to be preventive or remedial in nature (Gaitz and Varner, 1980); (4) concerns over service delivery, costs, insurance coverage for mental health care (Cohen, 1980; NIMH, 1979a); (6) concerns over mental health needs of the frail elderly and minority aged (Cohen, 1980; Kobata, Lockery, and Moriwaki, 1980); (7) professional training in the field of mental health and aging, to include attitudes of care givers (Cohen, 1980; Gatz et al., 1980; Lawton and Gottesman, 1974; NIMH, 1979b; Smyer and Gatz, 1979); and (8) factors affecting the utilization of mental health services by the aged (Cohen, 1980; Gatz et al., 1980; NIMH, 1979c).

Whether one is a potential (future) consumer of mental health services, is caring for an elderly parent, or is a provider of such services for today's aged, mental health issues like those discussed here must be of concern if old age is to be a truly fulfilling time of life—not only for those who are old now but also for those who will inevitably become tomorrow's aged—us. Old age can then be confronted with a sense of dignity and purpose.

REFERENCES

Baltes P., Reese H., Lipsitt L.P.: Life-span developmental psychology. *Annu. Rev. Psychol.* 31:65–111, 1980.

Bengston V., Treas J.: The changing family context of mental health and aging, in Birren J.E., Sloane R.B. (eds.): *Handbook of Mental Health and Aging*. Englewood Cliffs, N.J., Prentice-Hall, 1980.

Birren J., Renner V.J.: A brief history of mental health and aging, in *Issues in Mental Health and Aging: Volume I. Research*. Washington, D.C., National Institute of Mental Health, 1979.

Birren J., Renner V.J.: Concepts and issues of mental health and aging, in Birren J.E., Sloane R.B. (eds.): *Handbook of Mental Health and Aging*. Englewood Cliffs, N.J., Prentice-Hall, 1980.

Birren J., Schaie, K.W.: *Handbook of the Psychology of Aging*. New York, Van Nostrand Reinhold, 1977.

Birren J., Sloane R.B.: *Handbook of Mental Health and Aging*. Englewood Cliffs, N.J., Prentice-Hall, 1980.
Botwinick J.: *Aging and Behavior*. New York, Academic Press, 1978.
Brubaker T., Powers E.: The stereotype of "old": A review and alternative approach. *J. Gerontol*. 31:441–447, 1976.
Butler R.N.: The life review: An interpretation of reminiscence in the aged. *Psychiatry* 26:65–76, 1963.
Butler R., Lewis M.: *Aging and Mental Health: Positive Psychosocial Approaches*. St. Louis, C.V. Mosby Co., 1977.
Cohen G.: Prospects for mental health and aging, in Birren J.E., Sloane R.B. (eds.): *Handbook of Mental Health and Aging*. Englewood Cliffs, N.J., Prentice-Hall, 1980.
Coleman J.C.: *Abnormal Psychology and Modern Life*. Glenview, Ill., Scott, Foresman & Co., 1976.
Comfort A.: Sexuality in later life, in Birren J.E., Sloane R.B. (eds.) *Handbook of Mental Health and Aging*. Englewood Cliffs, N.J., Prentice-Hall, 1980.
Corby N., Solnick R.: Psychosocial and physiological influences on sexuality in the older adult, in Birren J.E., Sloane R.B. (eds.): *Handbook of Mental Health and Aging*. Englewood Cliffs, N.J., Prentice-Hall, 1980.
Davison G.C., Neale J.M.: *Abnormal Psychology: An Experimental Clinical Approach*. New York, John Wiley & Sons, 1978.
Donnan H.H., Mitchell H.: Preferences for older versus younger counselors among a group of elderly persons. *J. Counsel. Psychol*. 26:514–518, 1979.
Eisdorfer C., Cohen D.: The cognitively impaired elderly: Differential diagnosis, in Storandt M., Siegler I., Elias M. (eds.): *The Clinical Psychology of Aging*. New York, Plenum Press, 1978.
Erikson E.: *Identity and the Life Cycle: Psychological Issues. Monograph I*. New York, International Universities Press, 1959.
Gaitz C., Varner R.: Preventative aspects of mental illness in late life, in Birren J.E., Sloane R.B. (eds.): *Handbook of Mental Health and Aging*. Englewood Cliffs, N.J., Prentice-Hall, 1980.
Gallagher D., Thompson L., Levy S.: Clinical psychological assessment of older adults, in Poon L. (ed.): *Aging in the 1980's: Psychological Issues*. Washington, D.C., American Psychological Association, 1980.
Gatz M., Smyer M., Lawton M.P.: The mental health system and the older adult, in Poon L. (ed.): *Aging in the 1980's: Psychological Issues*. Washington, D.C., American Psychological Association, 1980.
Gentry W.D.: Psychosomatic issues in assessment, in Storandt M., Siegler I., Elias M. (eds.): *The Clinical Psychology of Aging*. New York, Plenum Press, 1978.
Gurland B.J.: A broad clinical assessment of psychopathology in the aged, in Eisdorfer C., Lawton M.P. (eds.): *The Psychology of Adult Development and Aging*. Washington, D.C., American Psychological Association, 1973.
Gurland B.J.: The comparative frequency of depression in various age groups. *J. Gerontol*. 31:283–292, 1976.
Gurland B.: Epidemiological research in mental health and aging, in *Issues in Mental Health and Aging, Volume I: Research*. Washington, D.C.: 1979.
Gurland B.: The assessment of the mental health status of older adults, in Birren J.E., Sloane R.B. (eds.): *Handbook of Mental Health and Aging*. Englewood Cliffs, N.J., Prentice-Hall, 1980.
Habot B., Libow B.: The interrelationship of mental and physical status and its

assessment in the older adult: Mind-body interaction, in Birren J.E., Sloane R.B. (eds.): *Handbook of Mental Health and Aging*. Englewood Cliffs, N.J., Prentice-Hall, 1980.
Harris L., and Associates: *The Myth and Reality of Aging in America*. Washington, D.C., National Council on Aging, 1975.
Hayslip B.: Suicide and the elderly, in Cimbolic P., Hipple J. (eds.): *A Systems Approach to Suicide Intervention*. Springfield, Ill., Charles C Thomas, Publisher, 1981.
Hilpert F.P., Selzer U., Barton R.L.: *Sex and Age of the Interviewer as Factors Influencing Response Omissions of Senior Interviewees*. Paper presented at the 28th Annual Scientific Meeting of the Gerontological Society. Louisville, Ky., 1975.
Jahoda M.: *Current Concepts of Positive Mental Health*. New York, Basic Books, 1958.
Jarvik L.: Aging and depression: Some unanswered questions. *J. Gerontol*. 31:324–326, 1976.
Kahn R., Miller N.: Assessment of altered brain function in the aged, in Storandt M., Siegler I., Elias M. (eds.): *The Clinical Psychology of Aging*. New York, Plenum Press, 1978.
Kasl S.V., Rosenfield S.: The residential environment and its impact on the mental health of the aged, in Birren J.E., Sloane R.B. (eds.): *Handbook of Mental Health and Aging*. Englewood Cliffs, N.J., Prentice-Hall, 1980.
Kastenbaum R.: Personality theory, therapeutic approaches, and the elderly client, in Storandt M., Siegler I., Elias M. (eds): *The Clinical Psychology of Aging*. New York, Plenum Press, 1978.
Kay D.W., Bergman K.: Epidemiology of mental disorders among the aged in the community, in Birren J.E.: Sloane R.B. (eds.): *Handbook of Mental Health and Aging*. Englewood Cliffs, N.J., Prentice-Hall, 1980.
Klerman G.L.: Age and clinical depression: Today's youth in the twenty-first century. *J. Gerontol*. 31:318–323, 1976.
Kobata F., Lockery S, Moriwaki S.: Minority issues in mental health and aging, in Birren J.E., Sloane R.B. (eds.): *Handbook of Mental Health and Aging*. Englewood Cliffs, N.J., Prentice-Hall, 1980.
Kramer M., Taube C., Redick R.: Patterns of use of psychiatric facilities by the aged: Past, present, and future, in Eisdorfer C., Lawton M.P. (eds.): *The Psychology of Adult Development and Aging*. Washington, D.C., American Psychological Association, 1973.
Lawton M.P., Gottesman L.E.: Psychological services to the elderly. *Am. Psychol*. 29:689–693, 1974.
Lawton M.P., Whelihan W., Belsky J.K.: Personality tests and their uses with older adults, in Birren J.E., Sloane R.B. (eds.): *Handbook of Mental Health and Aging*. Englewood Cliffs, N.J., Prentice-Hall, 1980.
Leiberman M.: Adaptive processes in later life, in Datan N., Ginsburg L. (eds.): *Life-span Developmental Psychology: Normative Life Crises*. New York, Academic Press, 1975.
Lowenthal M.F., Robinson B.: Social networks and isolation, in Binstock R., Shanas E. (eds.): *Handbook of Aging and Social Sciences*. New York, Van Nostrand Reinhold, 1976.
Maddox G, Douglas E.B.: Aging and individual differences: A longitudinal analysis of social, psychological and physiological indicators. *J. Gerontol*. 29:555–563, 1974.

Marsden C.D.: The diagnosis of dementia, in Isaacs A.D., Post F. (eds.): *Studies in Geriatric Psychiatry*. New York, John Wiley & Sons, 1978.

Miller E.: *Abnormal Aging: The Psychology of Senile and Presenile Dementia*. New York, John Wiley & Sons, 1977.

Miller E.: Cognitive assessment of older adults, in Birren J.E., Sloane R.B. (eds.): *Handbook of Mental Health and Aging*. Englewood Cliffs, N.J., Prentice-Hall, 1980.

Miller M.: *Suicide After Sixty: The Final Alternative*. New York, Springer Publishing Co., 1979.

National Institute of Mental Health. *Issues in Mental Health and Aging. Volume I: Research*. Washington, D.C., 1979 a.

National Institute of Mental Health. *Issues in Mental Health and Aging. Volume II: Training*. Washington, D.C., 1979 b.

National Institute of Mental Health. *Issues in Mental Health and Aging. Volume III: Services*. Washington, D.C., 1979 c.

Neugarten B.: Personality and aging, in Birren J.E., Schaie K.W. (eds.): *Handbook of the Psychology of Aging*. New York, Van Nostrand Reinhold, 1977.

Peterson J.A.: Social-psychological aspects of death and dying and mental health, in Birren J.E., Sloane R.B. (eds.): *Handbook of Mental Health and Aging*. Englewood Cliffs, N.J., Prentice-Hall, 1980.

Pfeiffer E.: Psychopathology and social pathology, in Birren, J.E., Schaie K.W. (eds.): *Handbook of the Psychology of Aging*. New York, Van Nostrand Reinhold, 1977.

Post F.: Paranoid, schizophrenia-like, and schizophrenic states in the aged, in Birren J.E., Sloane R.B. (eds.): *Handbook of Mental Health and Aging*. Englewood Cliffs, N.J., Prentice-Hall, 1980.

Raskin A.: Signs and symptoms of psychopathology in the elderly, in Raskin A., Jarvik L. (eds.): *Psychiatric Symptoms and Cognitive Loss in the Elderly: Evaluation and Assessment Techniques*. New York, Plenum Press, 1979.

Raskin A., Jarvik L.: *Psychiatric Symptoms and Cognitive Loss in the Elderly: Evaluation and Assessment Techniques*. New York, Plenum Press, 1979.

Redick R.W., Taube C.A.: Demography and mental health care of the aged, in Birren J.E., Sloane R.B. (eds.): *Handbook of Mental Health and Aging*. Englewood Cliffs, N.J., Prentice-Hall, 1980.

Riegel K.: The dialectics of human development. *Am. Psychol*. 31:689–700, 1976.

Salzman C., Shader R.: Clinical evaluation of depression in the elderly, in Raskin A., Jarvik L. (eds.): *Psychiatric Symptons and Cognitive Loss in the Elderly: Evaluation and Assessment Techniques*. New York, Plenum Press, 1979.

Schaie K.W., Schaie J.P.: Clinical assessment and aging, in Birren J.E., Schaie K.W. (eds.): *Handbook of the Psychology of Aging*. New York, Van Nostrand Reinhold, 1977.

Seligman M.E.P.: *Helplessness: On Depression, Development and Death*. San Francisco, W.H. Freeman & Co., 1975.

Simon A.: The neuroses, personality disorders, alcoholism, drug use and misuse, and crime in the aged, in Birren J.E., Sloane R.B. (eds.): *Handbook of Mental Health and Aging*. Englewood Cliffs, N.J., Prentice-Hall, 1980.

Sloane R.B.: Organic brain syndrome, in Birren J.E., Sloane R.B. (eds.): *Handbook of Mental Health and Aging*. Englewood Cliffs, N.J., Prentice-Hall, 1980.

Smyer M., Gatz M.: Aging and mental health: Business as usual? *Am. Psychol*. 34:240–246, 1979.

Stenback A.: Depression and suicidal behavior in old age, in Birren J.E., Sloane R.B. (eds.): *Handbook of Aging and Mental Health*. Englewood Cliffs, N.J., Prentice-Hall, 1980.

Storandt M., Siegler E., Elias M.: *The Clinical Psychology of Aging*. New York, Plenum Press, 1978.

Sussman M.: The family life of old people, in Binstock R., Shanas E. (eds.): *Handbook of Aging and the Social Sciences*. New York, Van Nostrand Reinhold, 1976.

Ullmann L.P., Krasner L.: *A Psychological Approach to Abnormal Behavior*. Englewood Cliffs, N.J., Prentice-Hall, 1975.

Wood W.G.: The elderly alcoholic: Some diagnostic problems and considerations, in Storandt M., Siegler I., Elias M. (eds.): *The Clinical Psychology of Aging*. New York, Plenum Press, 1978.

11

DENTAL PROBLEMS IN OLDER ADULTS

Sherryl Short Wesson, R.D.H., M.A.

THE ORAL CAVITY plays a vital role in the daily life of every individual, regardless of age. The state of a person's oral health can affect communication, mastication, social acceptance, and general physical and mental health.

All the structures of the oral cavity are used in producing speech. Thus, the presence of broken or missing teeth may interfere with communication. Whether learning to wear a new set of dentures or coping with an older, ill-fitting dental prosthesis, many people encounter speech problems. If a whistling noise is produced by badly fitting dentures, the wearer finds it embarrassing to talk.

The individual who is unable to masticate food due to an unhealthy mouth is in jeopardy both physically and mentally. If chewing is difficult, a person may not only reject certain foods but may also have less desire to eat. When oral health is poor, eating can become a chore; and if food intake is restricted, the results are obvious.

Social acceptance is based on many factors, but certainly one of the most important is a person's appearance. If the results of oral disease are obvious, the affected individual will most likely have a less than pleasing appearance, possibly resulting in rejection by peers. A person's self-image may suffer if the mouth is in a poor state of health.

The appearance and state of health of the oral cavity mirrors the person's general health. Most systemic diseases manifest themselves in the tissues of the mouth, while oral diseases may be the direct or indirect cause of disorders in other parts of the body (Hall, 1971).

Oral disease exists throughout the life span of most people. In fact, 98% of the United States population experience oral disease at some point. Despite the fact that oral diseases are not always life-threatening, they are more common than other chronic and acute diseases.

Although the elderly do not exhibit any oral diseases that cannot be seen in other age groups, the need for oral care among our nation's aged is acute. National statistics reveal that 51% of people 65 years of age and older have lost all of their teeth; the other 49% have an average of 15 missing teeth. In addition, 80% of the remaining teeth are afflicted with periodontal (supporting tissue) disease. Although nearly 50% of people 60 years of age or older report that they are satisfied with the condition of their dentition (teeth) or dentures, oral diseases—particularly periodontal disease and oral cancer—increase in both incidence and severity with advancing age (Gift, 1979; Wesson and Bullard, n.d.).

An encouraging fact, however, is that studies conducted by the National Family Opinion Poll for the American Dental Association in 1960 and 1975 showed a reduction in the percentage of those age 60 or over wearing at least one complete denture (from 62.5% to 40.8%). These reductions are related to such factors as water fluoridation, improved dental materials and practice procedures, and more extensive dental health education (Gift, 1979).

Oral Diseases

Two of the most prevalent diseases that afflict humans are located in the oral cavity. They are dental caries (tooth decay) and periodontal disease. The suggested etiology of both diseases is multifactorial. Contributing factors include, but are not limited to, environment, genetics, host resistance and response, microorganisms, oral hygiene, and diet and nutrition. (See Figure 11-1 for identification of dental structure.)

Dental Caries

Only a very small proportion, less than 2% of the population of the United States, never experience dental caries (Randolph, 1981). Even though children are highly susceptible to this disease, adults are not immune, especially older people (Fig 11-1).

A contributing factor in the development of tooth decay is dental plaque, a dense aggregation of bacteria on the tooth surface. The microorganisms responsible for tooth decay are acid-producing, however, they could not produce acid without the presence of food, in particular sucrose. Numerous studies have confirmed the role of sucrose in tooth decay (HEW, 1979). In fact, tooth decay is generally absent in citizens of developing countries until sucrose is introduced into the diet. The microorganisms in plaque ferment sucrose, resulting in acid production. Additionally, these same organisms proliferate during sucrose ingestion (Loesche, 1980); therefore, the consumption of sucrose has a twofold effect on oral health.

The ingestion of sucrose is not the only dietary factor in tooth decay. The frequency of consumption and the retention of the sucrose-containing food are of prime importance. How often the sucrose-containing food is eaten is much more important than the amount consumed. For instance, a

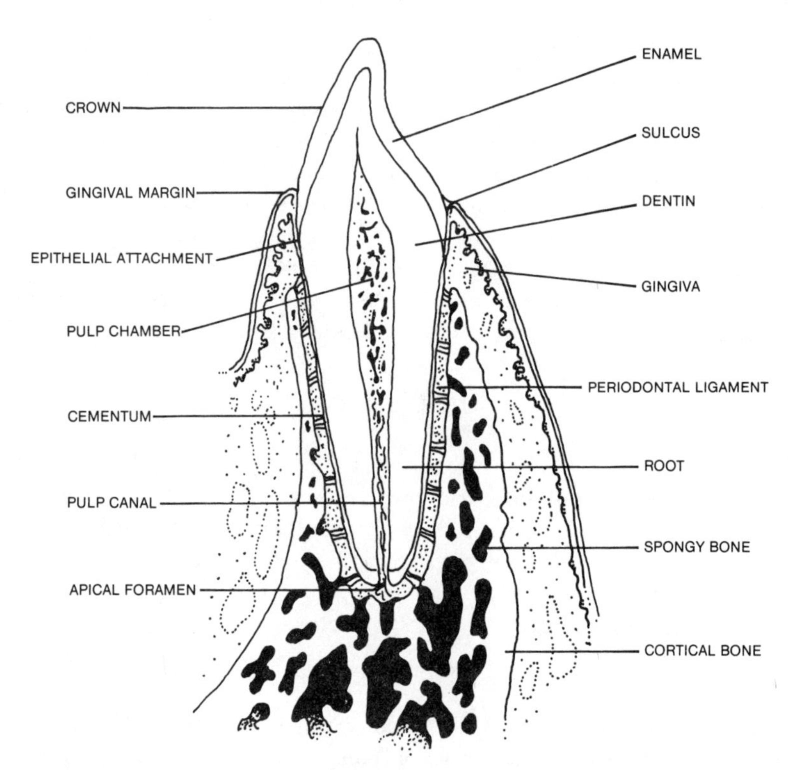

Fig 11–1.—Healthy tooth structure. (From Morrey L.W., Nelson R.J.: *Dental Science Handbook.* Chicago, American Dental Association, 1970. Reprinted by permission.)

person ingesting sugary snacks several times daily causes the production of acid around the teeth on a regular basis. Additionally, the physical form of the food determines how long it will be retained in the oral cavity. The difference in the retentiveness of a caramel and a soft drink, for example, is quite obvious. The longer the sucrose-containing food is retained in the mouth, the longer the period of acid production.

Acid production by dental plaque causes the pH of the mouth to drop to 5.5. The pH that remains at this acidity level for 20 to 30 minutes is capable of dissolving the minerals of the enamel. Once this happens, decay can progress into the dentin and, subsequently, into the pulp, which contains the vascular and nerve supply of the tooth. The results are usually pain and tooth loss. Saliva's buffering effect helps to control acid production to some degree. During meals, sufficient saliva is usually produced to buffer the acid, this is not true of between-meal snacks. Aside from its buffering effect, saliva also contains proteins that act as antibacterial agents.

The mouths of older people generally reflect the results of dental caries, such as missing and restored (filled) teeth. Usually the treatment for decayed teeth in the "old days" was extraction, creating the large number of totally or partially edentulous (toothless) older adults today. As mentioned, even though dental caries is linked to childhood and adolescence, many older people develop problems with tooth decay, some of which are rampant. Factors influencing the increase in caries in advancing years include changes in the diet, decreases in oral hygiene self-care, and diminished salivary flow (as well as changes in the content of the saliva).

Alterations in the diet are common among the elderly. Whether retirement, economic factors, loneliness, chronic disease, changes in taste and the ability to masticate, or a combination of these factors are to blame, the result can be devastating to oral health (Cutter, 1979; Chauncey and Wayler, 1981). For example, an older person who has always chosen a fresh apple as a snack now finds that applesauce, containing added sugar, is less expensive. Other influencing factors in this choice might be the level of ability to masticate with badly fitting dentures and/or a diminished ability to taste sweetness.

Oral hygiene self-care, the mechanical removal of dental plaque from the tissues of the mouth, plays a vital role in controlling dental caries. Often, older people decline in their ability to practice good oral hygiene, for various reasons. Physical impairments, such as arthritis, limit movement in the hands and arms. A decline in visual acuity might interfere with optimal oral cleanliness. Depression or decline in memory have been found to be barriers to personal oral hygiene. All these factors and others directly influence oral disease experience in older people.

Another difficulty, diminished salivary flow, is related to changes in the salivary glands due to disease or is a side effect of certain medications. The resulting xerostomia (dry mouth) increases caries by diminishing the natural cleansing and buffering effects of saliva. Root or cervical caries can be a significant problem in older adults. Decay of the exposed root surface of the tooth spreads rapidly, and this situation is aggravated by general depression, decreased salivary flow, and inadequate oral hygiene measures.

Periodontal Disease

Disease of the tissues that support and surround the teeth is known as periodontal disease and is the major cause of tooth loss in adults (Fig 11-2). "Periodontal disease includes an array of 'infections' that cause an in-

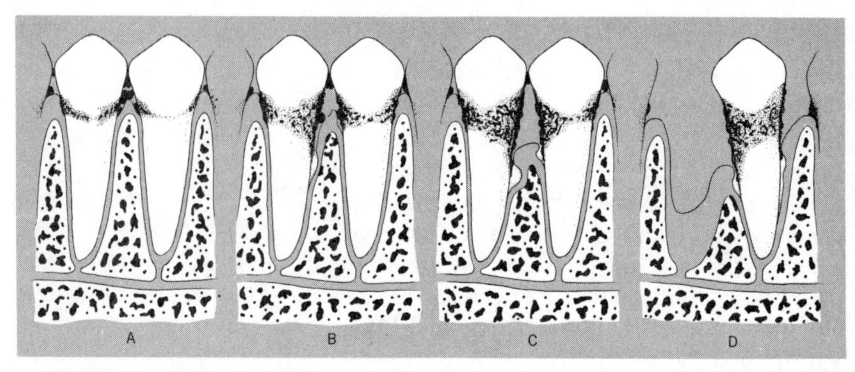

Fig 11–2.—Periodontal disease. *A,* calculus formation gingivitis. *B,* epithelial attachment destroyed; pocket formation; bone loss. *C,* further progressive periodontal tissue loss. *D,* tooth loss as a result of periodontal disease. (From Morrey L.W., Nelson R.J.: *Dental Science Handbook.* Chicago, American Dental Association, 1970. Reprinted by permission.)

flammatory response in the gingival and periodontal tissues" (Loesche, 1980). Even though this inflammatory response is a protective one, it causes destruction of tissue that cannot be replaced by the body. Thus, we see elongated teeth in adults. And if the disease is not treated and prevented from causing further damage, the tooth becomes mobile and is eventually lost as a result of the lack of supporting tissue, including the gingiva (gums), periodontal ligament, and alveolar bone.

Studies reveal that over 80% of adults who are 20 years of age and older exhibit gingivitis (inflamed gums)—the forerunner to destructive periodontal disease. An increase in the prevalence of destructive periodontal disease with age has been observed in numerous studies (Kelly and Van Kirk, 1965). Damage and destruction resulting from periodontal disease is reflected in the mouths of most older people. This oral disease may be chronic throughout the life span. Although the exact etiology is not known, one of the contributing factors is dental plaque. The bacteria causing irritation to the periodontal tissues do not invade the tissues, but rather produce toxic substances that penetrate the gingiva (Loesche, 1980). Additionally, the dental plaque involved in periodontal disease calcifies on the tooth surface; this calculus acts as a local irritant and can only be removed by a dentist or dental hygienist, not by self-care procedures.

Even though the diet is thought to be insignificant in periodontal disease, nutrition or the systemic role of nutrients is a factor in chronic inflammation. An individual's response to disease is determined by his nutritional status. The body's natural immune system, which is related to nutrition, is vital in the prevention of periodontal disease (Randolph, 1981; Slavkin, 1981).

Vitamin C, ascorbic acid, plays a significant role in the health of the gingival tissue. While scurvy (the deficiency disease of this vitamin) is rarely seen in the United States, bleeding gums, a symptom of insufficient amounts of vitamin C, are very common. This is not to say that vitamin C deficiency is the only cause of bleeding gums; poor oral hygiene and the presence of disease are also factors.

Oral Cancer

While not as prevalent as dental caries and periodontal disease, cancer of the oral cavity dramatically increases in incidence with advancing age. Of the nearly 15,000 cases of oral cancer recorded annually, approximately 7,000 deaths result, and only 34% will survive five years (Bednarsh, 1979; Siskind-Houle, 1979). Of all malignancies diagnosed in the United States, 6% are found in the oral cavity. Oral cancer is primarily a disease of the older adult; approximately 75% of all oral cancers occur in people over the age of 55. Additionally, oral cancer is predominantly a disease of men.

Squamous cell carcinomas, which start as an ulcer or area of thickening, account for 90% to 95% of oral cancers. Poor oral hygiene, neglected teeth, ill-fitting dentures, chronic irritation, and use of tobacco have all been associated with these carcinomas. Although cancers can occur at various sites in and around the mouth, a large percentage are found on the tongue, which is not only highly muscular and vascular but also has abundant lymphatic drainage. In addition, the constant movement of this organ increases the chance of metastasis (Keough and Niebel, 1973).

Because the mouth is an accessible part of the body, self-examination is highly recommended to detect early signs of oral cancer. Oral cancers are fast to metastasize, so individuals cannot rely on regular six-month to one-year dental appointments to detect them. With proper instructions and motivation, most people find self-examination relatively simple (Bednarsh, 1979; see "Warning Signs and Procedures").

Other Oral Problems

Dental Prosthesis

As previously mentioned, the majority of people have lost some or all of their teeth by the time they reach old age. Many of these partially or totally edentulous people have replaced missing teeth with removable partial or full dental prostheses (dentures). A few have had fixed prostheses (bridges) constructed. A fixed bridge is just what it indicates: a replacement for missing teeth that is permanently fixed, or cemented, to the remaining natural teeth. Partial or full dentures also replace missing teeth, but they are removable (Fig 11-3). Because dentures fit next to teeth and soft tissue, they must be kept immaculately clean. Dental plaque, food debris, and calculus can accumulate on these appliances. Obviously, if left uncleaned, the dentures could be a source of irritation, inflammation, infection, or halitosis.

Some people mistakenly believe that dentures herald the end of oral problems. However, for many, oral problems begin when they receive their dentures. Throughout life, the structures of the mouth are constantly changing, while dentures remain the same. For instance, a change in body weight can result in a denture no longer fitting properly. Another cause of ill-fitting dentures is bone resorption. The osseous (bony) ridges that the dentures should rest on may completely disappear, leaving a flat area where a ridge should be. It is apparent, then, why denture wearers have mastication and communication problems, and it is not surprising to find that many dentures are worn in "back pockets" or in "jars on the shelf." Adhesives are frequently used to alleviate the problem of poor fit; however, they are not recommended for continuous use because of their irritating nature. Even though dentures may not fit properly, many elderly people continue to wear them for several decades.

Even dentures that fit over healthy osseous ridges are not necessarily easy to wear. Relatively few individuals have trouble wearing an upper full or partial denture. An upper denture, constructed properly, is held in place by suction, and partials are stabilized by attaching them to natural teeth. However, a lower denture must be held in place by the tongue, cheeks, and lips—especially when chewing and talking.

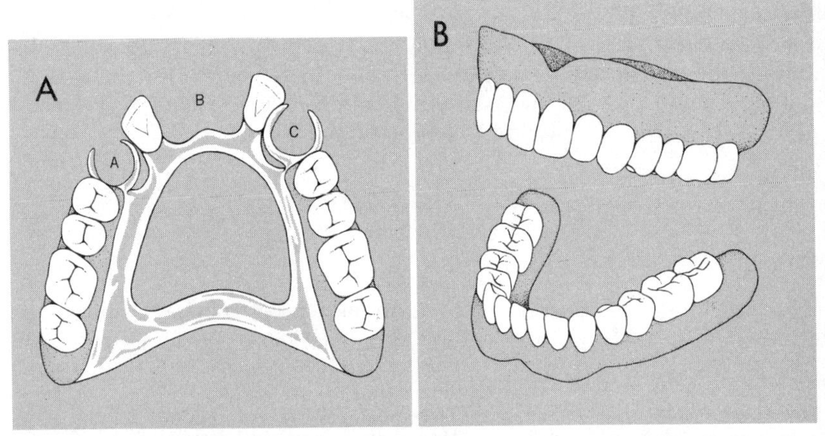

Fig 11–3.—Partial **(A)** and full **(B)** dentures. (From Morrey L.W., Nelson R.J.: *Dental Science Handbook.* Chicago, American Dental Association, 1970. Reprinted by permission.)

Broken or cracked dentures are common problems encountered by denture wearers. Older dentures that have worn thin tend to break easily when used to chew hard food. Dropping dentures while they are out of the mouth can result in breakage. Special care must be taken when cleaning dentures to prevent such damage. Many older people postpone denture repairs, relining, or reconstruction because of the cost involved in such procedures. This partially explains why some people either do not wear their dentures or wear dentures that cause irritated areas on the soft tissues of the mouth.

Oral Manifestations

While many changes may occur in the mouth of an individual over a lifetime, not everyone experiences all of them. Oral manifestations can often be attributed to environmental factors, chronic systemic disease, or poor oral hygiene habits. Research in this area is insufficient; therefore, exact etiology of many oral problems associated with aging is as yet unknown.

While dental caries and subsequent tooth loss are the major problems affecting dentition, the teeth of many older adults show marked attrition. This wearing of the crowns of the teeth may be due to the forces of mastication, especially from chewing abrasive foods. In addition, such habits as chewing tobacco or grinding the teeth (bruxism) result in acutely worn teeth. Most attrition is compensated for, up to a point, by passive eruption of the teeth (Freedman, 1979).

Abrasion of the tooth structure is also seen in many older adults. Toothbrush abrasion is common among people who use nylon bristle toothbrushes that are not specially processed to reduce abrasion. This abrasion manifests itself as notches worn into the neck or exposed root surface of teeth. Sensitivity to thermal changes may result from this wearing close to nerves. If the sensitivity is severe, these notched areas must be restored with a filling material. Wearing may also be the result of such habits as holding a pipe between the teeth, or using them for such things as opening hairpins or holding nails. Clearly, then, the occupation of a person may affect dentition.

Fractured or broken teeth may occur in older people, not only as a result of the undermining effect of dental caries, but also because teeth may become more brittle with age. This brittleness is often the result of a diminished blood supply to the tooth. When the tooth fractures, parts of it—usually the root—may be retained. Retained roots are a source of infection and should be removed. However, because pain does not always accompany these fractures, many people do not have the roots removed. If sharp edges result from these fractures, a source of constant irritation to the soft tissues is established. Left untreated, these irritated areas could develop into a much more serious situation.

The oral mucosa (soft tissue) may undergo changes in older adults. As mentioned, these changes are usually the result of disease, medication, habits, and/or nutrition. This thin epithelial lining is subject to constant trauma such as rough foods, chemicals, bacteria, extreme temperatures, and even bites by adjacent teeth. Because the tissue is highly vascular, there is natural protection against trauma. However, poor circulation may occur in these tissues in many older people. Thus, hyperkeratosis of the mucosa may result. This whitish, scar-like tissue can initiate a malignancy; but these areas may be just a protective covering. Seventy-five percent of these hyperkeratotic lesions are found in people aged 50 or older (Hall, 1971). Even though most white lesions of the mucosa are benign, they should not be ignored. At the very least, white or gray lesions should be kept under observation by a dentist.

Color changes of the mucosa other than the whitish lesions, oftentimes in older people, are a result of systemic disease. Heart and lung diseases or polycythemia can manifest in the oral tissues as a generalized cyanosis. Oral varicosities may also be found underneath the tongue, and are related to varicosities in other areas of the body (Nizel, 1976). Purplish or blue raised areas may be due to accidental biting, but if these lesions appear in areas that cannot be bitten, tumors might be suspected. Brown areas may be the normal pigmentation found in dark-skinned people, or could be the result of Addison's disease (hypoadrenalism). Fordyce's spots or ectopic sebaceous glands are quite common in adults. These yellowish spots, usually located on the mucosa of the cheeks and inside the lips, do not require treatment.

The mucosa covering the hard palate is thicker and is attached to the underlying bone. Rugae (ridges) transverse the front of this area. These hard ridges are used by some edentulous people in combination with the tongue to masticate. Nicotine stomatitis is seen in the mouths of many heavy smokers; inflammation of the tissue occurs, with the epithelium becoming hyperkeratotic. A raspy voice may accompany this condition. Another condition that mimics nicotine stomatitis, but is not the result of smoking, is inflammatory papillary hyperplasia of the palate. This situation results from ill-fitting dentures. Lesions of the palate can also result from injury by a denture or from foods, such as seeds, trapped between the denture and the mucosa. In this case, the lesion will be red with a ragged border. An osseous tumor known as torus palatinus may be observed on the palate of some people. These benign tumors appear early in life, usually in women, and grow slowly through the years. If a full denture is needed, it may have to be designed to fit this growth, or the growth may need to be removed.

The tongue can manifest many diseases or systemic problems. Black hairy tongue may be due to a local irritant, but it is most often associated with moniliasis. This condition, also known as thrush, is related to prolonged doses of antibiotics; the color is derived from food stains, caused by such substances as coffee, tea, or tobacco. A coated tongue may be the result of poor oral hygiene or it may accompany systemic disease, such as gastrointestional conditions. Mouth breathing or dryness of the mouth may also cause a coated tongue. In addition to becoming coated, the tongue may become enlarged or it may atrophy, with obvious resulting problems. Both conditions are related to disease, and the appearance of the tongue surface may also be altered. The papillae may enlarge or atrophy. For example, a B-complex deficiency can result in a balding or shining tongue; and glossitis, a painful condition associated with B_{12} deficiency or pernicious anemia, may also be characterized by a burning sensation.

Angular cheilosis, also common in B-complex deficiencies, causes sores in the corners of the lips. These lesions may also result from a collapse of the tissue after tooth loss; the folds in the skin can hold bacteria and moisture, resulting in cheilosis. The lips in an older person may also become dry and lose much of their elasticity.

Salivary function may be altered in many older people. While it has been shown that diminished salivary flow does not occur in healthy individuals, many older adults do suffer from the effects of decreased salivation in the salivary glands, resulting not only in hyposalivation, but also in a change in the content of the saliva. As mentioned earlier, these changes can result in increased dental caries experience. Xerostomia (dry mouth), an extremely uncomfortable condition, causes pain and a burning sensation. As might be suspected, xerostomia is also related to poor denture retention, swallowing problems, reduced taste sensation, and a decrease in self-cleansing action. Many medications taken by the elderly patient, such as life-sustaining drugs prescribed for hypertension, have xerostomia as a side effect. Artificial saliva (Xero-lube) is one method of combating this problem. Too often, however, hard candies or gums containing sugar are prescribed for this condition, resulting in an increase in tooth decay.

Effects of Other Chronic Health Disorders

Older people have a higher incidence of health problems and, at the same time, oral problems related to these disorders. A patient who has suffered a stroke may no longer have the ability to masticate bilaterally as a result of hemiplegia. Not only is this person more likely to retain food on the afflicted side, but the natural stimulation and cleansing effect of chewing will cease. Clearly, this patient is at a much higher risk for oral disease. Similarly, the person suffering from the effects of Parkinson's disease is more likely to retain food in the oral cavity because rigidity of the laryngeal and pharyngeal muscles makes swallowing more difficult.

Postmenopausal women may have a marked decrease in salivary flow resulting from hormonal changes. This condition can be aggravated by mouth breathing.

Diabetes, while not directly linked to oral health, contributes indirectly to oral problems. The tissues in the mouth of a diabetic are much less resistant to infection and trauma, and they show an exaggerated response to plaque, calculus, and other irritants. In addition, healing is much slower, particularly when the diabetic condition is not under control.

Problems affecting memory and recall, ranging from depression to chronic brain syndrome, may be responsible for oral disease. While persons suffering from such a problem may be able to recall events of long ago in detail, they may forget to practice oral hygiene self-care daily. Such people will need to be reminded of self-care regularly (Hall, 1971).

The high incidence of oral cancer among older people has been discussed previously, but one of the side effects of cancer treatment can have a devastating effect on oral health. Cancer patients receiving radiation treatment to the head and neck area will experience rampant dental caries. Radiation treatment, while a life-saving measure, destroys the action of the salivary glands, and all the problems, including dental caries, associated with diminished salivary flow will then occur.

Tardive dyskinesia, an irreversible condition characterized by profound involuntary movements of the orofacial musculature, is a complication of long-term neuroleptic therapy. Phenothiazine drugs are associated with this condition. Symptoms that first appear in the orofacial region may resemble the effects of long-term L-dopa therapy for parkinsonism. If symptoms are related to phenothiazine, the condition can be reversed (Kamen, 1975).

Effects of Diet and Nutrition on Oral Health

Poor oral health and poor nutrition compound each other. While proper intake of nutrients enhances the health of the mouth, the condition of the mouth is vital to proper nutritional status. Many oral problems, mentioned previously, have been related to diet or nutrition, including dental caries, glossitis, and angular cheilosis.

Inadequate amounts of nutrients, in association with other factors such as poor oral hygiene, result not only in glossitis and cheilosis but also in fragile, friable tissue with a loss of adaptability and tolerance to irritants and a loss of repair potentiality (Cutter, 1979). For example, a vitamin C deficiency not only results in bleeding gums, but also in delayed healing after extractions and prolonged and/or exaggerated postoperative swelling (Massler, 1971). Osteoporosis, experienced by many older women in particular, can be another factor in the health of the mouth. Not only do calcium, phosphorus, and vitamin D play a significant role in this disorder, but systemic intake of fluoride seems to be directly related to the prevention of osteoporosis. In all, oral osteoporosis affects support of the natural dentition as well as the ridges vital to a denture wearer.

Any factor that interferes with biting, chewing, and swallowing foods results in inadequate nutrition. Pain in the oral cavity will clearly affect the intake of food, both in texture and amount. Naturally cleansing foods are required for health of the oral cavity. Therefore, a diet of only soft-textured foods over an extended period can be detrimental to oral health.

Proper nutrition and nutrition counseling for the elderly are important from the standpoint of optimal oral health.

Long-Term Care Patients

While oral problems are prevalent among the elderly population as a whole, the conditions are even more serious in the elderly who reside in institutions. Numerous studies have indicated the acute need for dental care by these residents (Smith, 1979). However, dental care for the institutionalized elderly, in general, is totally inadequate. Lack of appropriate oral screening and treatment, combined with neglected oral hygiene measures, increases the chance of oral disease and/or other related oral problems (ADA, n.d.; Wilson, 1977).

Clearly, oral care can improve the quality of life and can also enhance general health. Left untreated, serious oral problems may accelerate the deterioration of the older patient's physical and mental conditions. However, in many cases the initial oral examination received by a patient admitted to a nursing facility could be the last one he or she ever receives (Hall, 1971). Unfortunately, many nursing homes do not have adequate funds allocated to dental care; only a minuscule number have dental facilities on site, and few have a staff dentist either full or part time.

Medicaid requires participating homes to have an advisory dentist. Unfortunately, this does not always ensure adequate oral care for the patients. Difficulty in treating the oral problems of the nursing home patient explains why many are left untreated. Equipment and supplies needed in oral care treatment are cumbersome and not easily transported; unless portable equipment exists, the advisory dentist may be unable to deliver needed service to a bedridden, nonambulatory patient.

A few complete portable dental units exist, such as the one designed and used by Dr. Jack B. Buck of Dallas City Dental Health Program. This equipment can be driven to the nursing home and easily transported inside for use with the patient who is unable to visit a dental office or clinic. It is hoped that in the future similar dental equipment will be available to more nursing homes.

Another problem influencing the oral health of a nursing home patient is the lack of oral hygiene procedures. Although many residents are capable of some oral hygiene self-care, neglect because of physical or mental impairment is widespread; it is therefore necessary for the staff to assist or remind the patient to perform these measures. Self-care, however, is important from a psychological standpoint and should be encouraged when feasible. Individual physical and mental differences should be considered and oral hygiene instructions adapted accordingly.

For special care patients, the acutely ill or disabled, oral hygiene will have to be performed by another person. The objectives of oral care for these patients are (1) keeping the mouth clean and free of odor and disease; (2) early detection of oral disease by observing for symptoms such as excessive dryness, pain, bleeding, or any unusual odor; and (3) providing for the comfort of the patient (Wesson and Bullard, n.d.). These objectives make it necessary for nursing home staffs to be trained in oral hygiene care and required to perform these duties as a necessary part of patient care. In states where laws permit, registered dental hygienists may be essential members of the nursing home staff, assisting in the promotion and maintenance of optimal oral hygiene among the patients. Another problem that is quite common in a nursing home situation is lost or misplaced dentures. It is therefore imperative that each person's dentures be permanently marked with his name or an identification number immediately upon admission to the facility. Denture marking kits are available and should be utilized to minimize the loss of expensive dental prostheses.

Prevention and Education

Control of the two major oral diseases depends largely on the control of dental plaque. Two approaches may be taken—to prevent it from forming or to remove it at regular intervals. Currently, toothbrushing and flossing are effective against plaque if used regularly and thoroughly. It is vital, in selecting a toothbrush, to make sure that it has bristles which have been specially processed to prevent abrasion. Generally, the package will say that the bristles are "rounded" or "round-end."

Löe believes that the "well motivated, properly instructed patient, who is willing to invest time and effort" can control plaque. Regrettably, most people do not fit in this category. Physical and mental impairments, such as those experienced by many elderly people, can be barriers to practicing plaque control. Futhermore, a lack of motivation and an unwillingness to commit the necessary time to oral hygiene measures influences prevention.

Some physical impairments may be overcome by simply adapting toothbrushes, floss holders, and denture brushes, using a variety of inexpensive material, so that they can be used by the impaired person. Problems with extension and/or mobility of the hands and fingers seen in patients with arthritis, for example, may be compensated for by enlarging the handles of these appliances; this can be done simply by embedding and securing the handle in a larger object, such as a bicycle handlebar grip or a rubber ball. A large rubber band attached to a handle may facilitate brushing for a person who is unable to close his hand. The handle of a toothbrush can be made longer or curved for the patient with limited arm movement. While manual brushes can be used by many, electric toothbrushes may be used to better advantage by physically impaired patients.

Even though brushing and flossing can be effective in preventing dental disease, the prevention of these diseases requires a combined approach. Diet control, regular professional examinations, and oral prophylaxis (cleaning) are of equal importance.

Denture Care

Uncleaned dentures are a hazard to the health of the wearer. Stomatitis, moniliasis, and hyperkeratinization can be prevented in many instances by maintaining a clean oral cavity and dental prostheses. Keeping the appliances clean will also prevent mouth odors and help maintain an attractive appearance (Garland, 1980). In cleaning dentures, the most important thing to guard against is breakage. Filling the sink or basin with water before beginning the cleaning can help to prevent breaking the denture by accidental dropping. This becomes more vital in nursing homes, where the staff is responsible for cleaning dentures for dependent patients.

Cleaning the soft tissues of the mouth, including the tongue, is imperative. The soft tissues not only need to have the bacteria and food debris removed, but they also need to be stimulated for improved circulation, which promotes healthy tissue. This can be accomplished by using a soft, rounded-bristle toothbrush or a sterile gauze sponge. Stimulation of the tissues may also be achieved by digital massage. Another achievable objective of oral hygiene is improved taste perception. It has been shown that the ability to detect sweet and salty taste significantly improves with a regular regimen of oral hygiene care (Langan and Yearick, 1976). Improved taste perception, in turn, promotes better nutrition and consequently better general health.

Clearly, optimal oral hygiene has many desirable results. However, preventive dentistry for the elderly has traditionally been ignored. While an individual never outgrows the need to practice daily oral hygiene, the thrust of dental health education has been directed toward the young. Dentistry, in general, has perpetuated a fatalistic attitude toward the oral health of older people; and older people have for the most part followed suit. Most dental health education material, including media advertising, is geared specifically toward the young. Fortunately, there is a trend now in the direction of promoting preventive care for the aged that encompasses self-care, even among nursing home residents.

Utilization of Dental Services

Although it is obvious that older people experience more oral problems than their younger counterparts, a study conducted by the American Dental Association reveals that nearly 47% of the elderly have not been examined by a dentist in five years or more. The percentage of edentulous persons not visiting a dentist in five years or more is even higher—72%. Utilization of dental care services declines after age 25, but this decline accelerates dramatically after age 65. Even though the dental service utilization rate of the elderly has nearly doubled since 1953 and this rate is increasing faster than the utilization of the population as a whole, the percentage of elderly receiving care is still lower than that of the total population.

The low utilization rate can be attributed to several factors. First and foremost, the issue of cost is paramount in the determination to seek dental care. Since most of the population views oral care as an elective procedure, it is not likely to be at the top of the list of items in a budget. In times of rising costs, people who live on low fixed incomes are not apt to spend money on dental care except in an emergency.

In contrast to other health services, 94% of the cost of dental care is paid by the older individual. Most elderly people are not coverd by private medical insurance that includes payment for dental services. Because of the predictability of oral diseases, insurance companies have been reluctant to include coverage for dental care; for example, Medicare covers dental care only for specific medical-related conditions. Medicaid, while listing dental care in its 15 types of health care, does not include it in its 5 mandatory services. Dental care coverage under Medicaid is at the discretion of each state. Consequently, coverage of dental care under Medicaid is very limited in most states and nonexistent in several (ADA, 1977). Many of the 23 million older people in this country have spent large sums of money on dental care in the past, yet at a time in life when oral diseases become more prevalent and severe, they can least afford this care (Kiyak, 1981).

A second barrier to oral care for the elderly is related to education. A lack of knowledge about preventive care as well as about modern treatments for oral diseases causes many older people to live with oral problems that they believe are normal and a part of getting older. At the same time, many elderly people fail to seek oral care because they do not believe they need it. Also, older people may base their understanding of oral care on past experience, which might have included painful extractions as a result of the lack of a local anesthetic. Clearly, a fear of dental treatment is not unfounded if these and similar horrendous experiences occurred. Advances in treatment procedures and dental equipment are not known to many elderly people.

Many other factors now make it more difficult for older people to obtain needed care. Living arrangements, unavailability of transportation, and lack of social support to provide help are just a few of the hindrances. In addition, many medical disorders create situations in which dental treatment would be contraindicated. For example, a patient receiving anticoagulant therapy could not have dental treatment, even his teeth cleaned, unless this drug therapy was terminated.

Negative attitudes held by the dental service provider can also present a barrier to appropriate dental care. It is hoped that the time is past when denture construction is the accepted treatment for the elderly (Epstein, 1981). However, the curricula of most dental and dental hygiene schools in the past have not provided adequate training for their students in the care of the elderly. Happily, this trend is changing, and an emphasis is being placed on geriatric dentistry in dental and dental hygiene curriculums.

Summary

Without a doubt, the well-being of the oral cavity is vital, for it affects nearly every aspect of an individual's life. Older people experience the result of a lifetime of oral disease. There are also factors that complicate their ability to maintain sound oral health. Physical, psychological, and sociological elements of an individual's life are interrelated with the status of oral health. For this reason, dental care, including both professional treatment and self-care, is necessary. It is not, as some believe, an elective procedure.

It is vital that health care personnel working with the elderly, especially in long-term care facilities, be aware of oral manifestations and their implications. In addition, oral health maintenance of the elderly, including oral hygiene, sound nutrition, and proper general health maintenance, should be promoted.

REFERENCES

Bednarsh H.S.: Oral cancer self-examination. *J. Tex. Dent. Hygienists Assoc.* 17:11–12, 1979.

Bureau of Economic Research and Statistics: *Utilization of Dental Services by the Elderly.* Chicago, American Dental Association, 1977.

Chauncey H., Wayler A.H.: The modifying influence of age on taste perception. *Spec. Care Dent.* 1:68–74, 1981.

Council on Dental Health and Planning: *Oral Health Care for the Geriatric Patient in a Long-Term Care Facility.* Chicago, American Dental Association.

Cutter C.R.: Nutrition in the advanced years. *J. Tex. Dent. Hygienists Assoc.* 17:5–7, 1979.

Epstein S.: Oral health care needs of the elderly. *Spec. Care Dent.* 1:5–9, 1981.

Freedman K.A.: *Management of the Geriatric Dental Patients.* Chicago, Quintessence Publishing Co., 1979.

Garland L.: *Oral Care for the Institutionalized Elderly, Problem in lieu of thesis.* Center for Studies in Aging, North Texas State University, Denton, 1980.

Gift H.C.: The seventh age of man: Oral health and the elderly. *J. Am. Coll. Dent.* 46:204–213, 1979.

Hall G.: Dental needs of the chronically ill and aged: As seen by the dental hygienist. *Arch. Foundation of Thanatology* 3:Winter, 1971.

Kamen S.: Tardive dyskinesia. *Oral Surg.* 39:January, 1975.

Kelly J.E., Van Kirk L.E.: Periodontal disease in adults by age, race, and sex. U.S. Department of Health, Education and Welfare, National Center for Health Statistics, series 11, no. 12. Washington, D.C., 1965.

Keough G., Niebel H.N.: Oral cancer detection—a nursing responsibility. *Am. J. Nurs.* 73:684–686, 1973.

Kiyak H.A.: Psychosocial factors in dental needs of the elderly. *Spec. Care Dent.* 1:22–30, 1981.

Langan M.T., Yearick E.S.: The effects of improved oral hygiene on taste perception and nutrition of the elderly. *J. Gerontol.* 31:413–417, 1976.

Latt B., Stowell B.S.: Dental care for nursing home patients. *Public Health Rep.* 93:90–92, 1978.

Löe H.: Mechanical and chemical control of dental plaque. *J. Clin. Periodontol.* 6:32–36, 1979.

Loesche W.J.: The bacteriology of dental decay and periodontal disease. *Clin. Prevent. Dent.* 2:18–24, 1980.

Massler M.: Oral aspects of aging. *Postgrad. Med. Applied Med.* 49:179–183, 1971.

Nizel A.E.: Role of nutrition in the oral health of the aging patient. *Dent. Clin. North Am.* 20:569–584, 1976.

Randolph P.M.: The role of diet and nutrition in dental health and disease. *Nutr. News* 44:February, 1981.

Siskind-Houle B.: The hygienist's role in care of the elderly. *Dent. Hygiene* 53:November, 1979.

Slavkin H.C.: The aging process and nutrition: Conception to senescence. *Spec. Care Dent.* 1:31–36, 1981.

Smith J.M.: How dental conditions handicap the elderly. *Community Dent. Oral Epidemiol.* 7:305–310, 1979.

U. S. Department of Health, Education and Welfare, Public Health Service: *Healthy People: The Surgeon General's Report on Health Promotion.* Pub. no. 79-55071A. Washington, D.C., 1979.

Wesson S., Bullard K.: Preventive oral care for the old and aged, in Harris N.: *Primary Preventive Dentistry.* Not yet published.

Wilson N.H.F.: The dental care of geriatric patients in hospitals. *Public Health* 11:97–102, 1977.

PART III

Health Care Science

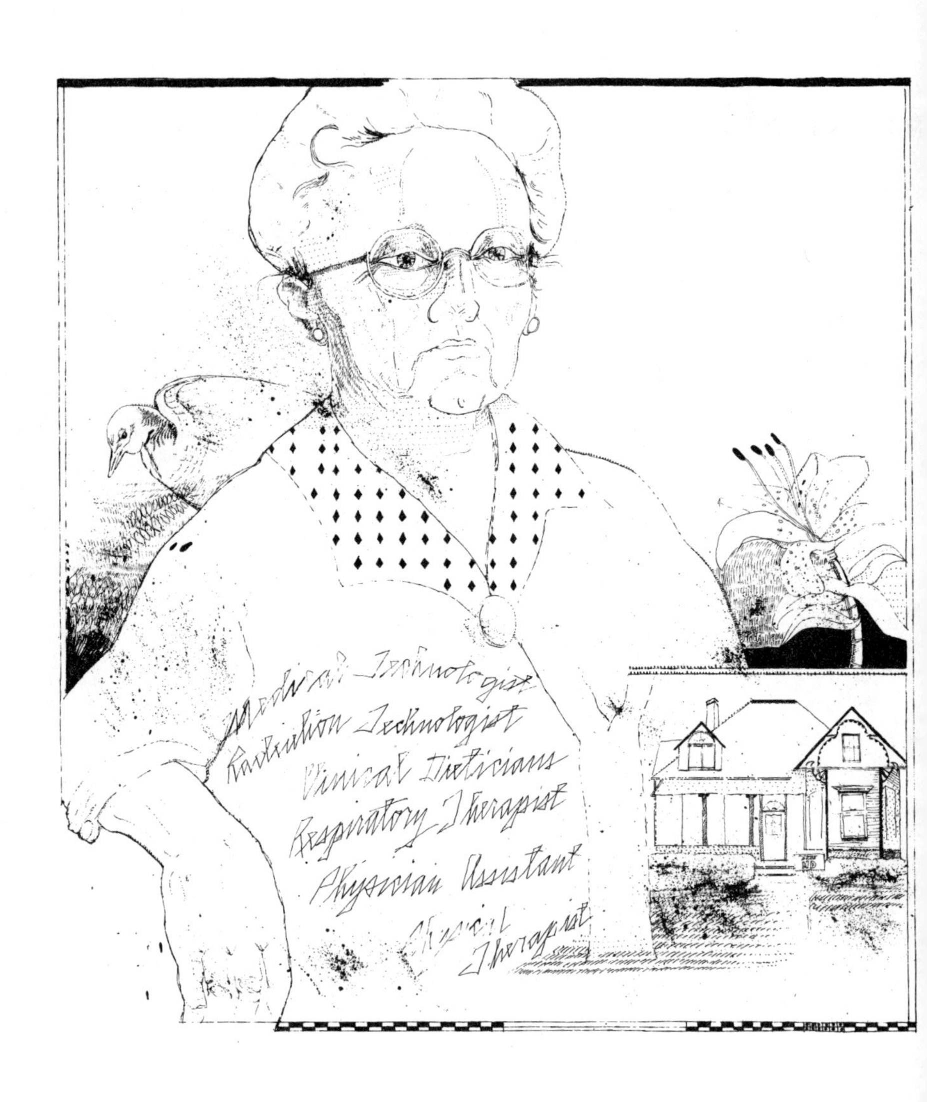
Medical Technologist
Radiation Technologist
Clinical Dieticians
Respiratory Therapist
Physician Assistant
Physical Therapist

12

INSTITUTIONALIZED ELDERLY

Gail House, Ph. D.

WHILE VARIOUS health-related services may offer long-term care, the term is typically used to refer to "care provided in an institutional setting over an extended period of time" (Cohen, 1974). The long-term care system has grown rapidly in just a few decades. This expanding system encompasses an array of supportive and caring services that may include medical, health, and/or social modalities (methods)—from the most restricted to least restricted. Such services may cover all levels of living arrangements, ranging from respite (temporary) and congregate (group living) care homes to chronic (continuing) and acute (crisis situation) care general hospitals (Brody, 1980). The forms of care provided can range from minimal assistance in dressing and bathing to sophisticated medical life-support systems. The most frequently recognized long-term care institutions include homes for the aged, private and public nursing homes, psychiatric hospitals, and chronic care hospitals. These facilities are operated in a variety of ways; they can be public, private-nonprofit, or profit-making organizations (Gelfand and Olsen, 1980). Institutions that specialize in providing care and other services to the elderly are relatively recent innovations. This rapidly growing phenomenon in our society can be tied directly to the ever-increasing numbers of aged persons who are the most predominant users of long-term care institutions.

History of Long-Term Care Institutions

Prior to the 1500s

Until the 16th century, very few needy persons, including the old, had any recourse for relief. Prior to this time, it was considered unethical to waste resources on persons who could not be completely restored. In fact, many primitive societies were likely to view the sick as afflicted by evil forces and they were thus subjected to abandonment (Sigerist, 1965).

1500–1799

During the religious and economic reformations of the 16th century, policies regarding care of the sick and the aged were redefined. Many able-bodied persons who did not work were given unusual punishment, for they were supposed to labor in order to provide for the needs of those unable to work. The sick and the old who did not have relatives capable of providing necessary resources for their care were placed in almshouses, or poorhouses. These have been described as places that combined the sick with the insane, deserted children with criminals, and prostitutes with the feebleminded (Stewart, 1925). Following the Revolutionary War, almshouses became increasingly popular. This almshouse philosophy of separating the infirm and the old from the rest of the community continued to be a prevailing social policy throughout the 19th century (Cohen, 1974).

The history of long-term care institutions began with the almshouses and the public poorhouses of early America. Colonial America patterned its philosophy of care of the needy and aged after the British model. The first American almshouse was built in Boston in the mid-1600s, and more were built in the other colonies shortly thereafter. This seemed to be the most efficient way to provide for the poor, the sick, and the old (Pumphrey and Pumphrey, 1961).

Persons residing in almshouses were frequently expected to work for very low wages as a means of paying a part of their expenses. Any additional financing of such facilities became the responsibility of the townships in which they were located. State or federal support was not forthcoming for at least another 75 years (Gelfand and Olsen, 1980).

1800–1899

The passage of the Poor Law Commission Report of 1834 was a result of the rapidly expanding labor needs of industry. This law was an attempt to put all paupers to work, which resulted in poor relief recipients being considered less desirable than the lowest-paid workers (Friedlander, 1961). While this law was not specifically directed at the aged, many elderly poor were subjected to the same discriminatory practices as the less ablebodied poor. Many of the aged were subjected to treatment that made them horrible examples in the workhouses (Gold and Kaufman, 1968).

The emerging medical technology of the 19th century was utilized by the aged who were fortunate enough to have resources to pay for available services. The remaining elderly were forced to accept a marginal existence, with little or no medical care available (Moroney and Kurtz, 1975). Until the 20th century, the majority of the poor aged were subjected to maltreatment and neglect. At the beginning of this era, the rise and concern of privately endowed foundations and philanthropists began to expand the types of institutional care available. For example, the Charitable Organization was part of this movement and was directly responsible for stimulating the development of alternatives to almshouses in the form of privately operated boarding homes (Drake, 1958).

The development of boarding homes provided residential alternatives for older members of families who could not or would not care for them. Very likely, the older family members were in generally good health upon admission to the boarding home, but as their health tended to decline and they required more assistance, the homes began to provide nursing services. As these facilities began to increase their nursing staffs, the nursing home concept emerged (Moss and Halmandaris, 1977). Few standards existed for the staff or the physical facility, and organized medicine showed little interest in intervening by developing regulations or standards for medical care. During this time, there were few relationships between nursing home operations and the medical care system (Moroney and Kurtz, 1975).

1900–1950

From 1900 to 1935, hospitals began to play a meaningful role in the treatment of the acutely ill, with the physician determining the course and degree of treatment. The central role of the acute care hospital was supported to a larger extent by the newly organized private insurance programs and was controlled by the ever-growing and powerful American Medical Association (AMA). While the acutely ill were able to receive relatively swift medical treatment, services for the chronically ill were minimal. Moreover, no systematic means for delivering services to the chronically ill, particularly those residing in almshouses, county houses, or boarding homes, had been developed. The primary care givers for residents of these establishments provided custodial services only and had little impact on the relationship of the medical profession to this constituency (Moroney and Kurtz, 1975).

By late 1929, major changes were beginning to occur. The Old Age Assistance Act had been passed and it offered a more general alternative to institutionalization. New legislation passed during the 1930s initiated such programs as the Works Progress Administration (WPA), a public works project which allowed many to obtain gainful employment during a severely depressed economic period. Enactment of the Social Security Act of

1935, which provided a new retirement income concept for the aged, had an impact that was to alter the course of medical care in this country (Cohen, 1974).

Through the 1930s and 1940s, institutional long-term care increased rapidly. During this period, an increase of over 45% was observed in the construction of boarding homes, convalescent homes, and nursing homes. Even with the passage of the Old Age Survivors Insurance (OASI) and the Old Age Assistance (OAA) programs, which provided the aged with some alternatives in choice of residence, the primary available facilities remained on the periphery of the medical care system (Cohen, 1974; Moss and Halmandaris, 1977).

1950 to the Present

Even though the income distribution programs for people over 65 years of age (SSA, 1935) had stimulated the growth of the nursing home industry, there was no fiscal incentive for the medical care system to become involved with chronic health problems of aged residents. Beginning in the 1950s, several federal acts authorized grants and loans for constructing and equipping long-term care institutions. The Hill-Burton Act, the Small Business Administration, and the National Housing Act provisions were the most prominent (Gelfand and Olsen, 1980). Passage of these federal acts was prompted by the severe bed shortages experienced by acute care facilities. These beds were frequently occupied by the chronically ill, many of whom were aged. Consequently, hospitals began to look for alternatives, and gradually the medical profession began to make more referrals to nursing homes. Such referrals were not always in the best interest of the elderly patient, for the aged were more likely to be poor and many could not afford the mushrooming costs of acute care hospital services (Moroney and Kurtz, 1975).

Passage of PL 89-97 (Medicare and Medicaid) is considered by many to be the most significant social legislation enacted since the original Social Security Act of 1935. The passage of Title XVIII (Medicare) in 1965 and Title XIX (Medicaid) in 1967 created new and major funding sources for long-term care institutions. These new funding sources set common definitions and basic national standards for service delivery for nursing homes, homes for the aged, convalescent hospitals, and chronic care facilities which until this time had been determined separately by each state (Winston and Wilson, 1977). Medicare, a health insurance program, and Medicaid, a welfare program, were designed to meet the medical needs of high-risk groups, the aged and the poor. By legislative intent, one program emphasizes comprehensive care and the other continuity of care; both operate on the assumption that health care will be improved if financial barriers are removed (Burns, 1966).

A major impetus for enacting Medicare and Medicaid legislation was concern over rising health care costs for the elderly and the poor. There is virtually no agreement on average cost of providing nursing home care, but the average monthly charge ranges from $600 to $1000 (1977 figures). Since the average Social Security benefit for a retired couple is about half this amount, most older Americans cannot afford long-term care (Horn and Griesel, 1977).

While 1 in 20 persons aged 65 or older is in an institution (principally nursing homes and homes for the aged) at any single point in time, perhaps 1 in 4 will be in a nursing home at the time of his or her death (Kastenbaum, 1973). The very old, those over 75 years of age, are the fastest growing of all population groups; and as people get older, their chances of being in a nursing home increase. Only 2% of those aged 65 to 74 are institutionalized, while 16% of those 85 and over are institutionalized (Moss and Halmandaris, 1977). The average nursing home resident is 82 years old, and 70% of the residents are over 70 years of age. Women outnumber men three to one in nursing homes (Gelfand and Olsen, 1980). Less than 50% of the residents are fully ambulatory, with 55% impaired and 33% incontinent. Only 20% of nursing home residents return to their own homes at some point (Moss and Halmandaris, 1977).

Long-term care institutions are closer to being chronic disease hospitals for physically and mentally impaired elderly than care centers and homes for ambulatory aged who are not self-sufficient (Tobin and Lieberman, 1976). Despite the expenditure of billions of tax dollars, new federal and state laws, and pronouncements of elected officials and representatives of the health professions and nursing home industry, a clear and progressive policy has not been initiated to meet long-term care needs of the elderly. The ex-chairman of the Subcommittee on Aging, former Senator Frank Church, has characterized long-term care as "the most troubled and troublesome component of our entire health care system" (U.S. Senate Special Committee on Aging, 1974).

Facilities for Institutionalized Elderly

The long-term care required by the old and disabled should be one of the most tender and effective services a society provides. Those with potential need of such caring services have increased significantly from 3 million in 1900 to approximately 25 million people over the age of 65 today. This elderly population is expected to reach 30 million in the year 2010, and 55 million, or approximately one in seven to one in five Americans, in the year 2030 (Butler, 1981). Moreover, the segment that is the greatest user of long-term care institutions—the elderly aged 75 or more—is growing faster than the elderly population as a whole (Reichel, 1978).

The enactment of Medicare and Medicaid legislation created a major demand for nursing home services, changing nursing homes from a service provided by religious and philanthropic organizations to a lucrative private industry. Unfortunately, the development of federal and state nursing home regulations has lagged behind industry growth and has been marred by industry pressure and administrative conflicts of interest.

The need for addressing the inadequacy of nursing home regulations led to major revisions in 1974, and the unification of Medicare and Medicaid standards. As a result, the extended care facility (ECF) of the Medicare program, the skilled nursing facility (SNF) of the Medicaid program, and the intermediate care facility (ICF) were identified and defined in terms of standards of care (Moroney and Kurtz, 1975). Facilities must adjust services to meet the criteria outlined in order to qualify for reimbursements at the national level. Facilities such as chronic care hospitals or domiciliary care homes may be under the authority of individual state regulations and are more difficult to compare with facilities meeting the more uniform national standards.

Extended Care Facilities

ECFs are defined almost entirely in terms of Medicare reimbursement and differ very little operationally from skilled nursing services. The concept of ECF has been elaborated in a directive to intermediaries:

> The term "extended" refers not to the provision of care over an extended period, but to provision of active treatment as an extension of inpatient hospital care. The overall guide is to provide an alternative to hospital care for patients who still require general medical management and skilled nursing care on a continuing basis, but who do not require the constant availability of physicians' services ordinarily found only in the hospital setting (Social Security Administration, 1969).

Skilled Nursing Facilities

Although the SNF concept differs slightly from the ECF definition, guidelines call for these facilities to meet basically the same need. Skilled nursing facilities are required to provide many of the same services as the ECF, such as emergency and ongoing physician services, nursing care, rehabilitative services, pharmaceutical services, dietetic services, and laboratory and radiologic services. However, some services may be provided by formal contractual agreement with resources outside the facility, such as rehabilitative, laboratory, radiologic, social, and dental services. SNFs call for a prescribed number of visits by attending physicians and for nursing staff requirements per patient day. In general, patients who are severely ill typically receive care at an SNF (Gelfand and Olsen, 1980).

Intermediate Care Facilities

ICFs were defined in conjunction with Medicaid legislation. The intent of the legislation was to remove the incentive to direct patients to more expensive and inappropriate bed placements. The initial goal was to reduce the costs of providing care to the aged. This "intermediate care facility" concept was developed for poor people who were not ill enough to require full-time attention by a professional staff (Senate Committee on Finance, 1970).

It should be noted that the definition of intermediate care is the level of care provided rather than the facility providing the care. Glasscote (1976) aptly described the regulations:

> Regulations for construction, sanitation, safety, and the handling of drugs are very similar. Theoretically and philosophically the difference is that the SNF is a "medical" institution and the ICF is a "health" institution. In the ICF, social and recreational policy is to be given near equal emphasis with medical policy.

The fallacy in the legislation is that the regulations are so general as to allow states to license any nursing home as an ICF that failed to qualify as a skilled nursing home. However, some states have attempted to administer, supervise, and control nursing homes to build an improved program. Other states have made an effort to define and classify ICFs and have set criteria of eligibility for different levels of care.

Life Care Homes

Life care homes, also known as continuing care homes, for the aging differ from other residential living primarily with regard to type of shelter and services offered. Many elderly opt for the continuing care arrangement rather than maintain their own homes. A "continuing care contract" is a generic term representing various types of agreements between the resident and the life care facility. These types of agreements may also be known as life care contracts, entrance fee arrangements, sustaining gift contracts, occupancy agreements, accommodation fee agreements, member trust fund contracts, founders' fee contracts, or community residence agreements. Such a contractual arrangement usually remains in effect for the life of the resident. If an older person can afford the fees and other requirements often requested by life care facilities, usually his worries are over concerning services that may be needed if he becomes disabled or infirm. Many are able to purchase necessary housing and services that they would otherwise be unable to afford over an extended period of time. However, before entering into a contract, the older person and/or other family members should make a careful evaluation of the life care facility and its requirements. Prospective older residents of life care facilities should thoroughly investigate the state law with jurisdiction over such a facility, since these laws vary considerably across the nation. Factors that a prospective resident should consider include procedures for governance and administration of the facility, how the fee will be determined, how this fee will be protected, refund policy for unused fees, termination rights of the resident, types of health and social services provided, and state regulations governing continuing care facilities (Wasser and Cloud, 1980).

Other Types of Facilities

The most common types of long-term care facilities for the elderly, not previously mentioned, include board and care, personal care, and domiciliary homes, as well as homes for the aged. Typically, these types of homes offer only personal and custodial care in a protected environment; residents are usually required to arrange their own medical care. In some instances, however, these homes may be attached to intermediate or skilled-care units. Some homes may go beyond state-regulated standards in providing comprehensive activities, social services, and personal care programs (Gelfand and Olsen, 1980).

Mental hospitals continue to care for the aged on a long-term basis, but there appears to be great variance in admission policies and criteria among these institutions. Often, admission procedures are complicated by difficulty in determining conditions related to organic brain syndrome.

The newest long-term care facility to emerge is the teaching nursing home concept. According to Dr. Robert Butler, director of the National Institute on Aging:

> It is time to gear up organizationally in research, training, and systems of health care and human services. In the area of long-term care, our society has lacked an institutional resource as powerful as the university-affiliated teaching hospital. Thus, an organizational focus for geriatric research and training should be developed: the academic or teaching-research nursing home. Affiliated with a university, teaching nursing homes would generate new knowledge about diseases affecting the elderly. They would furnish concepts and procedures for application in the nation's 18,000

nursing homes. Their effectiveness, quality, ability to attract and hold professionals, and public image would thereby be improved. The facility would serve as an educational crossroads for health and social service disciplines. The entry of research and teaching forces into the nation's nursing homes would do much to counteract the general view of geriatrics as the medical-nursing nadirs, and of old age as societal abandonment (1981).

Federal Agencies and Long-Term Care For the Aged

Health Care Financing Administration

HCFA is responsible for the Medicare, Medicaid, and Professional Standards Review Organization (PSRO) programs. The Medicare Bureau administers a health insurance program for the aged, Title XVIII of the Social Security Act, commonly referred to as Medicare. This insurance package has two components: hospital insurance (Part A) and medical insurance (Part B). Part A covers long-term care at a skilled nursing facility (SNF) for a specified period of time.

Title XIX of the Social Security Act is federally funded and administered by the states. It is commonly referred to as Medicaid. All states participating in Title XIX must include both skilled and intermediate long-term care.

The Office of Program Integrity, an investigative arm of HCFA, is responsible for detecting and managing cases of fraud and abuse by any long-term care provider receiving Medicare or Medicaid funds.

Social Security Administration

SSA's Bureau of Hearings and Appeals is the final arbiter of disputes involving Medicare claims and decisions of PSROs. The Supplemental Security Income (SSI) program is also administered by the Social Security Administration. SSI provides a federal payment program for individuals who are aged, blind, or disabled, and whose income falls below a federally established level. The most important distinction between SSI payments for any type of long-term care and payments made for long-term care under Medicare and Medicaid is that whereas SSI payments are made to the individual beneficiary, Medicare and Medicaid payments are made to the care provider.

Veterans Administration

Former members of the armed forces may receive aid from the Veterans Administration (VA) to pay for limited-duration skilled nursing care.

Administration on Aging

AoA has developed and administers the Nursing Home Ombudsman Program. Under Title III, AoA has encouraged development of local advocacy groups by its network of state and area agencies on aging.

Department of Justice

A special arm of this agency, the Office of Special Litigation, is charged with developing and protecting the constitutional rights of mentally and physically handicapped persons of all ages.

Federal Trade Commission

The FTC is primarily concerned with business practices and regulations that involve federal funds and interstate transactions. Recently, this agency has been investigating whether nursing home "owners, administrators, and others engaged in the sale of health care and other patient services may be engaged in unfair or deceptive acts or practices" (Holmes and Holmes, 1979).

State Agencies and Long-Term Care for the Aged

State Agency on Aging

The State Agency on Aging, in many states, sponsors the Nursing Home Ombudsman Program. Otherwise, the SSA usually has no formal or specialized role in long-term care programs for the aged. However, SSAs usually work diligently as an advocate of all older persons in the state. Many of these SSAs have adopted the stated goal of serving as an advocate to help in avoiding unnecessary institutionalization.

Public Health

The health department is generally the state licensing agency for health facilities. State licensing is a requirement for Medicare and Medicaid participation. Also, this agency may be responsible for issuing certificates of need so that long-term care facilities may proceed with construction.

Social Services and Public Welfare

This department may carry a different name in a given state. The primary function of a department of social services or a department of public welfare or a department of human resources concerning the aged is to administer or supervise the administration of the Medicaid program.

Quality of Care: A Critical View

While good nursing homes do exist, many older Americans and their families have found that most long-term care facilities for the institutionalized elderly offer minimal care at best. All too often inadequacies become obvious only after bitter experiences by elderly consumers.

How well long-term care facilities meet the mandate of federal and state requirements and provide the level of care agreed to under contract with funding sources is evaluated through an inspection system. Two major problems with current inspection systems are: (1) quality of care is more difficult to assess and evaluate than the physical plant, which many inspectors tend to focus on because it is easier to check a laundry list of physical facility requirements; and (2) the primary weapon for noncompliance is revocation of the license to operate, which is usually difficult to enforce because the need for nursing home beds is frequently so acute in many communities. Usually, state or local enforcement bodies will not impose the revocation of license to operate unless flagrant abuse has been observed over several years. Key areas to explore when evaluating a nursing home include: (1) fire safety, (2) nutrition, (3) patient care, (4) sanitation and environment, and (5) staffing and administration.

Fire Safety

In order to make nursing homes more fire resistant, certain architectural features should be incorporated. Emergency exits are absolutely essential for a building that houses many people who cannot move easily or quickly. Halls and doors should be wide enough to accommodate the passage of wheelchairs and beds. Most homes are required to have fire doors and working sprinkler systems.

Impressive strides have been made in the area of fire safety. During the Nixon administration, legislation was passed to provide federally insured loans to help nursing homes buy and install fire safety equipment. Health Care Financing Administration (HCFA) certification standards assure that buildings are not firetraps. Group fires, in which three or more residents perish, have been increasingly rare in recent years. As a matter of fact, none has been reported in federally regulated homes since 1976. In contrast, there have been group fires in personal care and boarding homes subject only to local enforcement. This problem seems to exist because local authorities, anxious to preserve needed local facilities, may in some instances become lax in enforcing the fire codes. Another problem in meeting fire safety codes involves many cases where homes have locked the exits to keep patients from wandering out.

Medicare standards also require a minimum number of fire drills each year so that the patients and staff become familiar with fire procedures. Inspection teams have uncovered any number of infractions—from no drills within the year to sprinkler systems that were not connected to water pipes.

Nutrition

Nutritious food is important at any age. Just because a person is old does not mean that he loses his love for food, his appetite, or past eating habits. Changing one's environment, particularly moving to a long-term facility, can produce severe mental shock. This may be compounded by poor food and food service that further serve to demoralize the nursing home patient. In a number of homes, meals are frequently scheduled according to nursing shifts. Many homes have no food available for their patients from 5:30 P.M. to 8:00 A.M.. Other mealtimes are scheduled at the nurses' convenience.

Even though regulations call for a dietitian to be retained, at least as a consultant, many nursing home staffs fail to control diets. For economic reasons, a high percentage of starchy foods are served instead of meats, vegetables, and fruits.

Esthetically appealing food service is often lacking in nursing homes. Prepared food may sit for hours without refrigeration, and kitchen sanitation may be questionable. Such procedures leave the door open to disease and food poisoning. And yet one of the basic needs of a person is a good nutritious diet every day of his life, preferably served with appeal.

Patient Care

Physicians, who could have a substantial impact on nursing home care, are often conspicuous by their absence. They protest, with some justification, Medicare and Medicaid regulations that require minimum visits on a fixed schedule, coupled with utilization screens that make reimbursement difficult for any doctor who visits a nursing home patient more times than the required minimum. Institutions frequently complain about being held accountable for visits by physicians over whom they have no control. At the same time, consumer groups object to any reduction in the number of required physician visits as a weakening of standards. All parties seem to agree that very sick and medically complex patients get less than ideal care.

The large quantity of drugs consumed by elderly patients in nursing homes requires special measures of regulation, but most government statistics reveal widespread carelessness. When staff is scarce and physicians are absent, the use of potent tranquilizers as invisible restraints is an easy management solution. Approximately 20% of the drugs bought for nursing home patients are tranquilizers. The average patient's drug bill is more than triple that of a noninstitutionalized elderly person. The current Health Care Financing Administration's requirement for monthly drug reviews by a pharmacist may be effective in some settings but is problematic where the reviewing pharmacist is also the drug supplier. To date, the major HCFA efforts in this area have been educational. This is one area in which physician peer review may foster improvements.

Sanitation and Environment

Bad nursing homes seem to be contagious. If enough homes in an area provide poor care, the other homes in the area also tend to decline, and when there is no good place to which a concerned family can move a patient, the incentive for a home to deliver quality care at fair rates may be destroyed.

Lack of privacy, inadequate visiting hours, no place to keep treasured mementos, and rigid and arbitrary schedules are common problems. Nursing home residents share with prisoners and soldiers the inevitable discomforts of the regimentation that characterizes large institutions. Certain areas can be improved; allowing personal pictures on the wall does not seem extraordinarily difficult, and more flexible visiting hours should be reasonably easy to arrange. However, institutions are institutions, and those who reside in nursing homes will continue to be faced with meals, baths, and bedtimes that are established for the organization as a whole rather than for each individual.

Staffing and Administration

Recruitment, retention, and training of staff are undoubtedly some of the most serious problems in staffing nursing homes. Nurse's aides, who are primarily responsible for direct patient care, are difficult to find and even more to difficult to retain. Frequently, aides are inadequately trained. An estimated 25% of all available positions are vacant at any one time; annual turnover estimates for aides frequently run as high as 75% annually. Most aides are paid only the minimum wage, thus adding to the retention problem.

Nurses are an integral part of the nursing home staff, but disproportionately few of the nation's registered nurses work in nursing homes. Those who do often devote their time to administrative duties. The severe nursing shortage faced by many hospitals has adversely affected long-term care facilities, which most nurses consider a secondary labor market. Such employment conditions have prompted nursing home administrators to rely on aides and orderlies to perform most of the jobs.

Nursing home owners are generally well removed from the public eye; and in some cases, state licensing inspectors have reported that they cannot determine exactly who is the owner. Most nursing home owners are corporations. There is, therefore, a problem of whom to hold responsible when a problem arises. The administrator is usually more accessible than the owner of a nursing home, although Medicare standards regarding nursing home administrators are minimal. Fortunately, regulations are increasing.

Good Nursing Homes

Nursing homes have a vital role to play in providing the elderly with skilled health care services. While good nursing homes are to be found, many people do not know what to look for when evaluating facilities. It would be helpful to carry a checklist when comparing nursing homes. One caveat to older persons and families searching for the appropriate long-term facility: compare skilled nursing homes with skilled nursing homes, and residential homes with residential homes.

CHECKLIST FOR COMPARING NURSING HOMES

If the answer to the first four questions is "no" do not use the home.

1. Does the home have a current state license?
2. Does the administrator have a current state license?
3. If you need and are eligible for financial assistance, is the home certified to participate in governmental or other programs that provide it?
4. Does the home provide special services such as a specific diet or therapy that the patient needs?

Physical Considerations

5. Location:
   a. Pleasing to the patient?
   b. Convenient for patient's personal doctor?
   c. Convenient for frequent visits?
   d. Near a hospital?
6. Accident prevention:
   a. Well-lighted inside?
   b. Free of hazards underfoot?
   c. Chairs sturdy and not easily tipped?
   d. Warning signs posted around freshly waxed floors?
   e. Handrails in hallways and grab bars in bathrooms?
7. Fire safety:
   a. Meets federal and/or state codes?
   b. Exits clearly marked and unobstructed?
   c. Written emergency evacuation plan?
   d. Frequent fire drills?
   e. Exit doors not locked on the inside?
   f. Stairways enclosed and doors to stairways kept closed?
8. Bedrooms:
   a. Open onto hall?
   b. Window?

c. No more than four beds per room?
d. Easy access to each bed?
e. Drapery for each bed?
f. Nurse call bell by each bed?
g. Fresh drinking water at each bed?
h. At least one comfortable chair per patient?
i. Reading lights?
j. Clothes closet and drawers?
k. Room for a wheelchair to maneuver?
l. Care used in selecting roommates?

9. Cleanliness:
   a. Generally clean, even though it may have a lived-in look?
   b. Free of unpleasant odors?
   c. Incontinent patients given prompt attention?
10. Lobby area:
    a. Is the atmosphere welcoming?
    b. If also a lounge, is it being used by residents?
    c. Furniture attractive and comfortable?
    d. Plants and flowers?
    e. Certificates and licenses on display?
11. Hallways:
    a. Large enough for two wheelchairs to pass with ease?
    b. Hand-grip railings on the sides of the hallway?
12. Dining room:
    a. Attractive and inviting?
    b. Comfortable chairs and tables?
    c. Easy to move around in?
    d. Tables convenient for those in wheelchairs?
    e. Food tasty and attractively served?
    f. Meals match posted menu?
    g. Those needing help receiving it?
13. Kitchen:
    a. Food preparation, dishwashing, and garbage areas separated?
    b. Food needing refrigeration not standing on counters?
    c. Kitchen workers observing sanitation rules?
14. Activity rooms:
    a. Rooms available for patients' activities?
    b. Equipment (such as games, easels, yarn, kiln, etc.) available?
    c. Residents using equipment?
15. Special-purpose rooms:
    a. Rooms set aside for physical examinations or therapy?
    b. Rooms being used for stated purpose?
16. Isolation room:
    a. At least one bed and bathroom for patients with contagious illness?
17. Toilet facilities:
    a. Convenient to bedrooms?
    b. Easy for a wheelchair patient to use?
    c. Sink?
    d. Nurse call bell?
    e. Hand grips on or near toilets?
    f. Bathtubs and showers with nonslip surfaces?
18. Grounds:
    a. Can residents get fresh air?
    b. Ramps to help handicapped?
19. Medical services:
    a. Physician available in emergency?
    b. Private physician allowed?
    c. Regular medical attention assured?
    d. Thorough physical immediately before or on admission?
    e. Medical records and plan of care kept?
    f. Patient involved in plans for treatment?
    g Other medical services (dentists, optometrists, etc.) available regularly?
    h. Freedom to purchase medicines outside home?

20. Hospitalization:
    a. Arrangement with nearby hospital for transfer when necessary?
21. Nursing services:
    a. RN responsible for nursing staff in a skilled nursing home?
    b. LPN on duty day and night in a skilled nursing home?
    c. Trained nurse's aides and orderlies on duty in homes providing some nursing care?
22. Physical therapy:
    a. Specialists in various therapies available when needed?
23. Activities program:
    a. Individual patient preferences observed?
    b. Group and individual activities?
    c. Residents encouraged but not forced to participate?
    d. Outside trips for those who can go?
    e. Volunteers from the community to work with patients?
24. Religious observances:
    a. Arrangements made for patient to worship as he pleases?
    b. Religious observances a matter of choice?
25. Social services:
    a. Social worker available to help residents and families?
26. Food:
    a. Dietitian plans menus for patients on special diets?
    b. Variety from meal to meal?
    c. Meals served at normal times?
    d. Plenty of time for each meal?
    e. Snacks available?
    f. Food delivered to patients' rooms?
    g. Help with eating when needed?
27. Grooming:
    a. Barbers and beauticians available for men and women?
28. Attitudes and atmosphere:
    a. General atmosphere warm, pleasant, and cheerful?
    b. Staff members show interest in and affection for individual residents?
    c. Staff members show courtesy and respect for residents?
    d. Staff members stop to chat with residents?

Future Trends

There is considerable evidence that most people in nursing homes need a significant level of services, even if these could be provided in other settings. Also there is concern that expanding coverage of alternatives to institutionalization under the existing open-ended, fee-for-service structure could increase governmental expenditures significantly, although the cost per beneficiary served may decline. It has been projected that governmental policy has been constrained to all but minor, often little more than cosmetic, changes since the ICF benefit was added to Medicaid in the early 1970s. Increased expenditures can be expected because the new benefits will primarily help currently unserved populations rather than substitute for care in institutions. Although some institutionalization may be prevented, the actual census of nursing home patients will not change significantly, particularly given the current shortage of beds for publicly financed patients.

From the early almshouse concept to the present-day nursing home concept, biases have been documented that favor nursing home use (inherent in public programs) with a concurrent fragmentation in the funding and delivery of noninstitutional services. The resulting discontinuity among programs that strive to serve the elderly is an artifical split between medical and social services that often makes it difficult for the individual to receive needed benefits. A nursing home is usually viewed as a medical institution; it can also be characterized as a housing arrangement that offers varying levels of supervision and support, medical service, and so on.

Still another problem, however, is the inherent problem of defining need based on age. Older people are a heterogeneous, not a homogeneous, group; therefore, age is becoming increasingly irrelevant as a predictor of lifestyle or need. Bernice Neugarten (1980) has asked the question: "Do older people deserve more support than young people because they are old? Or, if government policies are restructured to support the poor or the isolated rather than to support persons who happen to be old, then what new definitions of need will become necessary?"

There is also the critical problem of distinguishing between need for services and the need for government-funded services. The major source of long-term care services for noninstitutionalized patients is family and friends. Need is as much related to the availability of family support as it is to medical or functional disability. This description of need supports the thesis that most problems of long-term care services are clearly not medical. As such, these problems should not be left solely to the decision-making powers of the physician and the present health facilities.

Health care professionals can assist in the move to discover how to improve the coordination of health care and social services at the point of client intake, for example. Some kind of mechanism is needed to increase the likelihood of clients being directed to the most appropriate kind of care or service. Our government, along with health care and social service professionals, should engage in a major policy review aimed at developing a long-range policy framework for the next decade to guide initiatives in long-term care. This review should take into account services for functionally impaired persons, including health, mental health, social services, and housing services. A critical examination of options is necessary to create incentives for family care of the elderly, as well as incentives for preventive care such as "well elderly clinics."

As a society, we need to overcome the collective reluctance to accept and prepare for aging. The focus in the next decade must revolve around the future needs of our aging citizens as long-term care policies are reviewed and developed further. More important, there is reason to believe that the aged, at any level of competence, will respond better if helped to play an active, participating role in their own care.

REFERENCES

American Council of Life Insurance: Health care: Three reports from 2030 A.D. *Trend Analysis Program*. Washington, D.C., Spring, 1980.

Barney J.: The prerogative of choice in long-term care. *Gerontologist* 17:309–314, 1977.

Benedict R.: The politics of long-term care: Directions for the future. *Final Report: National Conference on Long-Term Care Issues*. Washington, D.C., Administration on Aging, September 1980.

Brody S.: Health care for the elderly: Doing it well vs. doing it poorly, in *National Journal's Conference Proceedings, Aging: Agenda for the Eighties*. Washington, D.C., Government Research Corp., 1980.

Burns E.: Some major policy decisions facing the United States in financing and organization of health care. *Bull. N.Y. Acad. Med.* 42:1072–1092, 1966.

Butler R.: The teaching nursing home. *J.A.M.A.* 245:1435–1437, 1981.

Cohen E.: An overview of long-term care facilities, in Brody E. (ed.): *A Social Work Guide for Long-Term Care Facilities*. Rockville, Md., National Institute for Mental Health, 1974.

Drake J.: *The Aged in American Society*. New York, Ronald Press Company, 1958.

Dudley C., Hillery G.: Freedom and alienation in homes for the aged. *Gerontologist* 17:140–145, 1977.

Friedlander W.: *Introduction to Social Welfare*. Englewood Cliffs, N.J., Prentice-Hall, 1961.

Gelfand D., Olsen J.: *The Aging Network: Programs and Services*. New York, Springer Publishing Co., 1980.

General Accounting Office (GAO), U.S. Comptroller General: Problems remain in review of Medicaid-financed drug therapy in nursing homes. Report no. HRD-80-56. Washington, D.C., 1980.

George Washington University, Department of Health Care Administration: *The Evolution of Long-Term Care in the United States*. Long Term Care Monograph Series, no. 1. Washington, D.C., 1969.

Glasscote R., et al.: *Old Folks at Home*. Washington, D.C., American Psychiatric Association and the Mental Health Association, 1976.

Gold J., Kaufman S.: Development of care of the elderly. Paper presented at the Gerontological Society Meeting, Denver, Colo., 1968.

Gottesman L., Hutchinson E.: Characteristics of the institutionalized elderly, in Brody E. (ed.): *A Social Work Guide for Long-Term Care Facilities*. Rockville, Md., National Institute of Mental Health, 1974.

Holmes M., Holmes D.: *Handbook of Human Services for Older Persons*. New York, Human Sciences Press, 1979.

Horn L., Griesel E.: *Nursing Homes: A Citizens' Action Guide*. Boston, Beacon Press, 1977.

Kastenbaum R.: The four percent fallacy. *Int. J. Aging Hum. Dev.* 4:15, 1973.

Koetting M.: *Nursing Home Organization and Efficiency*. Lexington, Mass., Lexington Books, 1980.

Mendelson M.A.: *Tender Loving Greed*. New York, Knopf Publishing Co., 1974.

Moroney R., Kurtz N.: The evolution of long-term care institutions, in Sherwood S. (ed.): *Long-Term Care: A Handbook for Researchers, Planners, and Providers*. New York, Spectrum Publications, 1975.

Moss F., Halmandaris V.: *Too Old, Too Sick, Too Bad*. Germantown, Md., Aspten Systems Corp., 1977.

Neugarten B.: Setting a new goal: An age-irrelevant society, in *National Journal's Conference Proceedings, Aging: Agenda for the Eighties*. Washington, D.C., Government Research Corp, 1980.

Percy C.: *Growing Old in the Country of the Young*. New York, McGraw-Hill Book Co., 1974.

Pumphrey R., Pumphrey M.: *The History of American Social Work*. New York, Columbia University Press, 1961.

Reichel W.: *The Geriatric Patient*. New York, H.P. Publishing Co., 1978.

Sigerist H.: The social history of medicine, in Katz A.H., Felton J.S. (eds.): *Health and Community*. New York, The Free Press, 1965.

Social Security Administration, Bureau of Health Insurance. *Letter No. 370*. U.S. Government Printing Office, 1969.

Stewart E.: *The Cost of American Almshouses*. U.S. Bureau of Labor Stat. Bull., 1925, p. 386.

The spreading scandals of the nursing homes. *U.S. News and World Report*. 78:21–23, March 31, 1975.

Tobin S., Lieberman M.: *Last Home for the Aged*. San Francisco, Jossey-Bass Publishers, 1976.

Tomlinson K.: Our shameful nursing homes. *Reader's Digest* 101:193–197, October 1974.

Townsend C.: *Old Age: The Last Segregation*. New York, Grossman Publishing Co., 1971.

U.S. Administration on Aging: *Nursing Home Ombudsman Program: A Fact Sheet and Program Directory*. U.S. Government Printing Office, 1977.

U.S. Congress, Senate Committee on Finance. *Medicare and Medicaid: Problems, Issues, and Alternatives*. Ninety-second Congress, First Session. U.S. Government Printing Office, 1970.

U.S. Department of Health and Human Services: *Long Term Care: Background and Future Directions*. Health Care Financing Administration, HCFA 81-20047. U.S. Government Printing Office, 1981.

U.S. Senate, Subcommittee on Long Term Care, Special Committee on Aging: *Nursing Home Care in the United States: Failure in Public Policy*, Introductory Report. U.S. Government Printing Office, December, 1974.

Wasser L., Cloud D. (eds.): *Continuing Care: Issues for Nonprofit Providers*. Washington, D.C., American Association of Homes for the Aging, 1980.

Willemain T., Mark R.: The distribution of intervals between visits as a basis for assessing and regulating physician services in nursing homes. *Med. Care* 18: 427–441, 1980.

Wilson S.: Nursing home patients' rights: Are they enforceable? *Gerontologist* 18:255–261, 1978.

Winston W., Wilson A.: *Ethical Considerations in Long-Term Care*. St. Petersburg, Fla., Eckerd College Gerontology Center, 1977.

13

HOME HEALTH CARE

Sharon Young Ward, M.A.

PROVIDERS OF home health care define their services as

> . . . that component of comprehensive health care whereby services are provided to individuals and families in their places of residence for the purpose of promoting, maintaining, or restoring health, or minimizing the effects of illness and disability. Services appropriate to the needs of the individual patient and family are planned, coordinated, and made available by an agency/institution, or a unit of an agency/institution, organized for the delivery of health care through the use of employed staff, contractual arrangements, or a combination of administrative patterns.*

Explicit in this definition is an awareness of the interrelated nature of the patient's medical and social needs. It asserts that home health care must be a comprehensive plan that treats the total needs of the patient, not just his medical symptoms.

The purpose of home health care is to provide an element in the health care delivery system that allows the individual to remain in a familiar environment as long as medically feasible. It is widely held that a familiar environment, especially for elderly patients, plays a critical role in the success of medical regimens. Home health care strives to establish and maintain the maximum obtainable level of independence for the patient, in accordance with the belief that individuals are most physically and mentally healthy in a familiar environment that encourages continued independence.

The History of Home Health Care: The First 200 Years

Home health care is the oldest formal mode of health care delivery in the United States. Its development can be traced back to the mid-1700s,

*The definition and statement have been developed and endorsed by the following organizations: (1) American Hospital Association, Assembly of Out-Patient Home Care Institutions; (2) National Council for Homemaker-Home Health Aide Services, Inc.; (3) National Association of Home Health Agencies; (4) National League for Nursing, Council of Home Health Agencies and Community Health Services.

when home health care was the only practical system for providing health care services in an undeveloped country. In 1796, the first organized system of home health care was established at the Boston Dispensary. At that time, hospitals were feared because of their exceptionally high mortality rates, a situation caused by both poor sanitation and rudimentary medical techniques. Consequently, home health care was viewed enthusiastically by the population as an alternative to hospitalization. During this early stage of its development, however, home health care consisted solely of nursing services and was provided exclusively to patients with acute conditions. Emergence of home health care as an organized component in the health delivery system actually accompanied development of the public health movement. In fact, many health departments in the United States can trace their inception to community awareness of the value of visiting community nurses.

The public health movement officially began in Liverpool, England, in 1859. It reached America in 1873, when Bellevue Hospital in New York City opened the nation's first nursing school. Bellevue's nursing program was founded on the principles of the Rathbone and Nightingale training school in England for community nurses. By 1877, the Women's Branch of the New York City Mission became the first voluntary community organization to employ visiting nurses. At this time, other communities were beginning to establish the nation's first health departments. These health departments employed the services of visiting nurses from voluntary agencies. In this capacity, visiting nurses carried out orders from the school medical inspector, visited homes to instruct mothers in general health and infant care, and took sick children to the dispensary (Waters, 1974).

The first Visiting Nurse Association (VNA) was established in Buffalo, New York, in 1885. Boston and Philadelphia followed soon afterward, establishing their VNAs in 1886. Early VNAs were supported primarily by community contributions; small fees were charged to patients who could afford to contribute. The VNA directors and board members were community lay persons.

The continuing development of community health departments paralleled the development of the VNAs. For years the health departments relied on the voluntary visiting nurse associations to furnish community nursing services. As the health department concept expanded, however, these agencies began to employ community nurses directly. Los Angeles led the way in 1898, when its health department employed community nurses to provide in-home nursing to the sick poor.

As community health nursing continued to expand, public health nursing care became more and more specialized, because it was easier to obtain community support and funding for individual medical problems. For several years there was controversy over the appropriate scope of care assigned to community health nurses. National associations organized to fight a specific disease, for example, the National Tuberculosis Association, called for specialized nursing. At the same time, the success of generalized county health units argued for generalized community nursing.

Eventually, the arguments for generalized community nursing skills prevailed. The goal of visiting nursing or public health nursing was care of the total person, not the specific disease. Community nurses strove to provide comprehensive in-home care to community residents (Hanlon, 1974).

By the beginning of the 20th century, advances in sanitation and fire control made hospitals physically safer places for treating the ill. Later improvements in infection control made them medically safer as well, and helped to erode their stigma. As the century progressed, further technologic innovations in medical care developed and were increasingly relied on in research, diagnostic procedures, and treatment. Hospitals actually became fashionable places for medical treatment as a result of these innovations (Hunt, 1962). With this movement toward hospital care, home health services diminished in their importance to the community.

But the continued reliance upon hospital care was, ironically, an important factor in the renewed development of home health care as a segment of the health services delivery system. The expanding capabilities of hospitals allowed them to provide a centralized and efficient delivery system for a broad array of services. The factor became more significant during World War II, when the relatively few civilian doctors were forced to utilize their time in the most efficient manner possible. They were no longer able to make numerous house calls to patients who did not require emergency care; rather, they turned increasingly to hospitals that could provide the latest technologic advances and sophistication in management of medical resources.

Such activity increased the efficiency and utility of physicians, but it created a substantial void in the provision of health care to those who found hospitals inaccessible or prohibitively expensive. This void in the health care delivery system was filled by visiting nurses and public health nurses, who continued to provide services in the home (Ricker-Smith, 1978). Because all medical services were reimbursed primarily by private fees-for-services or charitable contributions, the scope of home-delivered services continued to be limited to essential nursing services received primarily by the poor, who could not afford the expense of hospitalization.*

---

*While home health care services in the United States were virtually limited to nursing services for the poor, an expanded model for home health care was developing in Great Britain. With governmental support accompanying their development and implementation, home help services that originally were designed to care for ill children were extended to include home care services for chronically and acutely ill adults (see Ricker-Smith, 1978).

Although the prestige of hospital care remained high, hospitals were often inappropriate care settings for many patients. The centralized, technologically efficient facility was designed to treat acute conditions rather than chronic problems that required long-term rehabilitative care or maintenance. By comparison, public health and visiting nurses were successfully caring for chronically ill patients. This success encouraged the establishment of the first hospital-based, postacute system of home health care delivery at Montefiore Hospital in New York City in 1946.

The Montefiore program was founded on the premise that the length of a hospital stay could be effectively shortened by providing home health care services to postacute patients. A prerequisite for this care was a special support system that would enable the patient to receive appropriate care at home. In such a system, the family provided the necessary domiciliary and unskilled services in conjunction with skilled hospital services that were now duplicated at home by nurses, physicians, home health aides, and therapists. This system changed the focus of patient care from consideration of available hospital resources to consideration of care in terms of individual patient needs (Hunt, 1962). The Montefiore home health program offered a wide range of services designed to maintain the postacute patient in his home. (Cherkasky, 1949). These services included the following:

1. Home medical services available 7 days a week, 24 hours a day, with specialists including orthopedists, ophthalmologists, and surgeons.
2. Social services provided by the same social worker who had served the patient in the hospital.
3. Nursing services provided by the Visiting Nurse Association.
4. Housekeeping services for 5 to 10 hours a week.
5. Transportation to and from the hospital for intermittent inpatient services.
6. Medications and medical equipment.
7. Occupational therapy.
8. Physical therapy.

The development of the Montefiore program was especially significant for several reasons. Most important, it modified the function of the hospital from delivery of both chronic and acute medical care to one of caring primarily for acutely ill patients. Second, the services provided in the home were expanded from strictly nursing services to a multiservice array, the model for the delivery of home health care services today. Finally, health care was delivered with consideration for both the medical and the social needs of the patient.

For many years following its establishment, Montefiore's home health care program remained a lone pioneer in the field. Public health nurses and visiting nurses also supported a multiservice array, but they were severely restrained by funding sources that were largely private and community contributions. Available financing, rather than the extent of the illness, usually determined the number of home health care visits made. Until federal funding first became available in the 1960s, home health care services continued to be limited to care for acutely ill patients.

Emergence of Public Financing for Home Health Care Services

Throughout the 1950s and into the 1960s, home health care services continued to consist primarily of nursing services for patients with acute conditions. A turning point for the home health field occurred in the 1960s with the development of a political climate that encouraged the liberalization of publicly financed health benefits. This political climate expressed the ideology that health care was a right to which all citizens were entitled. There was also a growing public demand that patients have access not only to quality health care, but also to options in health care. The rise in medical care costs increased the public's insistence on less expensive health care options. Concurrently, interest groups sprang up that aroused public sensitivity to the special needs of low-income groups, the elderly, and the handicapped.

A legislative action by Congress accompanied this increased public sensitivity to health issues. Home health care was included in the array of health options under legislative consideration in the 1960s. The first major federal legislative initiative in home health care occurred in 1960 with passage of the Kerr-Mills Act, Medical Assistance for the Aged. The Kerr-Mills Act established the precedent for a continuing distinction between "skilled services" and paraprofessional services. Although the two are highly interrelated, this differentiation between professional and paraprofessional services has continued throughout the legislative history of home health care (Ricker-Smith, 1978).

Home health care became a joint federal and state project in 1961, with passage of the Community Health Services and Facilities Act. Under this act, matching funds were provided to states for the development of services for the noninstitutionalized aged and the chronically ill (Ricker-Smith, 1978). With the Kerr-Mills Act, this legislation established the foundation for the home health components of the major, publicly funded health programs that are still active today.

The development of subsequent state and federally funded home health programs has had a tremendous impact on the growth of the home health care field. Today, home health services are almost entirely funded by public programs. The following discussion presents an overview of these major programs. Although each has evolved since its initial enactment, we shall focus on the programs as they exist today. As with most segments of the health services delivery system, the passage of Medicare and Medicaid, Titles XVIII and XIX of the Social Security Act, had a particularly strong impact on the development of home health care as it is known today.

Medicare

During the 1960s, increasing health costs and a heightened public sensitivity to the health care needs of the aged and disabled contributed to the 1965 passage of Medicare, health insurance for the aged and disabled, Title XVIII of the Social Security Act. Medicare, a federally funded, nationwide health insurance program, provides benefits to the elderly and disabled. It is primarily financed by payroll taxes contributed by both employers and employees and the focus of its home health benefits is on acute care. In accordance with this focus, skilled professional services are provided to rehabilitate the acutely ill patient to independent status.

Medicare coverage is provided primarily to people aged 65 and over who have contributed sufficiently to the Social Security system during their years of employment. Medicare Part A, or hospital insurance, is the basic form of coverage to which all Medicare-eligible recipients are entitled, whereas Part B is an optional and supplemental health insurance plan that is partially financed by beneficiary contributions. Part A is financed by Social Security taxes and covers inpatient hospital services and some posthospital care—the latter provided either in skilled care nursing homes or in patients' homes. At the present time, prerequisites for home health care benefits under Parts A and B are medically oriented and include each of the following:

1. The patient must be homebound (confined to his or her residence).
2. The patient must be diagnosed by a physician as needing part-time or intermittent skilled nursing services and/or physical, speech, or occupational therapy.
3. The home health care services must be provided by an organization that has fulfilled Medicare standards for participation and is thus "Medicare certified."

If these three conditions are met, Medicare benefits will cover 100% of the charges for an unlimited number of home health care visits (Public Law, 1980).

Nursing is the primary home service covered by Medicare. In order to qualify for home health care benefits, the patient must be diagnosed as in need of skilled nursing care provided by, or under the supervision of, a registered nurse, or in need of physical, occupational, or speech therapy.

If one of these three services is required, any combination of the following services may be integrated into the home health care program:

1. Medical social services that are necessary to assist the patient and his or her family in adjusting to social and emotional conditions related to the patient's health problem.
2. Part-time or intermittent home health aide services, including help with bathing, self-administered medications, and exercise.
3. In the case of a home health agency affiliated with a hospital, medical services provided by an intern or resident of the hospital.

Federal administration of Medicare is delegated to the Department of Human Services' Health Care Financing Administration (HCFA). HCFA establishes guidelines for home health agencies that allow them to participate in the Medicare program. Included among these regulations is the requirement that all participating agencies must offer skilled nursing care and at least one additional service. Additional services offered most frequently include physical therapy (offered by 73% of all certified home health agencies), home health aide services (48%), speech therapy (22%), medical social work (20%), and occupational therapy (16%) (Ryder et al., 1969).

Rather than reimbursing the home health care agency directly, HCFA contracts with public and private intermediaries who then carry out reimbursement procedures between HCFA and the agency. Fiscal intermediaries are responsible for:

1. Paying the provider for services rendered.
2. Providing information and instructions about HCFA guidelines, and serving as a communication channel between HCFA and the home health care agency.
3. Assisting home health agencies to establish and apply safeguards against unnecessary use of services.
4. Reviewing claims for appropriate reimbursement criteria.
5. Establishing reasonable cost figures for provider services (GAO, 1977).

Medicaid

Another major legislative expansion of home health care benefits was established in 1965 with the passage of Medicaid, Title XIX of the Social Security Act. The purpose of Medicaid was to expand health care services to low-income groups through a program that shared costs between the states and the federal government.

Under the funding formula established for this program, the federal government contributes 50% to 80% of Medicaid program costs, based on the per capita income of the state, and it establishes legislative guidelines and regulations for the state programs. The states, however, have broad discretion in setting income eligibility requirements; establishing the benefit package, including scope and duration of services; and determining reimbursement rates for providers of Medicaid services.

Today, all states except Arizona participate in the Medicaid program, and federal guidelines are applied evenly to all states. Each state is allowed to develop an individual plan to meet its particular needs. Federal regulations require Medicaid programs to serve all income-eligible recipients of Aid to Families with Dependent Children, Supplementary Security Income, and welfare recipients of the Aged, Blind, and Disabled Program. States may individually decide to extend coverage to additional needy groups.

When Medicaid was first enacted in 1965, home health care was an option available to the state plans. In 1967, however, an amendment to Medicaid required that all states participating in this program provide, by 1970, a package consisting of seven services. One of the required services was home health care.

Home health care services provided by Medicaid are less medically oriented than are those provided under Medicare coverage. Unlike Medicare, Medicaid does not require that recipients be either homebound or in need of "skilled" nursing care. The only federal Medicaid requirements regarding health care status are the following:

1. Home health care services must be necessary on a part-time or intermittent basis.
2. A physician must certify the need for home health care.
3. Delivery of home health care services must be supervised by a registered nurse.

Federal guidelines also mandate that the Medicaid state home health care program contain, at a minimum, nursing services; provision of medical supplies, equipment, and appliances; and home health aide services. Many states supplement these required services by providing prescription drugs, dental services, mental health care, personal care services supplied by individuals not employed by the home health agencies (for example, family members, relatives, and neighbors), physical therapy, occupational therapy, speech therapy, and medical social services.

Many agencies that provide home health care services under the Medicare program are also participants in the Medicaid program. In fact, to be eligible for participation in Medicaid, an agency must first meet the federally established administrative and quality standards for Medicare participation. Although this certification process is the same for Medicare and Medicaid, reimbursement for the same service under each program often differs dramatically. Because the states have complete autonomy in setting reimbursement rates for Medicaid services, they often set these rates lower than would be allowed for the same service under the federally administered Medicare program. Some states set their rates so low that the allowed reimbursement is significantly less than the actual costs incurred for providing the services. As might be expected, this inadequate reimbursement has produced several problems, including the following:

1. Development of agencies that will provide services only to Medicare participants, often called "100 percenters" or "Medicare-only" agencies.
2. Quotas for Medicaid recipients in agencies that will provide services under the Medicaid program.
3. Most important, a resulting inaccessibility to home health care services for many needy individuals who are not eligible for services under other programs.

Older Americans Act

The Older Americans Act, passed in 1965, created the Administration on Aging (AoA) in the former Department of Health, Education, and Welfare. The AoA is the nation's primary agency for dealing with the special needs of the aged. One focus of the Older Americans Act, expressed in Titles III and IV, is the homebound elderly. These titles have a social rather than a medical focus. The total number of in-home services provided by this act is small when compared with those given under Medicare and Medicaid, but they fill an important gap in the delivery of in-home services.

In-home services provided under Title III are designed for individuals who can employ these aids to maintain maximum independence and dignity in their own homes. Five basic in-home services authorized by Title III are the following:

1. Home-delivered meals for homebound elderly and their spouses.
2. Homemaker services—trained and supervised homemakers assist older persons in the home to perform activities such as cooking and housekeeping, thus helping them to retain their independence.
3. Home health services—these may include part-time bedside nursing, occupational therapy, speech therapy, physical therapy, special services for the visually handicapped, and home health aide services.
4. Residential repairs and renovation—these services assist the elderly in maintaining their homes to conform with minimum standards or in adapting their homes to their special needs (e.g., equipping homes with safety features such as safety rails in bathrooms, carpeting slippery floors, etc.).
5. Additional support services that promote independence—including shopping, reading, and chore services.

Title IV funds also affect the development of in-home service delivery by supplying discretionary funds for model projects, training, and research in the home health care field. The purpose of these funds is to support the development of a comprehensive and coordinated system of community long-term care that successfully matches older people with the long-term care services they need (Norman, 1979, 1981).

The enactment of Medicare, Medicaid, and the Older Americans Act triggered rapid development and expansion among home health care agencies. This growth over the past 15 years, however, has been accompanied by federal indecision concerning a national policy for home health care. Regulatory changes made to the Medicare program since its inception in 1965 exemplify this indecision and an absence of federal commitment to home health care.

Each of these acts influenced the evolutionary development of the home health care field. However, because Medicare is administered completely at the federal level and provides a specific and uniform array of services nationally, its impact on the field is the most easily discerned. The impact of Medicaid and the Older Americans Act, although certainly important and contributory to the success of home health care, cannot be comparatively measured. Each state's autonomy in allocating these funds has caused such a divergence in state programs as to preclude comparative studies.

As federal money was funneled into home health care through Medicare, agencies providing these services expanded from 1,256 certified agencies (those that have met all standards for Medicare participation, as established by the Health Care Financing Administration) in 1966 to 2,365 certified agencies in 1977 (Gerson, 1978). This dramatic growth of almost 100% in the number of agencies providing home health care services can be directly linked to federal involvement in reimbursement.

Federal involvement has also precipitated reactionary changes in the composition of home health agencies, the main types being:

1. Public—an agency located in the official health department of the state, county, or city that is tax supported. Public agencies participate in both Medicare and Medicaid programs.
2. Visiting Nurse Association (VNA)—a freestanding, nonprofit private agency administered by citizens' groups. The VNA is supported by earnings and community contributions in addition to reimbursement from public programs. All VNAs participate in both the Medicare and the Medicaid programs.
3. Hospital-based—home health agencies that are extensions of services offered by the hospital. Hospital-based programs usually participate in both Medicare and Medicaid programs and are supported additionally by taxes, community contributions, and fees for service. The Montefiore program mentioned earlier is one example of a hospital-based home health agency.

4. Private, nonprofit agencies—privately controlled, nonprofit organizations. Often, these agencies do not participate in Medicaid programs, which frequently do not reimburse providers for the full cost incurred in rendering the service. In contrast, the Medicare program reimburses the provider agency for approximately 100% of its cost; thus these agencies are frequently called "100 percenters," or Medicare-only agencies.
5. Proprietary—profit agencies primarily supported by fees-for-service.

Despite numerous changes from 1965 to 1974, the largest growth in home health agencies has occurred among the hospital-based variety. During this period, the number of hospital-based, home health agencies care programs increased (Hammond, 1978), which can be attributed to the hospitals' growing confidence in the Medicare system and its liberalization of benefits.

The major providers of home health care services, VNAs and public home health agencies, have also undergone changes since the inception of Medicare. Before Medicare, 90% of all home health agencies were operated by these providers.

VNAs provided nursing care before the passage of Medicare, but the public agencies' in-home services consisted exclusively of health education and referral. VNAs now represent 25% of all certified home health agencies, have expanded to include direct care, have dramatically increased in number, and now compose 50% of the field of certified care providers (Hammond, 1978).

Medicare reimbursement for in-home services has created a new provider in the home health care field, the "Medicare-only" agency. Many of these new agencies developed in response to Medicare's total reimbursement of costs incurred in providing in-home services. These agencies frequently serve only private, fee-for-service patients or those eligible for Medicare coverage. Although relatively small in number when compared with other providers in the field, Medicare-only agencies are active home health care providers. Medicare has also precipitated growth in the proprietary sector. In addition, as funds became available through Medicare for the provision of in-home health services, other health care providers began to experiment with the delivery of home care. Today, home health care programs are found housed in such settings as rehabilitation centers and long-term care facilities.

The creation of Medicare affected not only the composition of providers of home health care but the range of their services as well. To fulfill the requirements for Medicare participation, all eligible agencies were required to offer skilled nursing care plus one additional in-home service. This requirement served to broaden the scope of services then available in the home. For example, at the time of Medicare's enactment, 41% of all certified home health agencies offered physical therapy and 44% offered home health aide services. But by 1974, as a direct result of the requirement for nursing-plus-one service, 74% of all home health agencies were offering physical therapy and 73% were offering home health aide services. The percentage of agencies offering the services of medical social workers, occupational therapists, and speech therapists also increased (Hammond, 1978). This widening of service scope was especially dramatic because it accompanied a rapid growth in numbers of home health agencies. Thus, not only did the absolute number of home health agencies increase by almost 100%, but the range of services offered by these agencies expanded significantly as well.

In summary, federal financing of home health care services made them accessible to many new segments of the population, including the elderly, those with specific diseases, and the poor. Federal financing of the home health care field, fragmented as it was, was the catalyst for the following changes during the years 1965 to 1975:

1. The number of home health agencies increased by almost 100%
2. Home health agencies that had been providing only indirect services (50% of all home health agencies in 1965) expanded to provide direct health care in the home.
3. The scope of services typically available was enlarged.
4. Utilization of home health care services grew substantially. In 1970, for example, there were 389 home health care visits per 1,000 Medicare recipients; by 1976, however, this figure had increased to 479 visits per 1,000 beneficiaries (Trautman, 1978).

Although there is no way of knowing which subgroups of the population were using home health care services before the inception of Medicare, Medicaid, and the Older Americans Act, it is apparent that targeted groups now have much greater access to home health care as a result of these pieces of legislation.

Title XX

Another major federal initiative, Title XX of the Social Security Act, has influenced further development of home health care services. Title XX, "Grant to the states for services," was implemented in 1975. It represented a consolidation of several earlier titles of the Social Security Act and was designed to provide social services to the states through matching grants. The federal government contributed 75% of Title XX funds and the remaining 25% was provided by each state.

The philosophy behind Title XX is self-determination, that is, each individual state can best assess its needs and resources and, thus, most effectively design the social services it needs. In compliance with this philosophy, the federal government has little control over the Title XX program. States determine what services the funds will provide and who will be served. The advantages afforded by this approach are partially offset by the fact that the federal government is unable to enforce minimum standards for providers.

Ten percent of all Title XX funds is spent on in-home services. The most common in-home services provided by these funds include:

1. Homemaker services—meal preparation, child care, and housekeeping.
2. Home health aide services—help with carrying out physicians' orders, assistance with bathing and exercise.
3. Chore services—repairs, yard work, shopping.
4. Home management—instruction in meal preparation, budget management, child care (Health Care Financing Admin., 1978).

The passage of Title XX marked the establishment of the last of the four major programs now providing home health care. Medicare, Medicaid, the Older Americans Act, and Title XX each contributed significantly to the development of home health care as it is known today. Although the programs have various foci, producing a fragmented pattern of coverage, the home health care field has grown dramatically under the sponsorship of these programs of public financing.

The following section will discuss the characteristics of the home health agency and its services as they exist today.

The goals of home health care today include the following:

1. *Rehabilitation of patients with acute problems*. Rehabilitation most frequently includes postoperative care, physical therapy, occupational therapy, and speech therapy. Its aim is to restore the patient to health or to stabilize his or her condition, allowing the individual to be maintained at home.
2. *Maintenance of patients with chronic conditions that can be managed solely in the home or in combination with inpatient services*. Maintenance services are most frequently provided for chronic disorders of the cardiovascular and central nervous systems. The level of maintenance in home care is also appropriate for cancer management. In such cases, patients often receive periodic intensive treatments in the hospital, followed by intervening periods of home care.
3. *Prevention of illness*. Preventive home health care services include prenatal and postnatal care, health education, and family counseling. Although preventive care is a goal, it is less frequently available than rehabilitative or maintenance care. Because acute and chronic condi-

tions are readily apparent and demand attention, they take precedence over potential health problems, both to the reimburser and to the potential patient.

Ideally, the scope of services available to patients requiring home health care should include:

1. Medical services
2. Dental services
3. Nursing services
4. Homemaker–home health aide services
5. Occupational therapy
6. Physical therapy
7. Speech therapy
8. Social work
9. Nutritional services (both preparation and delivery of meals to homebound patients, and nutrition education)
10. Health education
11. Laboratory services
12. Pharmaceutical services
13. Transportation
14. Medical equipment and supplies (Gordon, 1974).

In actuality, however, this range of services is rarely available. When such a system of home health care services does exist, it is usually confined to large agencies in urban areas that have both a large clientele and the necessary resources to implement a broad range of services. The development of home health care services has closely followed the dictates of the reimbursement methods available for these services. Consequently, most home health agencies offer a core of skilled nursing care, physical therapy, and home health aide services. These services are required most frequently by patients who are eligible for reimbursement. Skilled nursing care and physical therapy are primary qualifying requirements for patients receiving Medicare coverage; services of home health aides are necessary complements to both the services and are reimbursable when employed in this way. Additionally, Medicaid requires that home health aide services must be available as one of the three basic services offered under the program.

Nursing has historically been central to providing in-home health services and it continues to occupy this position today (Ryder, 1977). The nurse has the primary responsibility for ensuring that patients receive the appropriate level of care in the home. In addition to providing direct care, the nurse is responsible for monitoring the progress of the patient, coordinating the optimal range of services, and determining the continued direction of the patient's program of home care. Nurses represent the largest number of home health care employees, with registered nurses constituting 70% and licensed practical nurses 18% of all employees of certified home health care agencies (Hammond, 1978).

Medicare regulations have strongly supported the nursing core of home health services by requiring all certified agencies to offer skilled nursing care. Additionally, Medicare-eligible patients must demonstrate a need for skilled nursing, speech therapy, occupational therapy, or physical therapy before other in-home services are allowed. Thus, home health care at present continues to rest on a medical foundation despite the appeal for a multidisciplinary approach.

The homemaker–home health aide follows the nurse as the most frequently employed staff member of home health care agencies. These paraprofessionals compose 18% of the home health care work force in certified agencies (Hammond, 1978). Homemaker–home health aides provide services that enable their patients to carry out basic tasks which allow them to continue to receive care in the home. Under the supervision of a nurse or social worker, homemaker–home health aides provide assistance in the following areas:

1. Grocery shopping, planning and preparing meals.
2. Housework.
3. Exercise routines.
4. Self-administered medications.
5. Budgeting for required expenditures.
6. Patient education.
7. Maintenance of personal hygiene.

The importance of the homemaker–home health aide in caring for the patient cannot be overemphasized, as these employees usually have the most direct contact with the patients. Their ability to monitor patient progress, in addition to performing duties of patient assistance, can greatly enhance the quality of patient care.

Other employees of home health agencies include physical therapists (4% of all home health employees), medical social workers (1%), and speech and occupational therapists (less than 1%) (Hammond, 1978). The numbers of employees in these disciplines are not indicative of the availability of their services. Most home health care agencies employ their own nurses and homemaker–home health aides, but other services are often contracted through outside community organizations. All certified agencies provide nursing services; 74% provide physical therapy; 73%, home health aides services; 38%, speech therapy; 26%, occupational therapy; and 24%, medical social work (Hammond, 1978).

Although most home health care agencies do not offer a full scope of services, the desired plan of patient care can often be achieved through integration with other community resources. Home health care services do not operate in a vacuum. They must be coordinated with all medical and social services available in the community.

Home health care operates optimally when consumers and providers of health and social services understand its function. Discharge planners of hospitals and patient coordinators of long-term care facilities should be well aware of the advantages of home health care services to appropriate patients. Conversely, home health care providers should recognize certain patients' needs for more intensive care. Effective integration allows establishment of a patient plan that is implemented in multiple settings. Cancer management, for example, is often successfully achieved through the collaboration of the hospital and the home health care agency; the hospital provides intermittent inpatient treatments in conjunction with maintenance services in the home. When home health care is the most appropriate method for the provision of medical or social services, it must be augmented by complementary services such as transportation and the delivery of prepared meals.

Directions for the Future

The continued growth of home health care in the United States is greatly dependent on the coordinative success of federal, state, and local authorities that govern public home health care programs. At this time, it can be unequivocally stated that there is no national home health care policy in this country. In fact, U.S. Department of Health, Education, and Welfare officials said in 1977 that home health care services defy coordination under current legislation (GAO, 1977).

The situation, as it stands at present, has evolved from the independent and uncoordinated development of myriad public programs, each having different goals and including some form of in-home services within its programmatic scope. Programs with home care components were developed initially to provide health, social, or income maintenance services. In addition to programmatic differences, each program focuses its efforts on a specific group of clients. The following information highlights this variation in program focus throughout the country's publicly financed programs for delivery of in-home services to the elderly:

1. Medicare, Title XVIII of the Social Security Act—federal legislation and regulations are enforced by state employees who are paid by the federal government. Programmatic focus: Health services. Population focus: The elderly and disabled.

2. Medicaid, Title XIX of the Social Security Act—federal legislation and basic regulations are enforced by individual states. Each state establishes standards and administers the program. Programmatic focus: Health services. Population focus: The poor and public assistance recipients.
3. Title XX of the Social Security Act—basic federal enabling legislation. Each state is free to administer the program and to determine the scope of services and eligibility criteria. Programmatic focus: Broadly defined social services. Population focus: Low-income individuals.
4. Title III of the Older Americans Act—federal enabling legislation and guidelines. State program administration and distribution of funds. Programmatic focus: Support services. Population focus: The elderly.

As illustrated by this brief survey of program characteristics, each of the public home care programs has been developed to meet the specific needs of a targeted population. Each program has its own requirements, criteria for eligibility, scope of services, method of reimbursement, and administrative relationship to federal, state, and local governments. Thus, each public program offering in-home services effectively has its own criteria for all areas of operation.

The absence of a coordinated and consolidated home care policy at the federal level produces havoc for providers. A home care agency's delivery of services in the community is complicated, and sometimes incapacitated, by various reimbursement mechanisms and procedures; specific programs' disparate client eligibility requirements that may be age- , health- , and/or income-related; and the regulations of numerous governing authorities. A provider of home care services must carefully monitor all regulatory changes in each of the programs in which his agency participates. When the provider offers both health and social home care services under the various programs, it must screen each client for reimbursement eligibility for specific services under the program in which he is enrolled. For example, while a Medicaid recipient is often entitled to receive home health aide services as a primary or entitling service, the Medicare recipient must first be in need of skilled health services in order to qualify for home health aide services.

A report by the U.S. General Accounting Office summarizes the confused state of service delivery in the home by citing the following characteristics of current public programs:

1. Overlapping constituencies.
2. Varied service definitions and regulations regarding the range and duration of services.
3. Distinctions between health and social services that reinforce fragmentation.

4. Regulations that vary from program to program.
5. Different reimbursement methods for each program.
6. Different federal, state, and local relationships (Department of Health, Education, and Welfare, 1979).

The ultimate level of confusion, however, rests with the consumer of home care services. A most difficult problem facing the potential consumer of services is finding a point of entry into the system. For an elderly individual in need of several health and social services, finding those that can meet his or her needs is often difficult and frustrating. If the required services are found, the client must then meet the complicated eligibility requirements for reimbursement under each program that provides the needed services.

Because of program differentiation between health and social services, one agency is often not equipped to assess the elderly client's needs and offer him or her the range of services necessary to meet those needs. The elderly client must then receive services from more than one provider. When this occurs, the client's services are usually not coordinated and evaluated as a package of interrelated services; each provider monitors only the services provided by his own agency. Delivery of health and related social services then becomes more fragmented as the client receives services from various programs and providers.

When a client is no longer eligible for services under one program, he or she must cope with an interruption in the delivery of services until he or she is again eligible or can meet the administrative and eligibility criteria for another program. This situation often produces a time lag in services for the elderly client and results in an expensive duplication of administrative responsibilities for the provider (Department of Health, Education, and Welfare, 1979).

Home health care has proved to be a valuable and often cost-effective component of the health care delivery system. It can be expected that utilization of current home health care programs will continue to expand as consumers and health care providers become more familiar with this service. While private reimbursement of home health care services has been conspicuously absent in the past, the insurance industry is beginning to implement home health care benefits since it also sees the potential cost-effectiveness of this mode of care. Congress also will continue to look to home health care services as a cost-effective alternative to institutional care. With this scrutiny should come an expansion of home health care benefits under existing public and private programs and a concomitant increase in regulation and investigation of fraud or abuse in the home health care field.

Conclusion

Home health care has had a rich history in the United States as the nation's oldest mode of health care delivery. In fact, the early development of the public health movement in this country can be directly traced to the home health services offered by voluntary community organizations. As the 20th century arrived, however, technologic advances and a shortage of physicians directed the public's attention toward hospital-based health care services.

Despite a rather slow development that continued through the 1960s, home health care has again vigorously emerged as a viable and vital component of the health care delivery system in the United States. Continued expansion of home health care services is largely dependent on the organizational achievements of all health care providers, regulators, and legislators. Continuity of patient care and coordination of the various reimbursement sources are the two major challenges facing the continued expansion of home health care today. If these challenges are met successfully, the future for home health care promises to be bright.

REFERENCES

Cherkasky M.: The Montefiore Hospital home care program. *Am. J. Public Health* 39:164–165, 1949.

Gerson C.K.: The team approach to home health care. *Am. Pharm.* 18:37, 1978.

Gordon G.: Statement in testimony of the American Public Health Association. Presented before the Subcommittee on Health of the Elderly, Senate Special Committee on Aging, July 9, 1974.

Hammond J.: *Medicare Home Health Care Benefits, Agencies and Utilization: 1966–1975*. Office of Planning, Evaluation, and Legislation, U.S. Department of Health, Education, and Welfare. Washington, D.C., April 1978.

Hanlon J.J.: *Public Health: Administration and Practice*, ed. 6. St. Louis, C.V. Mosby Co., 1974.

Health Care Financing Administration: *HR-3 Report*, draft. Washington, D.C., October 1978.

Hunt T.E.: Care and rehabilitation of patients in their homes. *Can. J. Public Health* 53:22, 1962.

Norman B.: Administration on aging. Personal correspondence.

Ricker-Smith K.: In-home health services in California: Some lessons for national health insurance. *Med. Care* 16:175, 1978.

Ryder C.: A broader view of American home care services. *Mass. Phys.* 36:31, 1977.

Ryder C., Stitt P.G., Elkin W.F.: Home health services—past, present, future. *Am. J. Public Health* 59:1724, 1969.

Trautman D.: Medicare utilization analysis—Part two. *Home Health Line* 3:February 1978.

U.S. Department of Health, Education, and Welfare, *Home Health and Other In-*

Home Services: Titles XVIII, XIX, and XX of the Social Security Act—A Report to Congress. Washington, D.C. November 1, 1979, pp. 26–29.

U.S. General Accounting Office: *Home Health—The Need for a National Policy to Better Provide for the Elderly*, Report no. HRD-78-19. U.S. Government Printing Office, December 3, 1977.

U.S. Public Law no.96-499, Section 930: *Omnibus Reconciliation Act of 1980*. December 5, 1980.

Waters Y.: *Visiting Nursing in the United States* (New York, Charities Publication Committee, 1909), cited by Hanlon J.J.: *Public Health: Administration and Practice*, ed. 6. St. Louis, C.V. Mosby Co., 1974.

14

PATIENT EDUCATION

Hilda R. Glazer-Waldman, Ed.D.

As human disease has grown increasingly more complicated in the past half century, so has the problem of educating the public about illness and how to prevent it. That education process, though, has never been more important.

Lehmann, 1979

HEALTH EDUCATION, of which patient education is a component (as defined by the Task Force on Consumer Education), is receiving an increasing amount of attention by both health care practitioners and consumers. This is partly due to concern about the rapidly mounting costs of health care (Lehmann, 1979). Even more important is the focus on disease prevention and health promotion as evidenced by the Surgeon General's report on this topic, *Healthy People* (1979).

Patient education, defined as both the formal and the informal teaching provided by health practitioners, is becoming an integral part of health care. It is considered part of the patient care services rendered by all health professionals (AHA, 1979). Lehmann (1979) states that there are predictions that patient education or counseling will be an accepted and expected part of family health care and will be delivered increasingly by interdisciplinary teams of health care professionals.

The 1972–1973 joint Committee on Health Education Terminology (1974) defined patient education as those health experiences designed to influence learning that occur as a person receives preventive, diagnostic, therapeutic, and/or rehabilitative services. Although patient education is primarily carried out in a hospital setting and the primary patient educator is the nurse (Lehmann, 1979), patient education can occur in any situation in which the health care provider and the patient interact. All health professionals who have contact with patients have a potential role in their education (AHA, 1979). There are many situations in which patient education can occur. It can occur at bedside or in special rooms (either individually or in groups). Some hospitals broadcast patient education programs over closed circuit television (AHA, 1979). Patient education is not restricted to the patient but can extend to family members and friends. Increased knowledge and awareness of this support group are important not only during hospitalization but also following discharge.

The goals of patient education are varied: it can inform individuals about health, illness, and disability; it can help individuals achieve a higher level of health through skill training; and it can help people learn how to use the health care system more effectively and efficiently, which can lead to a reduction in health care costs. For the elderly patient, the most important goals may be to stabilize the level of health, stabilize or reduce dependency, and achieve and maintain an improved state of health (Filner and Williams, 1979).

One important aspect of patient education is learning. Patient education can be useful in helping the individual to develop or change habits so that he or she can take an active role in preventive care and/or health maintenance. One can gain knowledge; being better informed enables one to begin taking a greater degree of responsibility for health care. Additionally, factual information can help the individual to better understand the information he or she receives on diagnosis, treatment, and prognosis. Health beliefs and attitudes can be changed to better enable an individual to adapt to illness and health care.

A second component of patient education is the interaction that occurs between the educator and the patient. Regardless of the teaching, the sessions provide support for individuals who may be going through a difficult period. For the elderly patient, unaccustomed to or overwhelmed by the diversified maze of the health care system, the educator may be the one individual with whom a trusting relationship can be developed and from whom support and encouragement can be gained.

One result of patient education is often an increased compliance with the health care regimen. Increased patient compliance is a result not only of increased knowledge but also of changes in both attitudes and behavior. Thus, patient education encompasses these three areas: knowledge, behavior changes, and the attitude change that occurs concomitantly. The next part of this chapter focuses on the process for developing patient education materials.

A Developmental Scheme for Patient Education

Generally, a particular task is set for the patient educator. This task might be in the area of preparation for surgery, rehabilitation, skill training (self-administration of insulin), prerelease training, and so on. Often, patient education is part of the health care plan for the patient (Redman, 1980).

All patient education programs are designed to meet the needs of a particular patient. Ideally, when a patient education program has been developed for a particular task, skill, or knowledge area, the program will become a prototype for similar patient needs, and can then be revised as needed for a particular patient. A diabetes education program for example, could easily be modified and used again.

An initial step in designing a patient education program for a particular individual is to develop a list of goals and objectives. The overall goal of patient education is health behavior change accompanied by attitude change. With this goal in mind, there are specific objectives that might be set. Behavioral objectives include increasing knowledge of disease, increasing compliance with specific instructions or procedures, moving toward a stable or less pathologic health state, developing more appropriate use of health services, adjusting to the reality of the present health situation, increasing use of preventive health practices, or becoming a better health care consumer. Attitudinal objectives might include developing a better attitude toward oneself and one's capabilities, or developing a more positive attitude toward the health care system or toward seeking health care. The goals and objectives that are developed should be ones that are important *for* the patient and important *to* the patient. If this is to be accomplished, the patient must be provided with the opportunity for input into the selection and sequencing of objectives. Often, what the patient perceives as important does not match what the health provider sees as important. Although a common perception is desirable, this is often difficult to accomplish, as in preadmission and presurgery education. Having the educator and the patient reach a consensus on the importance of goals and objectives is one of the first steps toward developing a trusting, therapeutic relationship. Each objective should be broken down into its component parts: the relevant skills required to achieve the goal. This task provides the patient educator with the basis for the instructional design.

Next it is important to consider those factors that can influence the effectiveness of learning on the part of the patient; that is, readiness. Readiness is indicated by the ability to profit from a learning experience (Ausubel, Novak, and Hanesian, 1978). Factors that can influence readiness include comfort, energy level, motivation, education, sensory functioning, and learning ability.

Anything affecting the level of physical or psychological comfort or discomfort can also affect the ability to learn. Stress on the body, whether pleasant or unpleasant, if sufficiently intense can have an impact and interfere with the ability to learn. The energy level is affected by the physical condition, reaction to illness, medications, stress level, biorhythms, time of day, and mental state. If too high or too low, energy level can affect the ability to profit from learning. Often, an elderly patient is highly anxious about his or her illness and the prospects of recovery; this high level of anxiety may make it difficult for the patient to benefit from teaching.

Motivation must be taken into account as one attempts to make an instructional system work smoothly; it can significantly facilitate learning whenever it is present and operative. Additionally, if what is being taught relates to felt needs, long-term meaningful learning is more likely to occur (Ausubel et al., 1978). In terms of patient education, this means that the process of learning can be facilitated by setting goals that are motivating to the patient, by designing the curriculum so that individuals meet success frequently, and by providing support for patients thoughout the teaching-learning process.

There is a psychosocial process of adaptation to illness that can affect motivation and receptivity to patient education. In early stages of adaptation, denial may be present that can interfere with willingness to learn about one's illness, diagnosis, and prognosis, and willingness to comply with the prescribed regimen. This denial may be accompanied by a refusal to believe what he or she is told or by a distortion of information. Patient educators can help the patient move toward a more realistic understanding of the illness; as the patient begins to adapt to the illness, becoming more aware and accepting, he or she becomes more receptive to patient education and is better able to participate in his or her own care (Redman, 1980). Thus it is important that the patient educator is aware of the psychosocial state of the individual in developing a patient education program.

The individual's past experiences with the health care system, the value system, and the health belief model operating will also affect readiness to learn and willingness to accept patient education. Harwood (1981) has identified five major factors that contribute to variation in the health behavior and health beliefs of ethnic group members:

Exposure to biomedical and popular standards of health
Ethnic concepts of disease and illness in clinical care
How patients' evaluations of symptoms affect treatment
Coping with illness outside the mainstream medical system
Ethnic factors in encounters with mainstream medicine

Harwood (1981) notes that the health practitioner should evaluate each patient in terms of these factors to determine individual needs and the degree to which ethnic health standards and behaviors are likely to be relevant to treatment. Discussions with the patient should help the patient educator determine whether the patient's attitudes and values will affect learning in a positive or negative fashion.

There are a number of factors related to education that affect the teaching-learning situation. The most important of these is reading level; it is important that any materials intended for use by the patient be at a level that he or she can comprehend. Unfortunately, much patient education material is written at the ninth-grade reading level, or even higher, which may make it too difficult for a large segment of the adult population (Vivian and Robertson, 1980). Health information handouts must be readable if the patient is to learn from them (Holcomb, 1978) and to follow procedures explained. A number of techniques have been developed to help the practitioner determine the appropriateness of printed materials and the reading level, such as the Fog Index, the Fry Readability Graph, and the McLaughlin Smog Grading Formula (Vivian and Robertson, 1980). Leeper (1979) has suggested a reading level of grade 6.0 to grade 8.0; using this as a guide the patient educator can determine the level appropriate for each patient, taking into account the individual's facility with English and years of schooling.

An assessment of physical ability should also be made if the objectives include the learning of psychomotor skills. Determination should be made of height, weight, strength, coordination, and dexterity in relation to the task, regimen, and equipment involved (Narrow, 1979).

Level of sensory functioning is an important consideration when working with another individual in a teaching situation; this is especially so with an elderly patient. If one is unaware of visual handicaps, hearing loss, decreases in dexterity, and so on, the benefits of the learning experience may be lost and both the teacher and the learner will experience unnecessary frustration. A number of techniques can be used to facilitate the patient teaching situation once the areas of sensory loss have been identified. (A detailed description of sensory loss can be found in chap. 9.)

Different individuals learn at different rates regardless of age. This should be taken into account when developing a patient education program. Not all patients will progress through a program at the same rate. Thus, the timing and sequencing of instruction must be tailored to individual patients and the educator must be prepared to make changes during instruction when necessary. In the area of learning ability, there are a number of factors that should be considered when working with the elderly.

First, a slowing of motor functioning is not to be automatically equated with decreased learning ability; when older people can pace their own learning, there are no significant age-related differences in this ability. The elderly as well as the young benefit from increased study time, and even more so when time is available to search for, recover, and produce a response (Arenberg and Robertson-Tchabo, 1977). Second, the response rate of the elderly is often lower and their reaction time slower; these are not the result of a lack of motivation (Welford, 1977). It is important not to rush the elderly patient; this may result in frustration and as a consequence may decrease motivation. Thus, there may be a reluctance to learn because of a fear of failure. Frustration and confusion can be reduced by simplifying the environment and the tasks demanded of the elderly person (Lidz, 1976). The amount and content of material should be set so as to reduce the potential for failure and increase the opportunity for success.

Studies have shown that some patients will not understand what is expected of them (Becker, 1979). The problem may be in the communication of information, recall of information, or both. There is a difference between true noncompliance and forgetting; it is necessary for the patient educator to distinguish between them. Remember, the elderly can learn but it may take longer. What you may perceive as slow learning could be a result of sensory loss that you have not taken into account.

An elderly patient may verbalize understanding even when he or she does not understand, simply to avoid the embarrassment of asking questions. Patient educators can determine the level of understanding just by asking the right questions; for instance, it is better to ask patients to repeat what they understand than to ask if they understood. Take time to deal with each question. The elderly tend to be overcautious so it is up to you to make them feel comfortable. Be sure not to rush through a session; this can diminish understanding and lead to confusion.

Self-image may affect readiness to learn. If the patient does not perceive himself as benefiting from patient education, then he will probably not be willing to participate. A negative view of one's abilities and potential for improvement will also be detrimental. For example, if a patient who is confined to a wheelchair feels that he will never be able to function adequately out of the wheelchair, or believes it is not important to function independently of the wheelchair, then in all probability that person will not be receptive to patient education geared toward rehabilitation and independence from the wheelchair.

Designing the Curriculum

Once objectives have been set and readiness examined, the educator can begin to design the curriculum. There are a number of excellent references to guide the patient educator in designing instruction (e.g., Dick and Carey, 1978; McCormick and Gilson Parkevich, 1979; Freedman, 1978). Rather than providing a step-by-step procedure, the following section will give the reader some general guidelines for instructional design as it applies to patient education.

Analysis of the objectives will aid in determining the content to be taught. The health care provider must keep in mind those factors that can negatively affect learning and try to minimize them when planning the curriculum. Sequencing of objectives is important to both smooth progression and the achievement of outcomes. The patient educator must be sure that objectives are sequenced in the correct order, taking into account necessary prerequisites for progressing from one aspect to the next. Sequencing should consider priority objectives of the patient. When felt needs do not match medical priorities, it may still be advisable to deal with the patient's priorities early on to promote a sense of visible success in meeting goals seen as important. The following factors should also be considered: the importance of the patient's performing an aspect of therapy, areas that produce a great deal of anxiety for the patient, the degree of difficulty of integrating the activity into daily living, the amount of time available for patient education, and support services available after discharge (AHA, 1979). Content relevant to each objective then becomes the basis for instruction.

Instructional Strategy

Dick and Carey (1978) list five major components of the instructional strategy: preinstructional activities, information presentation, patient participation, evaluation, and follow-through.

Preinstructional Activities

Preinstructional activities are those designed to motivate the student. The practice of reaching agreement on objectives with the patient is a part of this activity, since through the objectives the patient will have an understanding of the tasks ahead. Another preinstructional activity may entail showing the patient what he or she will be able to do when the learning tasks have been completed; a demonstration film or slide-tape might be shown here as a means of demonstrating the course of activities and expected outcomes. These and similar activities are motivating and attention-getting and can serve as a positive initial experience in patient education.

Information Presentation

Information presentation involves making final decisions on sequencing and on the amount of material to be presented at each session. In determining the size of the "chunk," a number of factors should be considered. The first is the type of learning activity and whether the activity can be varied; regardless of age, if information presentation is varied and combined with other learning activities, individuals do not seem to tire of the activity as quickly (Dick and Carey, 1978). Knowledge of the patient will also help the educator make decisions about chunking. It may be necessary to alter the schedule during a particular session in response to the way the patient feels or responds at the time.

Information can be presented through a wide variety of teaching methods used either singly or in combination, such as handouts, lectures, independent study, discussion, demonstration, role-playing, and audiovisual aids. Choice of method is determined by the type of information being presented. For example, if training is on self-injection of insulin, a film might be shown, followed by a detailed step-by-step description, followed by a demonstration, and then reinforced by handouts detailing the procedure in words and diagrams.

Handouts should also be developed, for example, stickers, information sheets, checklists, wallet-sized cards. They can include a step-by-step explanation of the task or skill, medication information, side effects the patient should be aware of, and a name and phone number to call if there are problems with the procedure (AHA, 1979). Vivian and Robertson (1980) have suggested the following guidelines to aid in developing understandable patient education materials:

1. Make sentences as short as possible.
2. Select words of one or two syllables rather than longer words.
3. Underline, capitalize, or highlight technical or difficult words.
4. Paraphrase technical terms into popular language.
5. Double-space rather than single-space.
6. Leave margins unadjusted to provide readers with a reference point for continuing to the next line.
7. Use large type to make the print more readable for sight-impaired patients.
8. Aim reading level at fifth grade or lower. Use a variety of formulas to determine reading levels.
9. Test materials on a sample population before general use.

Patient Participation

The next component of the instructional strategy is patient participation. This must include both the opportunity for practice and feedback about performance. Repetition enhances learning. Shortly after initial learning has occurred practice enables the patient to consolidate the material and ensures that he will learn the various components in the proper sequence. This is extremely important in skill learning, where it is essential that all steps are carried out in the proper order, such as learning the steps for performing bronchial drainage. During practice, the patient educator provides feedback to the patient, reinforcing correct responses and retraining incorrect ones. The importance of positive reinforcement cannot be overemphasized; without it, the patient is unlikely to continue. Positive reinforcement increases the likelihood that the behavior in question will be repeated. Its use must be justified and should follow closely the correct response. Early in practice, the educator should reinforce behaviors that more closely approximate the desired response than previous ones did. Knowing that some responses are correct will be helpful to the patient. All individuals need to feel that they are doing at least some things correctly if they are to continue with a task. Continual frustration and disappointment may lead to a negative attitude toward patient education and the ability to learn.

Another important consideration is that initial learning often takes place in the hospital or clinic, whereas the patient will be performing the newly learned skill in another setting, probably without the patient educator present. A good example of this is insulin injection and urine testing, which are part of diabetic education. The patient should have an opportunity to practice in a variety of situations so that he or she is comfortable performing the skill wherever he or she may be. If a family member or friend is to assist the patient, that individual should also be given the opportunity to practice with him; for example, training a coach (relative or friend) to assist a COPD patient with breathing exercises (Schneider, 1980). Involving family and friends will often increase compliance. Continued opportunity for practice, review, and feedback should be provided—these activities help ensure learning. The amount of practice that occurs will have to be determined individually to meet the needs of the patient, as will the duration of a particular session. Practice is most effective when sessions are relatively short and there is rest between them. In designing the program, it may be beneficial to provide for a few short practice sessions interspersed with other activities.

The matter of prompting and guidance during practice is another consideration. Prompting is more necessary and effective in the earlier stages of learning, where it can prevent guesswork and the learning of errors. It is important that the conditions of practice gradually begin to approximate the desired end product; thus, as the amount of correct learning increases, the number of prompts should be reduced and replaced by feedback (Ausubel et al., 1978).

Evaluation

Evaluation is an essential component of any instructional unit. Primarily, there are two types of evaluations that should be performed. The first is formative evaluation, which is the process to increase the efficiency and the effectiveness of instructional materials; that is, make necessary revisions (Dick and Carey, 1978). There are numerous kinds of information that the patient educator can collect to aid in this process, including comments made by patients on areas that were particularly difficult to understand, ability to understand directions, and general reactions to the program (sequencing, relevance of objectives, and so on). The reactions of other health care practitioners to the instructional materials are also helpful. It is often beneficial to have some other health care provider review the instructional materials before using them; another person can often help isolate potential problem areas. In the course of instruction, the patient educator will often identify areas that need revision. Some revisions may be made during instruction—such as timing, sequencing, and rewording of instructions—and later incorporated into the instructional design. Any audiovisual aid used in instruction should be evaluated as to effectiveness and appropriateness both prior to and following instruction. Stein (1979) has developed a system (MERL) to select and evaluate media for patient education. The primary components of media evaluation are quality of the message, congruences with patient needs and characteristics, appropriateness of the learning environment, and effectiveness in eliciting a specific response. Additionally, the American Hospital Association (1979) has developed worksheets for media review that can easily be adapted for use in any setting. Ongoing evaluation of media will aid in developing quality patient education programs.

Assessment of the patient's progress is an important component of the evaluation of any patient education program. This is generally achieved by comparing the patient's results of instruction with the desired results as defined by the objectives. The following evaluation questions can be asked: Was the patient able to achieve the objectives in the time allotted? Were there any objectives that the patient was unable to achieve due to lack of readiness, poor instruction, and/or medical reasons? Were any of the objectives not met due to noncompliance on the part of the patient?

An evaluation checklist can assist the patient educator to review and revise instruction. The checklist might include the following questions: Was instruction interesting? Did the patient understand the goals and objectives? Was the reading level appropriate for the patient? Was there suffi cient opportunity for practice and feedback? Was the medium appropriate? Were any instructional areas unclear? Were timing and sequencing appropriate?

Follow-Through

Follow-through activities in patient education are very important. If the patient has not met the objectives, the patient educator may have to follow the initial instruction with remedial activities, which should be presented in a different way in order to optimize learning. Learning activities may need to be repeated at a later date when the patient or the family is less anxious or under less stress and can benefit from the session (Narrow, 1979). Additionally, the patient, in the course of medical treatment, may have setbacks that can interfere with participation in patient education and make it necessary for the educator to review or reteach certain areas.

When implementing the patient education program for an elderly person, there are a number of tactics that can be used to enhance the probability of success. An elderly person's sense of security, control, and orientation to the environment can be heightened if there is a set schedule of appointments, little variation in the appointment time from day to day, and the routine is stabilized (Purtilo, 1978).

When beginning a session, it is important to develop rapport with the individual. A few minutes of conversation can help relieve anxiety and show the patient that the educator is someone who has a genuine interest in her or him. Once rapport has been established, it will be easier to motivate the patient and to progress through the activities of the session.

Learning Through Patient Education

A number of different types of learning may occur in patient education: factual information, habits (skills), and attitudes.

The learning of factual information is an important educational objective (Klausmeier and Ripple, 1971). Information can be obtained directly through observing environmental objects and events, gained verbally by hearing what others say, absorbed by reading (Klausmeier and Ripple, 1971), or acquired through a variety of media. Patient educators should check for the accuracy of factual knowledge and be quick to correct misconceptions. It is important to help patients acquire new information relative to their illness, health maintenance, the health care system, and so on. Increased knowledge enables us to function more effectively.

Most of the training that will occur in the context of patient education will be the teaching of psychomotor skills. The reestablishment of skills lost through stroke, training in self-administration of insulin, or the taking of blood pressure may be the primary goals of patient education. There are a number of principles that relate to the teaching of motor skills:

1. Observing and imitating a model facilitates initial learning of skill movements.
2. Verbalizing a set of instructions enhances the early phase of skill learning.
3. Practice facilitates the learning of skills through eliminating errors and strengthening and refining correct responses and form.
4. Securing feedback facilitates skills learning by providing knowledge of results.
5. Evaluating one's own performance makes possible the continued improvement of skills (Klausmeier and Ripple, 1971).

Narrow (1979) suggests that the patient's perception of how he or she learns is important to the educator teaching a psychomotor skill. A patient's self-knowledge will help the patient educator to develop the most efficient and effective teaching method for that individual

Attitude learning and attitude change are important objectives in patient training. An attitude is an acquired, internal state that predisposes action toward a particular class of objects, events, or persons (Gagné, 1975). Attitudes may be acquired or changed as a result of acquiring factual information; some information will strengthen the attitude and some will support an alternative position (Travers, 1977). When a person reassesses his or her attitude toward an important issue such as the health care system, the assessment may involve a review of the relevant information the individual has acquired (Travers, 1977). By checking the accuracy of the patient's information, the patient educator can help foster positive attitudes. Attitudes may be acquired directly as the result of successful experiences on the part of the learner (Gagné, 1975). One effect of this is generalization. A positive attitude toward a patient education experience may generalize to a positive attitude toward health care.

Attitudes are acquired indirectly through modeling, where the patient observes the behavior and attitude of another and views this model as being rewarded for the behavior. The learner is reinforced indirectly, "vicariously." This increases the likelihood that the learner will perform in a manner similar to that of the model (Gagné, 1975). The implication of this for the patient educator is that by demonstrating a positive attitude toward patient education and health care he can have a positive effect on the attitude of the patient.

The patient educator will, in all likelihood, be the primary agent of attitude change. Travers (1977) has suggested some of the characteristics of effective communication for producing attitude change. The more the communicator is perceived as being an expert and as being trustworthy, the greater is the immediate effect on attitudes. A clear presentation of the facts is important. Messages should attract attention if they are to have an impact. The patient educator should be aware of the effects of his or her communication on the patient and how the nature of the communication will affect attitude change.

The emotional support of family and friends is also important. When the patient leaves the hospital, he or she for the most part is leaving behind a support network. Family and friends will, it is hoped, be able to fill this gap, providing encouragement, reinforcement, and support for the patient following discharge. This is particularly important for the elderly.

The family may need to help the patient to follow the regimen established in the hospital, for example, by reminding him to take drugs or to follow dietary restrictions. It may be difficult for the individual to remain on a diet if the person who prepares the meals is unaware or uncooperative.

There are a number of community-based agencies that can provide support services for both the patient and the family, such as visiting nurses and home health agencies. These people work with the patient in the home to maintain the level of skill performance gained in the hospital and can check on compliance with prescribed regimens. The hospital-based patient educator should initiate contact with the community-based health professionals.

At-Home Care

Final evaluation of most patient education rests on the ability of the patient to function adequately following discharge. There are a number of factors that can influence this, including the effectiveness of the teaching, the availability of family and friends to assist the patient, and the use of community resources available to the patient.

Perhaps the most crucial aspect of the use of family and friends to assist the patient is selection. Talabere (1979) suggests the following guidelines: willingness of the person to participate in patient care, geographic proximity of the patient and potential helper, the person's resources (time, energy, and transportation), and the patient's feelings about having this individual involved. Unfortunately, gains toward self-care made in the hospital can be lost if the person who assists does for the patient the things he or she can do without help. The patient educator should help those who are assisting the patient to gain an understanding of their role, and advise them of the prescribed regimen and other information necessary for follow-up.

On return clinic or hospital visits, the patient educator has an opportunity to personally follow up with a reevaluation of knowledge, skills, or performance of a procedure. In some instances retraining may be necessary. Narrow (1979) suggests use of a follow-up questionnaire mailed 1 or 2 months after the end of the sessions and again after 6 or 12 months. She suggests that the questions be designed to reveal changes in lifestyle or attitude, compliance with prescribed regimens, adherence to procedures, and areas of difficulty and concern. This information can be used in planning additional sessions with the patient and in revision of patient education programs. One effective follow-up procedure is for the health provider to ask for a telephone report at one- or two-week intervals. This can be an opportunity to both answer and ask questions and to check on compliance. The telephone calls can be arranged in advance, with the patient being told to have questions ready.

Compliance

Generally, 30% to 35% of patients fail to comply with therapeutic regimens (Redman, 1980). Failure to follow a diet and failure to take medications are two common areas of noncompliance. With the elderly, a great deal of noncompliance may be due to faulty short-term memory; the patient may not remember if he or she has taken the drugs. Visual problems may also be a factor. The individual who is unable to read labels on cans may be unable to determine whether the food inside is on the diet. When possible, the patient educator should devise methods for helping the patient to remember to take medications and should try to enlist the aid of family members, friends, and community support services. Hour-by-hour activity schedule boards can be set up for the patient so that he can check off columns if necessary; time for medications, physical therapy, meals, recreation, and so forth, can be included. Nut cups might be used to hold medications; these can be made up for a number of days at a time so the patient can see at a glance if all medications were taken or if a day was missed. Continuing contact by health practitioners is one way to increase adherence and to avoid or resolve problems.

Conclusions

Patient education is integral to health care. An interdisciplinary approach to patient education is necessary and should be based on sound educational principles. The importance of health education, and therefore of patient education, as one part of health education has been recognized by the American Hospital Association (1975):

> The major emphasis of health education is health promotion, which includes health maintenance, disease and trauma management, and the improvement of the health care system and its utilization. Through health education programs, hospitals and other health care institutions can contribute to important health care goals, such as improved quality of patient care, better utilization of outpatient services, fewer admissions and readmissions to inpatient facilities, shorter lengths of stay, and reduced health care costs.

REFERENCES

American Hospital Association: *Health Education: Role and Responsibility of Health Care Institutions*. Chicago, American Hospital Association, 1975.

American Hospital Association: *Implementing Patient Education in the Hospital*. Chicago, American Hospital Association, 1979.

Arenberg D., Robertson-Tchabo E.A.: Learning and aging, in Birren J.E., Schaie K.W. (eds.): *Handbook of the Psychology of Aging*. New York, Van Nostrand Reinhold, 1977.

Ausubel D.P., Novak J.D., Hanesian H.: *Educational Psychology: A Cognitive View*, ed. 2. New York, Holt, Rinehart & Winston, 1978.

Becker M.H.: Understanding patient compliance, in Cohen S.J. (ed.): *New Directions in Patient Compliance*. Lexington, Mass., Lexington Books, 1979.

Dick W., Carey L.: *The Systematic Design of Instruction*. Glenview, Il., Scott Foresman and Co., 1978.
Filner B., Williams T.F.: Health promotion for the elderly, in *Healthy People: The Surgeon General's Report on Health Promotion and Disease Prevention, Background Papers*. U.S. Department of Health, Education and Welfare, Public Health Service, Publication No. 79-55071A. U.S. Government Printing Office, 1979.
Freedman C.R.: *Teaching Patients*. San Diego, Courseware, Inc., 1978.
Gagné R.M.: *Essentials of Learning for Instruction*, expanded ed. Hinsdale, Ill., Dryden Press, 1975.
Harwood A. (ed.): *Ethnicity and Medical Care*. Cambridge, Mass., Harvard University Press, 1981.
Holcomb C.A., Ellis J.K.: The cloze procedure. *Health Educ*. 9:8–10, 1978.
Klausmeier H.J., Ripple R.E.: *Learning and Human Abilities*, ed. 3. New York, Harper & Row, 1971.
Leeper E.K.: Writing a helping hand: The art and technique, in McCormick R.D., Gilson-Parkevich T. (eds.): *Patient and Family Education: Tools, Techniques and Theory*. New York, John Wiley & Sons, 1979.
Lehmann P.: Health education, in *Healthy People: The Surgeon General's Report on Health Promotion and Disease Prevention, Background Papers*. U.S. Department of Health, Education and Welfare, Public Health Service, Publication no. 79-55071A. U.S. Government Printing Office, 1979.
Lidz T.: *The Person: His and Her Development Throughout the Life Cycle*, revised. New York, Basic Books, 1976.
McCormick, R.D., Gilson Parkevich T. (eds.): *Patient and Family Education: Tools, Techniques and Theory*. New York, John Wiley & Sons, 1979.
Narrow B.W.: *Patient Teaching in Nursing Practice*. New York, John Wiley & Sons, 1979.
Purtilo R.: *Health Professional/Patient Interaction*, ed. 2. Philadelphia, W.B. Saunders Co., 1978.
Redman B.K.: Report of the 1972–1973 Joint Committee on Health Education Terminology. *J. School Health*, January 1974.
Redman B.K.: *The Process of Patient Teaching in Nursing*, ed. 4. St. Louis, Mo., C.V. Mosby Co., 1980.
Schneider G.N.: Using audiovisual aids in COPD—patient-education programs. *Respir. Ther*. 81–84, September, 1980.
Stein D.: Selecting and evaluating media for patient education. *J. Biocommun*. 6:22–26, 1979.
Talabere L.R.: The challenge of patient and family teaching, in McCormick R.D., Gilson-Parkevich T. (eds.): *Patient and Family Education: Tools, Techniques, and Theory*. New York, John Wiley & Sons, 1979.
Travers R.M.W.: *Essentials of Learning*, ed. 4. New York, Macmillan Publishing Co., 1977.
U.S. Department of Health, Education and Welfare, Public Health Service. *Healthy People: The Surgeon General's Report on Health Promotion and Disease Prevention, Background Papers*. Publication No. 79-55071A. U.S. Government Printing Office, 1979.
Vivian A.S., Robertson E.J.: Readability of patient education materials. *Clin. Ther*. 3:129–136, 1980.
Welford A.T.: Motor performance, in Birren J.E., Schaie K.W. (eds.): *Handbook of the Psychology of Aging*. New York, Van Nostrand Reinhold, 1977.

15

THERAPEUTIC INTERVENTIONS WITH THE ELDERLY

Helen L. West, Ph.D.

THE NEED FOR institutionalized care has been changing in character. Historically, society has arranged to care for the poor and the sick who had no one to care for them, through either bed and board in exchange for work or extended hospital care for those with incurable diseases. Social reforms at the beginning of this century attempted to improve this situation. During the depression of the 1930s, public assistance became a necessary way of life. Congress passed the original Social Security Act in 1935. Since World War II, long-term care of the aged has been the object of legislative enactments, including Title XVIII (Medicare) and Title XIX (Medicaid) of the Social Security Act.

These legislative developments resulted in care and treatment that are primarily medical, even when the older person has many needs for care and treatment in other areas. This is the natural consequence of Medicare's definitions of the kinds of care that are reimbursable, since nonmedical needs are not covered by the program. Many persons are now living to age 80 and 90 and require long-term care; this group often presents the health care provider with complex medical and social problems. Often, the quality of life depends as much on ancillary care as on medical treatment. Quality of medical care is improving, therefore longevity increases, but the general degenerative processes of the very old continue and the extra years of life are often spent as a patient.

What is true of the institutionalized individual is true to a relative degree of the community-based older person needing care. There are numerous semimedical interventions that not only improve the quality of life greatly for many elderly, but can help prevent some problems and work to facilitate medical care. The work of Abraham Maslow serves to illustrate this quite well. Patients need care or service related to where they perceive themselves to be on a hierarchy of needs (1962). This perception may or may not be congruent with the health professional's assessment of the patient. The physician may be concerned with an individual's high-risk status for stroke while the older patient may be far more concerned with the psychological impact of resorting to use of a hearing aid.

Rehabilitation medicine is one large area of care where this thesis holds true. It is a social phenomenon that developed from enlightened approaches to man and his disabilities. The word "care" comes from the Latin *caritas,* meaning respect, esteem, affection, and value. It represents the shift from viewing the impaired person as an impediment to the good of the group, and therefore to be avoided or abandoned, to a concern for the well-being and social integration of the disabled. This parallels the modern movement in traditional medicine from treating the disease to treating the patient. Thus, current health care interventions assist the patient in making optimal psychological, social, and economic adjustments. It is now more than a philosophy, it is a dynamic process of restoring the capacity of the disabled person to sense and participate in the environment and communicate with others; to adapt to the physical world and its requirements of physical energy expenditure while resuming the activities of daily living; to utilize fully intellectual, social, and vocational potentials. It is the process of functional restoration of the chronically ill or disabled to a normal life style. The major components of rehabilitation are medical restoration and maintenance of health along with social, psychological, and economic adjustment. Not all patients benefit equally. Rehabilitation depends on thorough evaluation and assessment of residual abilities and compensatory adaptation. Complicating potential treatment is the fact that chronic disease can bring to the surface personality problems that were masked or controlled before the onset of illness but which may increase to the point of being major obstacles to satisfactory adjustment during illness or disability.

Secondary gains to the patient from remaining ill or disabled may also interfere with optimal recovery of functional capacity. In this regard, one must consider a host of variables surrounding the family and community in which patients exist. Patients are an integral part of a system of human interaction and role assignment, and health status plays an important part in their homeostasis. For example, older persons may perceive themselves as very ill and thus require family members to provide large time commitments for social interaction and physical health. As illness recedes, the older person may continue to demand the time by not recognizing improvement in health and by not attempting to return to normal status.

Geriatric rehabilitation is essentially the same as rehabilitation of the general population—with one important difference. This process must be modified to comply with the physiology and the psychosociology of the aging patient. The natural decline in physiologic functions must be considered in both assessment and expectation. Aging is not a disease process;

there is no illness exclusive to old age. Older people, however, have more than a proportionate share of disabling diseases. In addition, they usually have one or more chronic illnesses along with some disability. Age-related changes in learning and perception make progress slow, but results are usually very encouraging for practitioners with understanding and patience. For older patients, restorative goals probably do not include vocational rehabilitation outcomes. Activities of daily living become primary areas of focus. When the older patient has attained maximum performance in self-sufficiency, as well as the best psychosocial adjustment possible, he or she may be considered rehabilitated. Maintaining this level of self-sufficiency and adjustment is the challenge. However, reaching such goals with the elderly may reflect a relatively greater gain than helping younger patients attain a goal of returning to work.

One of the major deterrents to successful intervention with the elderly patient is the nonspecific therapeutic tool called *bed rest*. It is very often prescribed and practiced despite its dangers to the elderly. These dangers include the threat of hypostatic pneumonia, thrombosis and thromboembolism, pressure points and decubiti, muscle contractures, osteoporosis, urinary calculi, dyspepsia, and constipation. In addition, mental changes occur, due to the demoralizing effects of staying in bed, along with the sensory deprivation suffered. Such adverse effects are much better prevented than reversed.

Let us look, now, at the major therapeutic interventions commonly used with older patients. These range from physical therapy, through occupational therapy, speech-language therapy, audiology, reality orientation and attitude therapy, to remotivation therapy and recreation therapy. Each has a special contribution to make to the well-being of elderly patients. Physical therapy begins the return to independence, as does occupational therapy. Speech-language therapy and audiology restore communication abilities. Reality orientation and attitude therapy improve mental functioning, while remotivation therapy and recreation therapy are concerned with general psychosocial good health.

Physical Therapy

Physical therapy is defined as the use of physical means to reduce pain and to maintain or improve physical function. Its purpose is to provide individuals with the opportunity to achieve and maintain the highest level of body functioning possible, in order to remain as independently mobile as their condition will allow.

The goal of physical therapy focuses on maintaining, improving, or restoring functions of the neuromusculoskeletal, pulmonary, and cardiovascular systems through physical procedures of intervention. Specific objectives include (1) providing active and passive exercise for increasing strength, endurance, coordination, and range of motion; (2) facilitating activities of daily living; (3) stimulating motor activity and learning; and (4) applying physical agents to relieve pain or alter physiologic status.

Generally, and especially for Medicare and Medicaid purposes, physical therapy services are provided as part of a treatment regimen designed by a physician after consultation with a qualified physical therapist. The services are performed under the supervision of such a therapist. If the supervision is not directly with the patient, then a qualified assistant is given initial direction and periodic review. Physical therapy services are provided with the expectation that the patient will improve, based on an assessment of restorative potential, or with the understanding that such services are necessary to proper management of a specific state.

The scope of physical rehabilitation of the elderly can provide a continuum of care, beginning with prevention, through screening in the community, crisis intervention, short- and/or long-term rehabilitation, and ending with maintenance in a long-term care situation. Emphasis is placed on mobility (i.e., walking, stair climbing, use of assistive devices, coordination, posture); response to chronic or ongoing injury or disease trigger points, pain patterns, substitution of one muscle group for another, and range of motion changes.

In working with the elderly, the most common problems are encountered as a result of disabilities associated with arthritis, amputation, neurologic problems, and orthopedics. Unlike the general population, less common areas of disability are also seen, related to oncology and psychiatry.

For the relief of pain, common agents used include heat, massage, and immersion. When improved function is the desired result, exercise, training, and stretching are employed. In some instances, ultraviolet radiation is used as a germicide and rubefacient (counterirritant). Cold is used to raise the threshold of pain, and water to ease motion by reducing the effect of gravity. Electricity can be used to contract or fatigue muscles.

Occupational Therapy

Occupational therapy is called "the art and science of directing man's response to selected activity to promote and maintain health, to prevent disability, to evaluate behavior and to treat or train patients with physicial or psychosocial dysfunction" (Wiemer and West, 1970). Its purpose is to provide patients with an opportunity to develop and maintain the capacity, throughout their life span, to perform with satisfaction to self and others those tasks and roles essential to productive living and to the mastery of self and the environment.

The goal of occupational therapy focuses on the development of adaptive skills and performance capacity in activities of daily living and in the goal-directed use of time, energy, interest, and attention. Specific objectives include (1) the selection of tasks to restore, reinforce, and enhance performance; (2) facilitation of learning of skills and functions essential for adaptation and productivity; (3) diminishing or correcting pathology; and (4) promoting and maintaining health.

Generally, occupational therapy services are furnished as the result of an evaluation, through the use of diagnostic and prognostic tests, of the patient's level of function. Depending on the evaluation, certain task-oriented activities are selected to be taught to patients. These individualized treatment programs are subsequently supervised, progress is noted, and re-evaluation is performed when required. Only a qualified occupational therapist has the knowledge and training necessary to evaluate the patient and develop a plan of treatment. Implementation of the treatment program may be carried out by a qualified occupational therapist assistant functioning under the supervision and review of a qualified occupational therapist.

Restoring physical function through selection and teaching of task-oriented therapeutic activities is a common procedure. In addition, it is often necessary to restore sensory-integrative function, where the occupational therapist selects tasks and activities that increase sensory input and improve response. Often this is done with a stroke patient whose functional loss has resulted in a distorted body image. Other areas of practice include teaching compensatory techniques to improve the level of independence in activities of daily living. Examples are teaching a patient who has lost the use of an arm how to peel potatoes and chop vegetables with one hand, and teaching a paraplegic or hemiplegic new techniques to enable him or her to perform feeding, dressing, and other activities as independently as possible. Another area of activity for the occupational therapist involves designing, fabricating, and fitting of orthotic and self-help devices. This might involve making a hand splint for a patient with rheumatoid arthritis to maintain the hand in a functional position or constructing a device that would enable him to hold a utensil and feed himself independently.

Since the elderly must adapt to decreasing functional ability because of the aging process itself, in addition to any losses due to disabilities, occupational therapy aids in the adaptation process as well as in the rehabilitative process. This is done through direct service to patients in hospitals and institutions and to the elderly in the community, and through indirect service in the areas of education, consultation, and political action.

Speech-Language Therapy

Speech-language therapy is defined as the scientific study of human communication and the evaluation and treatment of communicative disorders. It is based on the belief that the ability of an individual to engage in reciprocal communication is vital to his psychological health and is often pivotal in the rehabilitation process.

The goal of speech and language therapy relates to individual communication, social, and emotional needs, and aims at helping patients cope with these needs while maximizing and maintaining communication skills for independent living, emotional adjustment, and effective environmental contact. Specific objectives include correcting or ameliorating dysfunctions of speech transmission and speech reception.

Speech pathologists are very often referred by neurologists or other physicians and specialists working in a hospital or long-term care facility. They evaluate the nature and severity of the speech and language impairment by measuring an individual's performance against "normal" communication behavior of the cultural community and/or against the patient's premorbid life. Treatment is performed by a qualified speech pathologist. The scope of speech-language therapy includes (1) assessment of linguistic behavior through diagnostic examination using formal tests of vocabulary, language comprehension and expression, and level of linguistic development; (2) assessment of linguistic behavior through evaluation of articulation, voice, and fluency; and (3) diagnostic assessments of speech-related health in terms of physical structures and functional speech adequacy, sensory-motor, perceptual, and learning responses, and psychosocial and environmental variables related to communicative functioning. These evaluative procedures result in the establishment and implementation of a comprehensive plan of treatment. When language disorders are considered, the pathologist will facilitate linguistic recovery of basic vocabulary and grammar and assist with problems of comprehension, short-term memory, judgment, verbal disinhibition, language production, and related impairments. Speech disorders usually involve modifying articulation, developing more efficient vocal behavior, and controlling or accommodating dysarthria. Common problems facing the elderly that require speech therapy include aphasia, apraxia or dysarthria, language disorders, articulation disorders, cerebral palsy, voice disorders, neurologic disorders, cancer-related disorders, and cleft palate. Patients are referred by a physician, but only those whose medical condition precludes participation in therapy would be excluded from an evaluation.

Audiology (Nonsurgical Aural Rehabilitation)

Audiology is the scientific study of hearing and its disorders, the evaluation of hearing impairments and habilitation or rehabilitation of the communication abilities of hearing-impaired individuals. It is based on the belief that individuals need to receive communication in order to enjoy psychological health and to retain the capacity for self-expression through speech. The goal of aural rehabilitation is to help the hearing-impaired individual adjust to the loss, to learn alternative methods of communicating, and to select and use a hearing aid if indicated. Specific objectives include hearing aid evaluations, hearing aid orientation and counseling, and communication rehabilitation, including auditory training and speech reading.

In most settings, the audiologist serves as a member of a clinical staff and functions through referral. The audiologist performs a basic audiometric evaluation that may include such tests as pure tone air-conduction and bone-conduction thresholds, speech reception thresholds, and speech discrimination measurements. Testing may be done to evaluate the site of lesion, for functional hearing loss, and to determine requirements for amplification. Reevaluation of user performance with recommended hearing amplification may consist of retesting in the manner of the original hearing amplification evaluation. Treatment procedures include individual or group habilitation sessions consisting of hearing-aid orientation, auditory training, speech reading, and speech conversation. The audiologist may also counsel patients and their family members.

Common problems encountered when working with the elderly include the following:

1. Sensorineural hearing loss.
2. Congenital disorders—anomalies and diseases.
3. Presbycusis—a progressive hearing impairment of the inner ear caused by deterioration of nerve ends, resulting primarily from the aging process.
4. Acoustic trauma—hearing impairments caused by accidents, exposure to excessive noise concentrations, and shock waves.
5. Ototoxic disorders—hearing impairments caused by exposure to chemical-industrial compounds, and diseases such as diphtheria, scarlet fever, dysenteries, and brucellosis.
6. Vascular disorders—vascular disruptions such as hemorrhages, thromboses, embolisms, including Ménière's disease.
7. Disorders of the VIIIth nerve—hearing loss caused by damage to the VIIIth cranial nerve (the prime conductive nerve of hearing to the

brain); diseases such as meningitis and tumors are frequent sources of these types of impairments.

Reality Orientation and Attitude Therapy

Reality orientation and attitude therapy are techniques used to rehabilitate elderly and brain-damaged patients with moderate to severe disorientation. These techniques have been developed to attempt to remedy the pathologic withdrawal and mental deterioration that are often features in the total aging process.

The primary goal of reality orientation is to reduce the confusion and disorientation experienced by some elderly. Specific objectives include continuous stimulation of patients by repetitive orientation to the environment and placing them in a group of people where they can meet and compete with other patients and can be taken out of their isolation.

Reality orientation is implemented on two levels. A patient's general environment offers a reality base in the form of signs, clocks, calendars, and nameplates that continually identify the place, date, time of day, next meal, and/or coming activity. The patient is always addressed by his/or her name and reminded of the name of the person that is talking. The other aspect of reality orientation consists of structured classes, conducted on a daily basis, that patients attend in very small groups for short periods of time. Exercises are provided to reinforce orientation for time and place, to assist in self-identification and recognition of others, and gradually to introduce other objects for identification. Sensory stimulation plays a major role in these exercises. Patients experience and identify different tastes, touch sensations, sounds, and visual stimuli. As an adjunct to reality orientation, attitude therapy is employed to provide a consistency of interpersonal approach and to modify behaviors. Attitudes are prescribed on an individual basis according to five major behaviors: "Kind firmness" is used with depressed or otherwise uncooperative patients who must be gently yet firmly coerced into action. The attitude of "passive friendliness" is used with patients who are fearful and suspicious of others. Since these patients often withdraw from any attempts to reach out, assistance cannot be pressed on them but must be made clearly available whenever needed. "Active friendliness" is appropriate with the apathetic and withdrawn patient, where the use of constant overtures and offers may spark some response. Patients who are demanding and querulous are treated with a "matter-of-fact" attitude that promotes the notion of taking responsibility for one's own behavior. Finally, there is the "no demand" attitude for the angry, frantic patient who has lost the usual defenses and is out of control. Ventilation and acting out are allowed, provided no harm is done to the patient or others, in a supervised but undemanding atmosphere.

Remotivation Therapy

Remotivation therapy is a technique of very simple group therapy. It is objective in nature and designed to make reality a pleasant experience and to restore a sense of self-worth to the patient. The rationale behind this form of therapy is that patients have healthy, untouched areas of personality that often have to do with everyday ordinary living. Sharing this objective world with the patient may make him or her open to more intensive therapy.

The overall goals of remotivation therapy include combating dehumanization; developing an interest in the objective, outside world; stimulating the healthy areas of personality; and developing constructive recall abilities. Specific objectives include building a sense of worth by drawing out past experiences and accumulated knowledge; slowing the "social dying" process by building bridges to other people; giving a sense of belonging to the patient, especially within a small group; providing opportunities to experience good feelings associated with good experiences; fostering self-expression; and arranging for new experiences.

Remotivation is usually a structured group program that follows five steps. The first step is to create a climate of acceptance. Participants are greeted cheerfully by name and something positive and honest is said about each one. Attention may be called to the day, season, or weather. In the second step, a bridge to reality is made through the use of articles and pictures from newspapers and magazines, through sharing objects of personal value or interest, or through discussion of poems or short stories. The materials used should appeal to the participant's sense of hearing, sight, taste, touch, or smell. The third step is to explore the world in which we live by drawing out participants regarding what they know about the nature of things, about their personal likes, and about historical events and experiences. Sharing the work of the world is a method of inviting participants to discuss the work they have done, how they have functioned in the past and in the present. During the fourth step, a participant may be asked to tell another person how to do something, or to provide new information; this gives the one who is sharing a sense of self-worth. The last step is to create a climate of appreciation. This lets participants know through word, touch, or a smile that being with them was enjoyable and that what they shared was interesting.

The program can readily be adapted to use with individuals while bathing, feeding, or helping them to bed. In either case, it is a "talking therapy" as opposed to a "doing therapy" (such as recreation therapy); it is drawing out as opposed to teaching, such as reality orientation, and is objective as opposed to subjective, such as most psychotherapy. Remotivation therapy is very often used with patients who have "graduated" from reality orientation and who need a bridge to normal social functioning.

Recreation Therapy

Recreation therapy is the strengthening of aspects of an individual's personality that have not been affected by disabling conditions in order to prevent further limitation or greater functional loss. It is based on the philosophy that, essentially, each individual is personally responsible for meeting his or her own recreative needs, which must be appropriate to the existential situation. Recreation therapy aims at strengthening unaffected aspects of personality, enabling individuals to maximize existing potentials in the face of limitations, and preventing secondary disabilities. Specific objectives include stimulating mental and physical abilities; encouraging a sense of usefulness and self-respect; inhibiting symptoms of physical and mental regression due to illness and/or old age; and providing the means for preventing or coping with isolation, dependency, helplessness, institutionalization, apathy, lowered sensory input, and general atrophy.

Recreation therapy is usually achieved through implementation of activities programs. General types of programs include social, diversional, work-type, service, creative, intellectual, and spiritual or religious. These may be offered as individual or group activities, with the best programs offering both options. Recreation therapy is an intervention at the nonpathologic level, and deals, therefore, with the unaffected aspects of an individual. Consequently, the therapist working in this mode is seen by the patient as essentially different from other health professionals. As a result, important avenues of communication are often discovered and are facilitated in the course of recreation therapy activities. Additionally, the wholesome message is conveyed that "You are more than a sick person; you are not just an invalid."

Summary

As more and more people become "very old," it is common for them to experience disabilities and chronic illnesses. Medical intervention alone is often not sufficient, and rehabilitative therapists are frequently an essential factor in a preferred plan of care and treatment. As Talcott Parsons (1951) claims, it is all too easy for the older person in our society to adopt the "sick role." There is no other easily identifiable role for the elderly, yet the social-medical system is at best minimally equipped to provide for the chronically ill. When this becomes the societal expectation, role identity often follows; therefore, good rehabilitative efforts are doubly important in negating the "old and feeble" stereotype of aging, while improving the quality of life for those who might otherwise accept a life of dependent invalidism.

Certainly, the restoration and maintenance of ambulatory functions, mobility, and ability for self-care are primary factors in combating the stereotype and its consequences. No less important is the ability to communicate, to interact with others, and thus remain a viable member of society. Inherent in this concept is the assumption of adequate mental functioning. If there were only one damaging stereotype that could be corrected, it might well be that "old equals senile." Any treatments or programs that can alter behaviors which add to this stereotype are worthy of our efforts. The types of therapy outlined in this chapter, properly administered, can work minor miracles in the lives of older people. An ever-increasing group of older people who function well can "speak volumes" to society concerning the viability of old age.

REFERENCES

Licht S. (ed.): *Rehabilitation and Medicine*. New Haven, Elizabeth Licht, Pub., 1968.

Maslow A.: *Toward a Psychology of Being*. Princeton, Van Nostrand, 1962.

Nichols P.J.R. (ed.): *Rehabilitation Medicine: The Management of Physical Disabilities*, ed. 2. Boston, Butterworths, 1980.

Parsons T.: *The Social System*. Glencoe, Ill., Free Press, 1951.

Pegels C.C.: *Health Care and the Elderly*. Rockville, Md., Aspin Systems, 1980.

Schow R.L., Christensen J.M., Nerbonne M.A.: *Communication Disorders of the Aged: A Guide for Health Professionals*. Baltimore, University Park Press, 1978.

Rusk H.A.: *Rehabilitation Medicine*. St Louis, C.V. Mosby Co., 1971.

Weimer R.B., West W.L.: Occupational therapy in community care. *Am. J. Occup. Ther*. 24:323-328, 1970.

16

NUTRITION

Don Mannerberg, M.D.

WITH THE PROGRESS of industrialization of the world, the environment has undergone numerous changes that are variables in the production of disease. People in Western cultures now live longer than those in former centuries due to the conquest of most infections and the advance of surgical technology. Therefore, nutritional effects, physical inactivity, pollution, cigarette smoking, consumption of alcohol and drugs—combined with the complicated, rapidly changing emotional stress of society—have more time to produce an effect on health.

Westernization and Degenerative Diseases

Chronic degenerative diseases of aging are those of civilization and are characteristic of the modern affluent Western technological communities of the world. These degenerative diseases are essentially man-made and are produced by a profound alteration of the environment, particularly in the area of nutrition. This discussion addresses appropriate guidelines for the content of the menu for the aging American as it relates to diseases most prevalent over 50 years of age: coronary artery disease, stroke, diabetes mellitus, cirrhosis of liver, arteriosclerosis, gallbladder disease, diverticulosis of the colon, and possibly cancer. What diseases can potentially be altered by nutritional intervention, and what are the guidelines for these therapeutic modifications? Epidemiology provides the greatest number of clues for determining a relationship between nutrition and disease. Since the turn of the century, for example, the American diet has changed, with a corresponding change in disease patterns and causes of death. The diet of this country around 1900 had a great deal of natural carbohydrate, with its high-fiber content, and little refined sugar. That diet composition has been transformed into the salty, refined, fatty, high-calorie diet of today.

Throughout the underdeveloped world, in countries such as Africa, modernization and the same accompanying changes in diet have occurred in a relatively shorter period of time. These modifications in the diet are very similar to the alterations in food patterns experienced by Americans along with the emergence of the same degenerative diseases. Among these are blood pressure rising with age and increased prevalence of hypertension; cerebrovascular disease; obesity; diabetes mellitus type II; coronary artery disease; and several diseases of the gastrointestinal tract, including gallstones, which did not exist until the Westernization of developing societies throughout the world. Blood pressure elevations with age or actual hypertension did not exist in the food gatherers or nomads of the world (Donnison, 1929). From 1930 to 1935, physicians in Kenya had never seen essential hypertension in Africa and no case was reported in either Kenya or Uganda until 1941 (Trowell, 1980). These populations had lifelong low blood pressure prior to 1941. Cerebrovascular disease was the first arterial disease of clinical significance to emerge in these Africans following modernization. The change in incidence of hypertension and associated cerebrovascular disease correlated with the introduction of salt into the diet of these native populations.

Genetic salt sensitivity varies considerably. There is evidence to suggest that low blood pressure exists when daily salt intake is below 3 to 4 gm. Above this level of sodium intake, an increasing percentage of salt-sensitive subjects develop blood pressure elevations with age. Above 6 to 8 gm per day, almost all salt-sensitive subjects develop blood pressure levels that rise with age and a fair proportion develop essential hypertension, especially if they are overweight. Recent evidence has shown that hypertensives vary considerably in their response to a decreased intake of sodium. This led Kawasaki et al. (1978) to classify hypertensives into two groups: those who were salt-sensitive and those who were not. These investigators reported that blood pressure fell in both groups when sodium intake was reduced, but that the decrease was greater in the salt-sensitive group than in the nonsensitive group. This reversal of hypertension or lowering of borderline blood pressure in a population with salt-limited intake has been found by other investigators (Morgan et al., 1978). In all the populations of the world where salt is not a part of the diet, essential hypertension does not exist.

More recently, Iocano (1980) and Wright et al. (1979) have implicated fat and fiber in the etiology of hypertension. Iocano produced remission of hypertension in 75 medicated hypertensive individuals by a reduction of fat intake with a one-to-one saturated to unsaturated fat ratio. There were no alterations in salt intake or weight changes during that particular study. Wright suggested that differences in the type and quantity of dietary fiber as well as fat may be responsible for lower blood pressure in vegetarians. These studies, then, indicate two possible effects of the modern diet on blood pressure other than excessive calories or excessive salt.

A survey of populations in Central America has reported increased incidence of diabetes associated with Westernization of the diet (West, 1971). Available evidence suggests that diabetes emerged in East Africans in the 1920s and 1930s, especially in urban communities where the earliest changes in diet occurred. Increasing diabetes paralleled changes in the diet such as the introduction of refined foods, decreased fiber content, and increased caloric density, that in turn lead to more prevalent obesity.

In the African groups, coronary heart disease was the last major cardiovascular Western disease to emerge (Walker, 1975). There was an absence of coronary heart disease reported in 1,000 autopsies during the 1930s. Coronary disease today is common in South African blacks. This is the emergence of another degenerative disease of advancing age in modern society, correlated with changes in the diet. In many other developing countries of the world, as well as in Africa (Vaughan, 1977), these same changes are duplicated.

In modern America, the Seventh-Day Adventist vegetarian's diet has a lower fat and higher fiber content than the typical nonvegetarian's diet (Phillips et al., 1978). The risk of fatal coronary heart disease is three times greater in the nonvegetarian from ages 35 to 64 years. This is an equivalent diet to disease correlation as described in the developing countries of the world.

The Role of Dietary Intervention

Epidemiology of the emergence of degenerative diseases of aging with modernization of the diet is certainly pertinent to preventive medicine. Does intervention by dietary means alter the natural history of degenerative disease in our Western society? Will changing the diet back to the pre-Westernization composition produce reversal of these emerging diseases associated with aging? If so, this would lend support to dietary intervention in these diseases as well as to a role in prevention.

Progression of atherosclerotic disease can be modified by dietary intervention. Morrison (1960) demonstrated this possibility in a 12-year study using proved coronary infarctions. In that study, the fat intake was restricted to 15% of total calories and the cholesterol to 100 mg daily. The normal control group had died in 12 years, but 30% of the low fat, low cholesterol group were still alive. Dodson and associates (1981) have added additional experience to provide credibility for dietary intervention in modern degenerative diseases. This clinical program used a low sodium, high potassium, low fat, high fiber, low sugar diet in management of hypertension and angina, as follows: 2.5 to 3.5 gm salt, 1,600 to 1,800 calories, 10%

to 13% protein, 15% to 20% fat, 50% to 60% starch, 5% to 10% sugar, 30 to 35 gm dietary fiber, and 500 to 600 mg cholesterol per day.

Improved control of blood pressure was achieved in 25 of 32 hypertensive patients for follow-up averaging six months. Twelve of those required no continued drug therapy, 13 others had reduced drug therapy, while the remaining 7 were not improved by dietary change. Eleven angina patients, average age 56 years, were given the same diet. After one month, a beneficial effect was witnessed that continued during a follow-up of a minimum period of six months. Seven angina patients became completely free of all angina pain while walking more than 3 miles per day. The remaining four experienced a marked decrease in angina or in the need for nitroglycerin while walking 0.5 to 2.0 miles daily.

Nutritional intervention in the treatment of diabetes, other than promotion of weight loss in the adult onset or type II diabetes, is very effective. Singh (1955) demonstrated this when 80 newly diagnosed diabetics were placed on a sugar-free, 12% fat diet that was high in complex carbohydrate. In six weeks, 62% no longer needed insulin, and by 18 weeks, 72% tested with normal blood sugar. Anderson and Ward (1979) reported the effect of a high fiber-carbohydrate diet on adult-onset insulin-treated diabetes. Of the 33 insulin-treated patients, 17 were treated with 14 to 20 units of insulin per day; on a high carbohydrate-fiber diet, the insulin was discontinued in 16 of the 17 patients after an average of 14 days. Eleven of the original 33 required 25 to 32 units of insulin per day, and on the dietary change 5 of these discontinued the use of insulin. After discharge from the hospital, all the patients responded well to this diet and with maintenance sustained their improvement. This is a diet containing 60% energy from complex carbohydrate and 50 gm dietary fiber per day. Follow-up was extended over a period of 6 to 48 months in the group. The effect of this particular diet was felt to be due largely to the high fiber content (Anderson, 1979).

Approximately 20 years ago, health surveys pinpointed risk factors for development of coronary heart disease such as elevated serum cholesterol, hypertension, and electrocardiographic changes. Since that time other risk factors such as cigarette smoking, physical inactivity, and other blood chemistries that can be affected by nutrition have been introduced. These risk factors have been shown to be emerging factors with the development of Western cultures (Kannel et al., 1961).

Further statistics suggest that the biologic norms of aging for Western adults are not the norms for health, but are average figures for a population that later develops degenerative diseases. This is reflected by the rising blood pressure, body weight, serum cholesterol, and triglycerides as well as decreased carbohydrate tolerance with age in our Western society. The

Coronary Drug Project (Stamler et al., 1978), a nationwide collaborative study, reported the relationship between fasting blood cholesterol and triglycerides over a four-year span. These men with previous myocardial infarction were up to 64 years of age on entry in the program. Results of the project indicate that after recovery from acute myocardial infarction, reduction of serum cholesterol improved the long-term prognosis.

Evidence of the potential for reversal of atherosclerosis in the arteries of humans has been demonstrated in a very limited fashion. Sonmarco et al. (1978) showed evidence to indicate that if risk factors for developing the disease are not altered, the majority of individuals show progression after four to five years. However, most studies indicate that with vigorous reduction of risk factors such as hypertension and hyperlipidemia, which are influenced by nutrition, there was a potential for stabilizing most lesions. One study of early atherosclerotic lesions of the femoral artery suggested that regression may follow the lowering of blood lipids and blood pressure. It must be emphasized that the evidence for these changes is not adequate enough to satisfy most scientists (Barndt, 1977). A prospective long-term study in humans with objective evidence in a large number of subjects will meet that requirement.

At this time, the only large human clinical experiment to incorporate all these elements is a short-term residential nutritional intervention program reported by Diehl (1981) and Mannerberg (1979). This was a study of 893 patients, mostly between 50 and 70 years of age, which primarily used nutritional intervention. The diet was an unrefined complex carbohydrate diet with about 70% of the daily energy from largely whole grain cereal products, potatoes, and legumes. Refined simple carbohydrates such as honey, molasses, and sugar were not permitted. Fat and oil intakes were very low, representing less than 10% of the daily energy. The diet was high in fiber content and low in salt, with less than 5 gm per day; no salt was added during cooking or at the table and salty foods were avoided. This was a copy of a diet used in the developing countries of the world where modern degenerative diseases did not exist prior to changes in diet approximating ours.

On admission to the program, the diseased status patients were as follows: coronary heart disease, 66%; hypertensives, 36%; intermittent claudication, 22%; obesity, 29%; diabetes mellitus, 12%; and gouty arthritis, 6%. After four weeks of the dietary program described, plus physical activity, the following results were obtained. After four weeks, of the 32 adult-onset diabetics using oral hypoglycemic drugs on admission, 26 had normal blood glucose levels and required no drugs. Eleven of the 22 adult-onset diabetics using insulin had ceased insulin therapy and were discharged with normal glucose levels. These were all classified diabetic patients of diabetes type II, or adult-onset, diabetes. Of the 324 patients who were hypertensive on admission, 218 were being treated with antihypertensive drugs. Of these 218, 186 (86%) left with normal blood pressure after discontinuance of antihypertensive drugs.

Of the 419 medicated angina pectoris patients, 60% no longer required drugs at the time of discharge and at the same time had improved function. Half of the 198 claudication patients were discharged, able to walk several miles daily with little or no pain while taking less or no medication. In claudication and angina patients, improved tolerance by a treadmill stress test was demonstrated. These short-term, dramatic results are evidence supporting the conclusion that nutritional intervention is scientifically valid.

Although a follow-up study is currently in progress, reports are only available on diabetics as a group. A 12-month evaluation of the 81 discharged diabetics has been tabulated. Seventy-four of these patients continued with a total fat consumption of less than 10% total calories. The group's main body weight during the 26 days at the center had decreased from 172 to 163 pounds. At one year following the residential program, the average weight has further decreased to 157 pounds. The therapeutic gains obtained while in the program continued during the 12-month follow-up. This is an indication that good adherence to this radically different diet is possible in well-motivated persons.

There has been no report of as large a number of patients as those in this study from the Longevity Center in Santa Barbara, California. No other therapeutic program has been as low in total fat, saturated fat, cholesterol, sugar and salt, or as high in unrefined complex carbohydrate with dietary fiber. There were significant clinical regressions evidenced by remission of the symptoms of disease or by discontinued use of pharmacologic treatment of these degenerative diseases. Therefore, it is possible for basic dietary intervention to have the potential for therapy in diabetes and vascular diseases common to the elderly.

Constipation and its damage to the gastrointestinal tract is one of the major problems of the aged. Again, as with other diseases, epidemiologic studies have implicated a dietary change—the removal of fiber from the diet (Burkitt, 1977). There is an inverse relationship between the prevalence of many diseases of the gastrointestinal tract and the amount of fiber consumed. Two diseases related to constipation are diverticulosis of the colon and hemorrhoids. Other diseases such as appendicitis, varicose veins, hiatus hernia, and large bowel cancer have been suggested on the basis of the same evidence (Brodribb, 1976). These diseases were rare in the African populations before 1940. Inhabitants of rural communities consumed over 20 gm fiber daily in their complex carbohydrate diet, while by contrast the refined diet of the Westernized countries usually contains less than 8 gm. It is possible to assume that these intestinal diseases are largely related to that change in fiber content in the diet which produces an alteration in the evacuation of bowel contents, intra-abdominal pressure, and intraluminal pressure of the bowel (Fedail et al., 1979). It has also been inferred that diluting and hastening the evacuation of bowel contents by added fiber reduces the potential effect of possible carcinogens produced in the bowel.

Large-bowel cancer is one of the major causes of death in the Western world; in this country, 90,000 new cases are diagnosed annually. An analysis of statistics from 23 countries shows a strong correlation between daily consumption of meat and incidence of colon cancer. This high beef intake with a fiber-deficient diet hypothesis is criticized since the postulated relationship is supported only by epidemiologic studies, with no confirming experimental evidence (Walker, 1976). As previously stated, there may be a possible correlation with the decreased fiber intake of the diet, which then allows the role of intestinal bacterial flora to convert chemical substances into possible carcinogens. Again, this is strictly hypothetical at present (Trowell, 1976).

The changing incidence of cancer due to modification of the diet is illustrated by the situation in Japan. In the 1960s, the most common cancer of both sexes in Japan was of the esophagus; cancer of the colon was not among the seven most common cancers in either sex. Changes that are now occurring in this pattern are those expected from the experience in other Westernized countries (Armstrong et al., 1975). Cancer of the stomach, the esophagus, and the biliary tract are declining, while the rates of cancer of the lung, pancreas, colon, and rectum are increasing. Following World War II, the diet in Japan underwent significant changes, becoming more like the Western diet. There is strong evidence that dietary changes such as excess caloric and fat intake are related to cancer of the breast and uterus. Dietary meat and fat contribute to the etiology of cancer of the colon and rectum; and, as previously stated, dietary fiber may act as a protective factor. Cancer of the colon is correlated more strongly with meat and animal protein than with fat (Cummings et al., 1979). Also, as the cereal and grain consumption decreases, the incidence of colon cancer increases.

Latto and staff (1981) evaluated the effect of added fiber (wheat bran, 50 gm per day; dietary fiber, 22 gm per day) on the incidence of deep vein thrombosis in surgical patients. Constipation reduction was the most rapid improvement, with a 42% reduction of hemorrhoidectomy during the 1970 to 1977 observation period. Resection of colon diverticular disease changed from one every two weeks to one each year. Brodribb (1976) reported from the same hospital symptomatic relief of colon diverticulosis. Reduction in colon pressure and normalization of transit times was found in 88% of 40 patients after six months' treatment with bran added to the diet.

Cholesterol gallstones are definitely a disease of civilization. This disease has increased everywhere in the last three decades, and in progressively younger age groups. Diets that induce cholesterol gallstones in animals are generally rich in refined carbohydrates, which replace the fiber containing complex unrefined carbohydrate. Also, there is a direct correlation between increased dietary fat and cholesterol content to cholesterol gallstones in humans.

Anatomical and physiologic changes in the gastrointestinal tract with aging produce problems with assimilation of food. In this afflicted group of elderly Americans, approximately 50% have lost their teeth and must depend on dentures. For this reason, many elderly avoid certain foods because of their consistency, which is not handled well by dentures. Muscle tone of the bowel decreases, leading to a delay of emptying from the esophagus on through the rectum. Chronic atrophic gastritis, leading to potential B_{12} deficiencies, has been estimated to occur in approximately 25% of elderly persons. The same atrophic gastritis often leads to the avoidance of citrus juices because of gastric distress on ingestion; this also increases the vulnerability for vitamin C deficiency.

Vitamin and Mineral Deficiencies

Supplementation of the diet with vitamins and minerals to prevent loss of function in the aged can be considered even more controversial than the nutritional intervention previously described. All surveys show that persons in advanced years consume far less food than is usually required for the vitamin and mineral standards for their age, sex, and weight (O'Hanlon et al., 1978). Such consistent evidence indicates that this must be an important area when considering nutrition of the elderly. The most common vitamins found to be deficient were vitamin C, vitamin A, and niacin, in addition to members of the B vitamin group.

The most common mineral deficiency was iron. A gradual depletion of body stores of various nutrients due to poor dietary habits, often secondary to disease or treatment of disease, can result in numerous preclinical symptoms. These can include malaise, irritability or somnolence, anorexia, and weight loss. Consequently, psychological and physical performance can be impaired in all aspects of life. The elderly are particularly vulnerable to vitamin and mineral deficiency because of the high incidence of illness or disability in the later years of life, or because of other common problems such as low income or social isolation.

Examples of effective intervention in this area of nutrition are best illustrated in a study reported by Mitra (1971). It was found that confusional states in the elderly were associated with deficiency of vitamin B complex and vitamin C. When these deficiencies were corrected by use of suitable vitamin supplements, there was reversal in 15 of the 17 cases studied. Leevy et al. (1965) determined nutritional status with reference to vitamins in a random group of patients in a municipal hospital, where they found that folic acid was deficient in the highest proportion of cases. Other deficiencies were of thiamine, niacin, vitamin C, and vitamin B_{12}. These deficiencies were shown to be corrected by supplements.

Osteoporosis, characterized by spontaneous fractures of bones, occurs in 30% of women over 60 years of age and also in men to a much lesser extent (Wachman and Bernstein, 1968). This bone loss is an age-related phenomenon. It coincides with reduced physical activity in later years of both sexes and is aggravated by age-associated hormone changes in women and chronic inadequate intake of calcium. Optimal bone density in women is reached at about age 40; after that the wasting process begins. The prevention and treatment of osteoporosis are not clearly defined at present, but several investigators believe that changes in dietary calcium and phosphorus intake are major factors. Milk as a dietary source of calcium is often limited by sensitivity to milk proteins or intestinal lactase deficiency in the elderly.

There is evidence that elevated phosphorus intake in the presence of calcium deficiency can lead to skeletal bone loss. The major problem of the modern American diet is a high phosphorus-low calcium intake that triggers bone calcium loss. This demineralization process, resulting from an approximate 2-to-1 phosphorus to calcium intake ratio found with the American diet, can be reversed with a calcium to phosphorus ratio of 1 to 1. The convenience of prepared foods in the diet that contain phosphate derivatives, as well as soft drinks that also contain phosphate additives, is responsible for high phosphorus intakes. Bell et al. (1977) found that individuals consuming a diet high in phosphate had high levels of circulating parathyroid hormone, which suggested a nutritionally induced hyperparathyroidism. This is in agreement with work on primates, which suggests the same effect on calcium homeostasis and normal bone (Anderson et al., 1977). Chronic alcoholism, high protein intake, glucose intolerance, as well as kidney and liver disease, can also produce secondary hyperparathyroidism, as can excess vitamin D ingestion. The ideal 1-to-1 ratio of calcium to phosphorus can be obtained by an alkaline-ash diet that is high in vegetables, fruit, and milk products. Animal experiments (Barzel and Jowsey, 1969) support the acid-alkaline hypothesis for maintenance of a healthy skeleton and for prevention of osteoporosis with aging.

Clinical studies have shown that postmenopausal women who supplement their diet with calcium for as long as eight years have had a reversal of bone loss with an increase in bone density and no adverse effects. A Department of Agriculture survey in 1968 of 5,500 normal women showed that in a group over 45 years of age, estimated calcium consumption was 450 mg per day (Albanese, 1978). This is about 50% below the recommended daily allowance of 800 mg established by the Recommended Dietary Allowances (RDA—National Academy of Sciences, 1980). This, coupled with a diet that has an increased phosphorus intake from processed foods, promotes the bone loss problem. Therefore, changes in the basic diet and supplementation with calcium would seem to be indicated in the prevention of osteoporosis.

It has been estimated that 50% of the 32 million people over 60 years of age have a chronic illness that requires continuous medical care. For this reason, the need for drugs and surgery for treatment of various degenerative disorders is greater in the aging and elderly. Frequently, many of the effects of drugs on nutritional status are not appreciated. When diuretics are used, there is awareness of the possibility of potassium deficiency. The interreaction of drugs should be considered at all times by physicians who prescribe medication; but since nutrition is not considered therapeutic, the same interreactions are not considered. A common example of this is alcohol, which decreases the absorption of thiamine and folic acid, and produces an increased urinary excretion of vitamin C. Penicillin is capable of producing a low-potassium level, while the antibiotic tetracycline is responsible for decreased absorption of calcium, iron, magnesium, amino acids, and fat. Also, broad-spectrum antibiotics can produce increased urinary excretion of vitamin C, riboflavin, folic acid, and niacin. In conjunction with this, there is a decreased synthesis of vitamin K by intestinal bacteria. Laxatives are frequently used in the elderly since constipation is a product of the low-fiber, processed American diet. These cathartics or laxatives can cause problems such as increased intestinal calcium and phosphate loss as well as decreased glucose absorption. Any laxative containing mineral oil will decrease absorption of carotene; vitamins A, D, E, and K; calcium; and phosphate. This list of examples can be quite extensive. March (1976) covers these interreactions and his study should be considered whenever nutrition of the elderly in the disease state is a consideration.

It has been found that individuals dying suddenly with ischemic heart disease have lower levels of tissue magnesium and potassium in the heart muscle than individuals dying from other causes (Johnson et al., 1979). An excellent review by Seelig et al. (1974) summarizes the usefulness of magnesium and explains its importance in preventing sudden death from ischemic heart disease by maintaining an intracellular balance of calcium and potassium. Sudden death risk exists most frequently in individuals who have had previous myocardial infarctions or who are presently having angina or are at increased risk for myocardial infarct. Many of these individuals are on medications that alter mineral status significantly, including a large number of elements other than potassium.

Dietary Guidelines

The evidence presented in this chapter, largely epidemiologic, can best be summarized by recommendations of the United States Senate Select Committee on Nutrition and Human Needs (1970). This committee collected evidence concerning coronary heart disease, obesity, and other degenerative diseases from medical experts at the National Institutes of Health and from doctors elsewhere in the United States and in other countries. In December, 1977, the second edition of their recommendations was published. The recommendations were as follows:

1. Reduce energy if overweight.
2. Reduce sucrose from 18% to 10% of total calories.
3. Reduce total fat from 42% to 30% of total calories.
4. Reduce saturated fat but increase polyunsaturated fats.
5. Reduce cholesterol to 300 mg/dl daily.
6. Reduce salt intake from approximately 12 to 16 gm to 5 gm daily.

These dietary guidelines were given as recommendations to prevent the "killer diseases" that are not only the most common diseases of the elderly but also the leading causes of death. These suggestions are similar to the therapeutic high-carbohydrate diets that have just been shown to aid in the regression of diabetes mellitus type II, hypertension, angina, and gastrointestinal diseases. Gastrointestinal diseases, including gallstones, hiatus hernia, diverticulosis of the colon, colon and rectal cancer, appendicitis, and hemorrhoids, can be added to that list of diseases subject to change by the same nutrition factors.

Although these dietary guidelines have received support from nutritional authorities (Hegsted, 1978), there has been a lack of enthusiastic endorsement from governmental agencies and the food industry. Evidence from population studies concerning the emergence of degenerative diseases with dietary changes in the present American diet cannot be disregarded. For cardiovascular disease, including hypertension and adult-onset diabetes, it would seem there is sufficient evidence to make changes. Scientific interest has been stimulated and future research will help clear up this controversy, but meanwhile there seems to be sufficient evidence for action. Making such modest changes in the basic diet as outlined above would seem appropriate at this time with no actual risk to the population.

Beyond a low-salt, low-fat, low-refined carbohydrate diet with its increased fiber intake, there is also adequate evidence for serious consideration of supplementation of the diet on an individual basis. The interreaction of drugs and nutrition should always be considered when designing a diet. Every effort should be made to assure at least the recommended daily allowances of all essential nutrients in the aged.

Prevention of osteoporosis, cancer of the large bowel, and sudden death from coronary artery disease are possibilities. Intervention by nutrition in these medical problems, which could also include arthritis, is too speculative to be reviewed at this time.

Conclusions

Guidelines for nutrition for the elderly as well as the whole population have not received the degree of effort required to answer the questions required for scientific validity. This deficit can be overcome by enhanced research and assessment of nutrition relating to disease of the aging. Therefore, at the present time, we depend on limited clinical studies and largely epidemiologic evidence.

REFERENCES

Albanese A.A.: Calcium nutrition of the elderly. *Postgrad. Med.* 63:167–172, 1978.

Anderson J.W., Chen W.L.: Plant fiber: Carbohydrate and lipid metabolism. *Am. J. Clin. Nutr.* 32:346–363, 1979.

Anderson J.W., Ward K.: High carbohydrate, high fiber diets for insulin-treated men with diabetes mellitus. *Am. J. Clin. Nutr.* 32:2312–2319, 1979.

Anderson M., Hunt R., Griffiths H.J., et al.: Long term effect of low dietary calcium:phosphate ratio on skeleton of Cebus albifrons monkeys. *J. Nutr.* 107:834, 1977.

Armstrong B., Doll R.: Environmental factors and cancer incidence and mortality in different countries with special reference to dietary practices. *Int. J. Cancer.* 15:651–665, 1975.

Barndt R.: Regression and progression of early femoral atherosclerosis in treated hyperlipoproteinemic patients. *Ann. Intern. Med.* 86:139–146, 1977.

Barzel U.S., Jowsey J.: The effects of chronic acid and alkali administration on bone turnover in adult rats. *Clin. Sci.* 36:517, 1969.

Bell R.R., Draper H., Tzeng D., et al.: Physiological responses of human adults to foods containing phosphate additives. *J. Nutr.* 107:42, 1977.

Broad W.J.: National Institutes of Health deals gingerly with diet-disease link. *Science* 204:1175, 1979.

Brodribb A.J.M., Humphreys D.M.: Diverticular disease: Three studies. *Br. Med. J.* 1:424–430, 1976.

Burkitt D.P.: Large-bowel cancer: An epidemiological jigsaw puzzle. *J. Natl. Cancer Inst.* 54:306, 1975.

Burkitt D.P.: Relationship between diseases and their etiological significance. *Am. J. Clin. Nutr.* 30:262–267, 1977.

Cummings J.H., Hill M.J., Bone E.S., et al.: The effect of meat protein and dietary fiber on colonic function and metabolism. *Am. J. Clin. Nutr.* 32:2094–2101, 1979.

Diehl H., Mannerberg D.: Hypertension, hyperlipidaemia, angina, and coronary heart disease, in Trowell H.C., Burkitt D.P. (eds.): *Western Diseases: Their Emergence and Prevention*. London, Edward Arnold, 1981.

Dodson P., Humphreys D.: Hypertension and angina, in Trowell H.C., Burkitt D.P. (eds.): *Western Diseases: Their Emergence and Prevention*. London, Edward Arnold, 1981.

Donnison C.P.: Blood pressure in the African native. *Lancet* 1:6–7, 1929.

Fedail S.S., Harvey R.F., Burns-Cox C.J.: Abdominal and thoracic pressures during defaecation. *Br. Med. J.* 1:91, 1979.

Hegsted D.M.: Dietary goals: A progressive view. *Am. J. Nutr.* 31:310–315, 1978.

Iocano J.: *U.S. Depart. Agri. Bull.* U.S. Government Printing Office, 1980.

Johnson C.J., Peterson D.R., Smith E.K.: Myocardial tissue concentrations of magnesium and potassium in men dying suddenly of ischemic heart disease. *Am. J. Clin. Nutr.* 32:967–977, 1979.

Kannel W.B., Dawber T.R., Kagan A., et al.: Factors of risk in the development of coronary heart disease: Six year follow-up experience. The Framingham Study. *Ann. Intern. Med.* 55:33–49, 1961.

Kawasaki T., Delea C.S., Bartter F.C., et al.: The effect of high sodium and low sodium intakes on blood pressure and other related variables in human subjects with idiopathic hypertension. *Am. J. Med.* 64:193–198, 1978.

Latto C.: Hemorrhoids, diverticular disease and deep vein thrombosis, in Trowell H.C., Burkitt D.P. (eds.): *Western Diseases: Their Emergence and Prevention*, London, Edward Arnold, 1981.

Leevy C.M., Cardi L., Frank O.: Incidence and significance of hypovitaminemia in a randomly selected municipal hospital population. *Am. J. Clin. Nutr.* 17:259–271, 1965.

Mannerberg D.: Rehabilitation of cardiovascular disease in a U.S.A. centre. *Chest Heart Stroke J.* 3:62–65, 1979.

March D.C.: *Handbook: Interactions of Selected Drugs with Nutrition Status in Man*. Chicago, American Dietetic Association, 1976.

Mitra M.L.: Confusional states in relationship to vitamin deficiencies in the elderly. *J. Am. Geriatr. Soc.* 19:536–545, 1971.

Morgan T., Adam W., Gillies A., et al.: Hypertension treated by salt restriction. *Lancet* 1:227–230, 1978.

Morrison L.M.: Diet and coronary atherosclerosis. *J.A.M.A.* 173:104, 1960.

National Academy of Sciences–National Research Council: *Recommended Dietary Allowances*, ed. 9. Washington, D.C., 1980.

O'Hanlon P., Kohrs M.B.: Dietary studies of older Americans. *Am. J. Clin. Nutr.* 31:1257–1269, 1978.

Phillips R.L., Lemon F.R., Beeson W.L., et al.: Coronary heart disease mortality among Seventh Day Adventists with differing dietary habits. *Am. J. Clin. Nutr.* 31:S191–S198, 1978.

Seelig M.S., Heggtueit N.H.A.: Magnesium interrelationships in ischemic heart disease: A review. *Am. J. Clin. Nutr.* 27:59–79, 1974.

Singh I.: Low-fat diet and therapeutic doses of insulin in diabetes mellitus. *Lancet* 1:422–425, 1955.

Sonmarco M.E., Blankenhorn O.H.: Atherosclerosis: Its progression and regression. *Primary Cardiology* 51–54, July/August 1978.

Stamler J., Forman S., Krol W.F.: Natural history of myocardial infarction in the coronary drug project: Long-term prognostic importance of serum lipid levels. *Am. J. Cardiol.* 42:489–497, 1978.

Trowell H.: Definition of dietary fiber and hypothesis that it is a protective factor in certain diseases. *Am. J. Nutr.* 29:417–427, 1976.

Trowell H.: From normotensive to hypertensive in Kenyans and Ugandans, 1928–78. *East Afr. Med. J.* 57:167–173, 1980.

United States Senate, Select Committee on Nutrition and Human Needs. *Dietary Goals for the United States*, ed. 2. U.S. Government Printing Office, 1977.

Vaughan J.P.: A brief review of cardiovascular disease in Africa. *Trans. R. Soc. Trop. Med. Hyg.* 71:226–231, 1977.

Wachman A., Bernstein D.S.: Diet and osteoporosis. *Lancet* 1:958, 1968.

Walker A.R.P.: The epidemiologic emergence of ischemic arterial diseases. *Am. Heart J.* 89:133–136, 1975.

Walker A.R.P., Burkitt D.P.: Colonic cancer: Hypothesis of causation, dietary prophylaxis and future research. *Am. J. Dig. Dis.* 21:910–917, 1976.

West K.M., Kalbfleisch J.M.: Influence of nutritional factors on prevalence of diabetes. *Diabetes* 20:99–108, 1971.

Wright A., Burstyn P.G., Gibney M.J.: Dietary fiber and blood pressure. *Br. Med. J.* 2:1541–1543, 1979.

17

THERAPEUTIC INTERVENTIONS—MENTAL HEALTH

Bert Hayslip, Jr., Ph.D.
Robert A. Kooken, M.S.

Mental Health Services and the Older Adult

Within the past several years, there has been growing interest in the clinical psychology of aging. Until the early 1950s, psychological services to older persons were largely absent (Birren and Renner, 1980). Even then, available approaches to treatment were largely pharmacologic (drug-related) and somatic (i.e., electroshock) in nature. Many investigators (Gatz, Smyer, and Lawton, 1980; Knight, 1978–79; Smyer and Gatz, 1979; Sparacino, 1978–79; Storandt, Siegler, and Elias, 1978) have documented the neglect of the mental health needs of older persons based on a model of biologic decline with increased age. Thus, questions such as "Why do psychotherapy with older people?" and "Can the elderly change?" have been raised (Ingebretsen, 1977) by clinicians prone to see elderly persons as "lost causes" therapeutically. Consequently, the field of counseling and psychotherapy with the elderly is in its infancy. Only recently have practitioners, counselors or therapists, and researchers become seriously concerned with the issues surrounding therapy with older adults (i.e., Birren and Sloane, 1980; Kastenbaum, 1978; Storandt, Siegler, and Elias, 1978).

In spite of common belief to the contrary, age per se has not been shown to be a predictor of psychotherapeutic success (Garfield, 1978; Smith and Glass, 1977). Luborsky and associates (1971), for example, conclude that "older patients tend to have a slightly poorer prognosis." The few research studies cited, however, did not employ older (beyond middle-age) patients, and many lacked controls. On the other hand, Smith and Glass (1977) found age to be uncorrelated with effect size of different therapies.

Gatz et al. (1980) suggest that the negative attitudes and stereotypes about aging contribute to the reluctance of therapists (many of whom are young) to treat the aged. Such biases have been termed "professional ageism" (Butler, 1975; Butler and Lewis, 1977), and rest on such factors as therapists' fears about their own aging and unresolved conflicts about their patients' aging, a belief that aging means inevitable decline, pessimism about the prospects for change in elderly clients, and views that suggest it is futile to invest large amounts of time and effort in someone with a limited life expectancy. Blum and Tallmer (1977) have discussed the phenomenon of "countertransference" that prevents many counselors from seeing their clients as real people—in terms other than those of physical decline, pain, disengagement from others, lessened intelligence, and rigidity. In other words, elderly clients do not fit the YAVIS syndrome: they are not *y*oung, *a*ttractive, *v*erbal; frequently are perceived as possessing low *i*ntelligence; or are perceived as being un*s*uccessful.

Consequently, the therapist's own fears relating to illness, mutilation, death and dying, rejection by parents, or any number of losses (monetary, psychosocial, physical) associated with being old may be aroused. The therapist becomes unrealistically critical and intolerant, and he tends to blame the older person for failure to show improvement (see Birren and Renner, 1980; Davis and Klopfer, 1977; Ford and Sbordone, 1980). Furthermore, a belief that most, if not all, symptoms have a physical basis strengthens the expectation that elderly clients are beyond treatment. At the same time, the use of such physical complaints by aged clients to mask underlying psychological distress (such as depression) is reinforced. Alternatively, an overconcern with psychogenic symptoms frequently leads the therapist to ignore genuine physical complaints. Thus, both domains (the physical *and* the psychological) must be carefully scrutinized.

The failure of elderly persons to use available psychological services is influenced by their attitudes toward and beliefs about counseling (Gatz et al., 1980). Many view therapists with suspicion, and feel that counseling is all right for other people but not for them. It may be that as future cohorts of elderly become "psychologized," they may be more receptive to available help and will tend to see their problems as treatable by some form of therapeutic intervention (Lawton, 1978). While this is possible, increased sophistication could lead to a demand for a more active role in treatment and a more critical view of service providers. Alternatively, improved health care, increased social services, and more education could result in a reduced demand for future psychological services. If the current preference for self-help among the elderly continues (Butler et al., 1979–80), such changes could be realities for allied health professionals who attempt to solve their problems.

Inappropriately designed services, staffed by ill-trained personnel, also contribute to the reluctance of the elderly to use available counseling services (Gatz et al., 1980). Efforts at training persons with expertise in counseling or psychotherapy, assessment, and diagnosis of the aged need to be markedly stepped up if future mental health service needs are to be met (Birren and Woodruff, 1973; Birren and Sloane, 1980; Storandt et al., 1978; Smyer and Gatz, 1979; NIMH, 1979b). While there is some debate on how to both structure such training and utilize current personnel (Lawton, 1978; Lawton and Gottesman, 1974; Smyer and Gatz, 1979), it seems clear that future elderly (whose demand for therapeutic services seems likely to increase) will require services that are accessible and that are staffed by those with training in multiple areas, such as clinical psychology and counseling, life-span development, and community psychology (Smyer and Gatz, 1979). Both the quality and the quantity of professional therapeutic services to the elderly must be maximized. Reimbursement for outpatient services remains a problem (Knee, 1979) for those who can be treated on this basis, but whose insurance plans do not pay for such treatment.

Gatz, Smyer, and Lawton (1980) have summarized the major variables accounting for underutilization of current mental health services by older persons and their families (see also NIMH, 1979a):

1. Timeliness—services are not used by elderly persons and their families until a problem reaches "crisis proportions."
2. Lack of information regarding services.
3. Attitudes of elderly toward the acceptance of services (to do so is demeaning and shameful).
4. Prohibitively expensive cost of services, frequently not reimbursable via Medicaid and Medicare.
5. Poor accessibility to available services, particularly where transportation is a problem, and where fear of crime is prevalent.
6. Duplication or gaps in service, resulting in inefficiency.
7. Poorly administered programs.
8. Paternalistic and/or hostile attitudes of staff.
9. Lack of programs geared to the special needs of minorities.
10. Lack of trained personnel.

Lieberman (1978), Lawton (1978), and Sargent (1980) have all pointed out that traditional psychotherapy is not a likely alternative for many elderly seeking some kind of assistance. Instead, more successful efforts could be organized around nontraditional approaches that facilitate coping with stress, emphasize self-improvement, enhance the prevention and/or avoidance of emotional distress, and foster a more positive self-image characterized by autonomy, assertiveness, and self-direction (Sargent, 1980). The acceptability of "therapy" might thus be enhanced in a less-formalized mode for use with older persons. Help provided by paraprofessionals, friends, volunteers, visiting nurses, and persons from the "natural helping network" (i.e., druggists, custodians, beauticians, peers), offered *outside* the loci of traditional institutional-private practice, may be just as effective as well as more accessible and acceptable to elderly persons as are traditional therapists and therapies. This possibility is particularly intriguing in light of the Parloff et al. (1978) review suggesting weak (at best) evidence for therapist experience as a determinant of outcome. Parloff et al. (1978) alternatively suggest that experience with a particular *population* may be *more* important in influencing outcome; thus, having helped older persons in the past may be the indicator of future success.

While little research on the matter exists (Donnan and Mitchell, 1979), it seems probable that therapist-client variables such as age, sex, social class, and similar value systems would affect the likelihood of therapy being effective with, and acceptable to, potential elderly clients (Garfield, 1978; Levy et al., 1980). Research on the effects of such factors, as well as controlled comparisons of traditional versus nontraditional therapies utilizing elderly clients, is as yet lacking, however. Approaches based on age-related normative considerations, that is, developmental tasks (Zimet, 1979), are moreover incomplete and conceptually misleading; it has been pointed out that such age-graded normative events are but *one* set of antecendent or causal factors that are responsible for developmental change throughout the life span (Baltes & Willis, 1977; Baltes, Reese, and Lipsitt, 1980). In this light, a nontraditional approach to counseling older persons seems to be most consistent with an emphasis on increased interindividual variability and with the increased impact that nonnormative events (such as death, illness, relocation, natural disasters, unforeseen unemployment) may have on the aged (relative to that of history-graded or age-graded occurrences). Thus, nontraditional therapies would seem to be a viable option for many aged.

Gatz and associates (1980) cite several research studies supporting the notion that *(a)* on the basis of current surveys, between 6% and 16% of elderly surveyed indicated a need for counseling services, but that *(b)* there are substantial differences in what service providers are offering and what older adults want. A sensitivity to subgroups of elderly "at risk" (homebound, the depressed, women, minority aged), as well as a recognition of the fact that mental illness is best treated when the interplay between health, stresses or supports in the environment, and life experiences of the elderly person is emphasized, will heighten both today's aged and future cohorts' awareness and use of mental health services.

Thus, as Levy et al. (1980) point out, therapeutic endeavors with older persons might serve the dual functions of enhancing the individual's growth and development and maximizing the interaction between the older person and his environment, whether it is the community or the institution. As such, environmental intervention (rather than person-oriented intervention) would *also* define the goals of counseling or psychotherapy for those frail elderly whose adaptive skills are limited by poor health, lack of funds, or social isolation. Levy et al. (1980) see intervention as based on a holistic view of human development, where *all* health problems are viewed as having a psychological component. Problems that are not strictly psychological, but are a mixture of the products of biologic-psychosocial change, would likewise be targets for intervention, such as being homebound or institutionalized, or experiencing malnutrition, loneliness, sensory impairments, or role losses (bereavement, retirement). Obviously, therapeutic intervention with the aged could take place in the community as well as in the institution.

Counseling Elderly Persons

What special or unique considerations need to be acknowledged when entering into a therapeutic relationship with an elderly person? Lawton (1976) advocates acquiring specialized knowledge about older persons. Thus, it is important to have a familiarity with characteristics common to *many, but not all,* elderly persons, such as sensory loss and intellectual and personality change. Moreover, in explaining the cognitive competence of older persons cohort differences, relative to age differences, are a central consideration. Thus, historical changes in health care, value systems, level of education, and attitudes toward assessment are *more* important than are age-causal (or biologic) factors (Baltes, Reese, and Lipsitt, 1980). Much of the current research in cognitive functioning of the aged rejects the notion of irreversible, universal decline.

There are a number of other important considerations. Discussing abstract ideas (such as dependency and conflict) in terms older persons can understand or in their own words can aid communication. Creating a supportive, trusting atmosphere to minimize anxiety, while proceeding at a pace slow enough to allow the older client to become comfortable, should encourage him to verbalize feelings that may not otherwise be shared for fear of criticism. An awareness of sensory impairments, which may be embarrassing and anxiety producing to the older person, is also vital. Sensitivity to both adaptive and socially appropriate behaviors, as well as those that are maladaptive and socially inappropriate, is very important. Despite a wish to be kind, therapists nevertheless need to give accurate feedback, whether it is critical or constructive, to the older person they are helping.

Distrust or hostility stemming from a kind of helplessness may be felt by some older persons. This helplessness may be triggered by anxiety of both real and anticipated losses of health, memory, finances, or interpersonal relations. Some may also feel hostility toward nonexistent "inevitable senility."

Lawton (1976) feels the elderly person should be permitted to hold onto defenses, such as denial, which have proved valuable in the past (McGee and Lakin, 1977; Wilensky and Weiner, 1977). To deny a person the use of such defenses is like taking a crutch away from someone who is physically handicapped, leaving him no other support. For example, a client's morale may be boosted by his denial of physical change, maintaining that "I'm just as good as I've always been." Such "psychological crutches" serve an important function for many aged, particularly if they are alone, or perceive a discrepancy between desired and actual lifestyles, or are in poor health. Insight into the more painful aspects of one's life, especially those beyond one's control, is not necessarily helpful. Some may be overwhelmed by the resulting self-criticism and guilt (Ingebretsen, 1977).

One need not attempt to completely "rework" the older person's personality in order to be effective. Short-term helping efforts to alleviate transient depression and anxiety can be of immense value to many elderly persons. Help in easing the transition from a work role to a semiretired one or from one's home to an institution, or in coping with losses of long-term relationships or a physical-sensory change is vital. Simply being able to express sadness, pain, anger, depression, or loneliness is an invaluable service to aged persons who have no one else in whom they can confide. It may be particularly important to emphasize that it is all right to be dependent and to encourage some elderly persons to give up goals that are simply beyond their resources, such as maintaining power over grown children or being totally independent.

Flexibility, honesty, the ability to listen, openness to others' experiences or values, a willingness to change established procedures, warmth, genuine caring, and treating each elderly person as an *individual* are central ingredients of a successful, *mutually* satisfying therapeutic experience with older persons. The following skills should be developed by those working with the elderly: an attention to nonverbal cues, the use of short frequent sessions, recognition of the importance of touching, slower expectation of change, knowledge of the person's environmental supports and resources, sensitivity to the need for changes in the home and family, the need for review or reminiscence in later life (Butler, 1975; Sussman, 1976), and a recognition that one may be perceived as an "expert" or a "professional" with whom highly personal, anxiety-evoking, threatening emotions and thoughts are to be shared. Whether the aged individual is referred for treatment by another health provider or the family or enters into therapy voluntarily obviously affects the initial motivation to change and his willingness to remain committed to a therapeutic relationship.

Lawton and Gottesman (1974) suggest several roles or skills that the "geropsychologist" might acquire. These involve:

1. A facility in different types of intervention—individual or group therapy, reality orientation, remotivation, cognitive skills training, milieu therapy, family therapy, and various other techniques (art therapy, pet therapy, music or exercise therapy).
2. Expertise in psychological test construction, administration, and interpretation.
3. Functional (life skills) assessment.
4. Psychosocial care planner (integration and coordination of available community or institutional services and personnel).
5. Ombudsman or advocate.

It is likely that effective diagnosis and treatment will involve the expertise of several professionals from *different* disciplines in order to arrive at a satisfactory care plan for the older person.

Of all these skills, that of advocate is perhaps the most ill defined, but yet the most effective. Many elderly persons are at a disadvantage in terms of power and it is important that their needs be recognized and acted on. The geropsychologist can perform this "consciousness-raising" function by being knowledgeable and willing to represent his clients' needs in an accurate yet forceful manner. Because many elderly have no one to depend on in this sense, the geropsychologist may be called on to document the need for mental health services for the aged and to convince others of its urgency; for example, in justifying the creation of a new program, or in the training and hiring of staff sensitized to the mental health concerns of the elderly.

At the present time, several alternatives to treatment exist for the disturbed elderly person, both in the community and in the institution. While specific models for the choice of treatment have been proposed (Gottesman, Quarterman, and Cohen, 1973), there are no established guidelines for choosing the "best" treatment for a particular disorder. Choice of treatment should always involve a consideration of the physical, emotional, and cognitive capacities of the elderly individual and societal demands regarding appropriate behavior. Expectations of family, friends, and other persons important to the aged person, as well as self-expectations, must be considered. Therapy reduces the discrepancy among any of the above factors and intervention focuses on altering what the person expects of himself. If, for example, an aged person wants to drive a car but is not physically able, the helper would encourage an awareness of his own physical limitations or would recommend a bus or a ride from a friend or family member. The source of the problem might also be societal, such as an age limitation on drivers' permits, or it may rest with family members who demand that the older person continue to be independent. Intervention, in this example, would be directed at changing laws allowing older persons to drive, or altering family expectations of an older member. In situations such as these a discrepancy exists that is causing the elderly person distress. Elements are more or less "brought into line" with one another to reduce the discrepancy.

One goal of therapy may be to "add life to the years instead of years to the life" (Gotestam, 1980). In therapy, we are primarily concerned with improving the *quality* of life, rather than merely its quantity. Specific goals in therapy with the aged are:

1. Aiding insight into behavior
2. Providing symptom relief
3. Providing relief to relatives
4. Delaying deterioration
5. Aiding adaptation to a present situation
6. Improving self-care skills
7. Encouraging activity
8. Facilitating independence

Each goal will be more or less important depending on the physical health and resources of the elderly person and the therapist's own biases. Whether to opt for a long-term or a short-term approach and whether community-based or institutional care is desired are individual decisions. Certain types of therapy such as individual, group, and family work better for some individuals and therapists than for others. Some are more acceptable to older persons than others.

There are many viewpoints one can take when trying to counsel an older person. A variety of theories exist concerning how people get over emotional disturbance, and most therapies that spring from these theories have been found to be effective. Reviews of the literature on psychotherapy outcome have shown that no one type of psychotherapy is significantly better than any other (Smith and Glass, 1977). The conclusion can thus be drawn that no *single* therapy is the right one to use, particularly in view of the enormous diversity of the older adult population with whom a therapist must work. How is a decision made about what therapy to utilize?

Often, paraprofessionals find themselves placed in the position of *acting* as a therapist or counselor to clients in a facility, and in this sometimes unavoidable position, preparation for such a role pays valuable dividends. The paraprofessional always should keep in mind that a great deal of training is necessary to justify serious therapeutic intervention. It is essential to familiarize oneself as thoroughly as possible with the more prominent theories of personality that have been advanced over the last 100 years. Since existing theories of personality have varying degrees of relevance for the aged (Kastenbaum, 1978), such familiarity is all the more important. Texts such as those by Hall and Lindzey (1978), Rychlak (1981), and Maddi (1976) are examples of such sources. Each theory uses its own particular view of the human mind to create a system of psychotherapy; without knowledge of these theories, study of various forms of therapy is impossible. Therapy should *never* be attempted without proper training and supervision by a professional.

Major Forms of Therapy

There is a great variety of forms of psychotherapy and this review is by no means intended to be exhaustive. The therapies considered here are major therapeutic movements that have been in existence for some time, and all have a great deal of support in the research literature. One should keep in mind that the number of experimental investigations that have been done with elderly clients is small compared to studies done with other age groups (Eisdorfer and Stotsky, 1977; Gotestam, 1980; Hartford, 1980; Storandt et al., 1978).

Psychoanalysis

It might be most appropriate to begin this review of psychotherapeutic intervention with Sigmund Freud's psychoanalysis. Psychoanalysis is an attempt to resolve conflicts that reside in the unconscious. Freud believed that there were different levels of consciousness and that the level that contributed most to how the person behaved was completely unknown to the individual—this was called the unconscious or subconscious. Freudian therapeutic technique involves helping the client uncover subconscious motivations and conflicts. Free association, which involves having the client speak freely, without prompting or inhibition, is often used for this purpose. Often, many hours of free association are required, with appropriate interpretations offered by the therapist. Freudian analysis is a very time-consuming affair, and change takes place very slowly. There are a few studies of the effects of psychoanalytically oriented therapy with the elderly in the literature, but flaws in their design make it difficult to evaluate the technique for this population. Freud himself was skeptical that his therapy would be effective with the elderly, reasoning that many of the elements of disturbance in a person of advanced years would be so well established as to be almost impossible to change. A great deal of training and supervision are necessary to become an analyst, as well as undergoing analysis oneself. For the paraprofessional, Freudian theory and therapy are not a fruitful area of study and practice. Classical psychoanalysis is not typically employed with elderly persons. Many modifications in technique, however, have been suggested (Davis and Klopfer, 1977; Ingebretsen, 1977) that make possible psychoanalytic approaches with older clients that previously would not have been utilized (Gotestam, 1980). Some theories and the therapies derived from them that are relevant to the paraprofessional working with the elderly are described below.

Client-Centered Therapy

Carl Rogers' "client-centered" approach begins with the central idea that man's nature is basically good and that in every person there is an innate tendency to develop and grow. Rogerian therapy is an attempt to facilitate this "actualizing principle" in each client. The Rogerian therapist is nondirective; in other words, he or she makes no attempt to lead or to "educate" the client in the correct way to lead his or her life. Instead, the client must be allowed for find his or her own way, and the therapist's task is simply to listen and to facilitate the expression of feelings and thoughts. This is difficult to do, as it requires the therapist to have what Rogers calls "unconditional positive regard" for the client. Unconditional positive regard involves taking a nonjudgmental attitude toward every aspect of the client's actions and attitudes, so that in this atmosphere of acceptance growth can begin. In addition, the therapist must "feel with" the client as he or she expresses feelings and thoughts; he must be able to see things through the eyes of the client, "feel" his feelings, inhabit his world. Nondirective therapy can be effective only when this empathy exists. Empathy is expressed to the client by accurately reflecting feelings and thoughts after their expression. Often older clients don't need anyone to tell them what to do, but instead need a therapist who can help them realize the growth potential that lies dormant within. A final ingredient necessary for client-centered therapy to be effective is that the therapist be genuine at all times. No pretense or facade can be allowed to intrude; the therapist cannot simply take on a "role." Attitudes and skills such as unconditional positive regard and accurate empathy must be ingrained and cultivated before client-centered therapy can take place.

It is difficult to say which clients will respond best to nondirective therapy. Very little research has been done with any therapy to specify certain client characteristics that predict the best outcome. Almost all schools of therapy claim that their techniques are effective with all clients, but this is not likely. There are general guidelines that can be applied when trying to choose the correct approach for a particular client; if the client *expects* to be told what to do and asks for advice, more directive forms of therapy may be appropriate. One might also speculate that socially isolated clients might benefit more from nondirective therapy than from other forms of treatment, as lack of social contact may have contributed a great deal to the problems with which the client is grappling.

Certainly, the therapist must be comfortable with the kind of therapy he or she is doing, and must have some faith in the theory that underlies the therapeutic process being used.

Behavior Modification

Behavior modification springs from a theory that views man's behavior as caused by an environment of positive reinforcers and punishers. B. F. Skinner (1953) developed this theory to a large extent, and behavior modification has been used therapeutically in many ways. The pattern of behavior that the client needs to change is broken down into discrete, quantifiable units of behavior. "Positive reinforcers" are any kind of perceived reward that increases the frequency of the targeted behavior.

Let us take as a hypothetical case an elderly woman in a nursing home who refuses to get out of bed, even though she is physically capable of doing so. In a behavior modification program, staff would be instructed to interact with the patient minimally while she was in bed, but on those few occasions when she left the bed, to be very warm and communicative. By making verbal reinforcement dependent on "out of bed" behavior, this program might be effective in making the patient more physically active. If the program did not work, another reinforcer could be tried. It is important to remember that different people respond to different rewards and reinforcers. The verbal reinforcement used in the above example might not be effective with another person who has had different experiences. Examples of other reinforcers are a touch, a smile, cigarettes, shopping privileges, or spending money. Of course, ethical problems can be encountered if the therapist has too much control over the client's environment. Collaboration with family members and other mental health professionals can help to avoid violations of the client's rights.

The use of punishment as a primary means to modify behavior is generally a poor second choice to positive reinforcement. Punishment can be defined as any perceived aversive (negative) stimulation that leads to a *decrease* in frequency of a targeted behavior. The phrase "aversive stimulation" is often associated with electric shock and other painful things, but it can also be a loss of television time, having to do the dishes, or donating $10 to a rival political campaign fund. If used at all, punishment can be self-administered or administered by the therapist in varying degrees; elimination of dangerous or severe behavior problems should be left to the professional behavior therapist. Punishment appropriate for such behaviors is generally severe and often involves painful stimulation. The nonprofessional should never utilize painful or severe punishments, even at the risk of losing treatment effectiveness.

However, milder forms of punishment can be effectively utilized in programs to eliminate problem behaviors of the elderly. This can be accomplished only if the client is allowed to participate in making decisions about the behavior to be modified and agrees to the positive reinforcers and punishments in the program and when they should be administered. In behavior modification programs set up by the paraprofessional, the client should have full knowledge of the program and all its aspects. A mild form of punishment will often be initiated by the elderly person in response to directives from the therapist, for example, when asked to come up with a self-imposed punisher, an elderly person might make a visit to an unpleasant acquaintance as the punishment for failure to live up to a behavioral contract.

Another technique that can be utilized by the behavior modifier involves positively reinforcing a behavior that competes with the unwanted target behavior. For example, if the goal is weight loss, the therapist might have persons who interact socially with the client reinforce eating diet food rather than eating chocolate cake or other high-caloric food.

Contracting is an important form of behavior modification. In this procedure, the client and therapist arrive at a clearly specified goal. The goal might be to exercise for weight loss and health reasons. The therapist and client specify in the contract the amount of exercise to be performed per day, the form of exercise used, the intensity of the exercise, and the kind of reinforcement that would be most effective for maintaining the exercise goal week to week. Punishment can be inserted into a contract—in the above example, if the exercises were not done.

A paraprofessional therapist must exercise great care in applying the very powerful principles of behavior modification to the aged. Professional therapists should be in consultation when any doubt exists about the ethics of the procedure to be followed.

While a complete review of the research on behavior therapy is beyond the scope of this chapter (Gotestam, 1980; Richards and Thorpe, 1978), short-term behavioral techniques such as those discussed above have been successfully employed with predominantly institutionalized aged to treat a variety of problems, such as antisocial behavior, speech difficulties, chronic pain, incontinence, self-feeding, and personal self-care skills.

Cognitive Behavior Therapy

Cognitive behavior therapy (Ellis, 1962; Meichenbaum, 1974; Beck, 1976) has recently been investigated with elderly persons (Kooken, 1981), and findings cast a hopeful light on the use of this technique. Cognitive behavior therapists believe that the way a person *thinks* largely determines the way he or she feels. In other words, thought causes emotional response. Cognitive behavior therapy is an attempt to help the client change his or her maladaptive thinking habits to relieve emotional disturbances such as depression, anger, and anxiety. Ellis (1962) views this process in an A-B-C fashion. *A* is designated as the event that the client thinks is causing the anxiety or the depression. The emotional disturbance lies at point *C*. A client might believe, for example, that her depression (*C*) is being caused by her getting old (*A*). Ellis insists that aging (*A*) is not causing the depression (*C*); instead, the depression (*C*) is attributed not to aging (*A*) but to the woman's *belief* (B) about her own aging as the culprit. In this case, the woman might erroneously believe that being old means that she is a horrible person, unworthy of respect or love. A cognitive behavior therapist would attempt to point out to this client that aging does not mean that she is worthless, and that no life event makes her unlovable and unworthy of respect. In this case, the client's irrational overgeneralizations caused her to become depressed.

Older persons make certain kinds of thinking errors more often than their younger counterparts. The thought "Because I am old, I can do less" may lead to self-doubt and self-derogation, and the older person may perform less capably because he attempts less. If indeed the older person is less capable due to health problems or other reasons (disuse of skills), the thought "Because I can't do now what I could do then, I am worthless" is often the cause of depression, anger, and other emotional disturbances.

The cognitive behavior therapist can teach the clients to dispute these thoughts and to substitute more rational statements in their place. For example, the client might be persuaded to alter his thoughts in the following way: "It is unfortunate that I can now do less than I could at one time. But this does not affect my worth as a person. I will simply try to develop my capabilities to their fullest, and to accept myself as I am." This more rational self-statement leads to adaptive change rather than to self-defeating depression.

Cognitive behavioral approaches to therapy have been successfully utilized to treat a variety of cognitive and emotional problems in the aged, such as depression, cautiousness, test anxiety, and response speed (Richards and Thorpe, 1978). As with all other forms of psychotherapy, cognitive behavior therapy takes time to learn, and requires practice and adequate supervision.

Reality Orientation

There are several other therapies that do not spring from complex theoretical formulations. Reality orientation, commonly known as RO, is a therapeutic technique based on the assumption that repeated orientations to the immediate environment will reduce disorientation and withdrawal from that environment (Folsom, 1967). Often RO is done in a group setting, and the therapist will ask each client in turn to recite simple orienting responses such as the day of the week, the name of the facility, and so on. Such participation may prevent withdrawal and social isolation, as well as cognitive deficits that may result from a lack of stimulation. Most often, this technique is utilized with rather deteriorated, institutionalized elderly persons, but the principles of the treatment could be utilized in any setting. The important principle to keep in mind is that of exposure to a demand for processing and retrieving information, or, in simplistic terms, thought practice. Thinking skills do not go unused for long periods of time without some deterioration occurring, whether such losses are experiential or organic in nature. Keeping the mind of the elderly person active is a prime objective of the paraprofessional therapist; and unlike psychotherapy with other age groups, it may require daily or twice-daily sessions if no other source of stimulation for the client exists or can be cultivated. RO, however, lacks consistent support as to its long-term effectiveness (Gotestam, 1980).

Other Forms of Therapy

Other approaches commonly used with elderly persons involve (*a*) group therapy, (*b*) family therapy, (*c*) organic (drug) treatment, and (*d*) a variety of approaches subsumed under the guise of "institutional therapy" (i.e., remotivation, milieu therapy, art therapy, exercise therapy).

GROUP THERAPY.—The distinguishing feature of group therapy with the aged is that dependency needs can be used to their best advantage. This approach can take many forms, ranging from issue-oriented discussion groups, to groups designed to stimulate verbalization and interaction among group members, to groups specifically geared to promoting independence and a positive sense of self. They permit a member to set realistic goals while focusing on each client's strengths, thereby building group cohesiveness. Groups are typically short term (when used within the institution) and informal in nature. Group therapy is often used in a variety of settings by those offering dance therapy, art therapy, or music therapy for elderly persons. Leading groups requires considerable training and skill and should not be undertaken lightly; a more complete discussion can be found in Hartford (1980). While group therapy has been used in conjunction with many social services for the aged, its utility is undocumented as yet. It does appear to possess potential in this regard as a therapeutic technique.

FAMILY THERAPY.—This is a very attractive alternative in treating older persons whose difficulties are communicative in nature. Changes in roles, such as retirement or grandparenthood, problems accompanying chronic or acute illness, institutionalization of one's parent(s) or spouse, or conflicts arising when an older parent is being cared for at home by a middle-aged child can be approached by bringing together all parties involved. Then it is possible to set up clear expectations for behavior, improve communication, lessen distrust and guilt, or deal with hostility and anxiety. Such an approach may also be used with elderly couples when issues regarding sexuality or resolution of past conflicts that have been intensified by illness or retirement are of concern. Family therapy can also be used when communication has broken down between parent and child, and thus may be appropriate when an older parent wishes to remarry but is opposed by a child, or where difficulties arise when an elderly parent must be institutionalized. It may be important to clarify a grandparent's role and responsibilities to avoid conflicts over child-care duties or over "who is to be the parent." Where an older parent is being cared for by a child at home, difficulties can arise when the adult child attempts to place the elderly parent in a submissive, dependent role, which the older parent explicitly rejects. Again, a "clearing of air" is helpful to allow both parties to express guilt, hostility, or anxiety and deal with manipulative behavior or withdrawal. "Filial immaturity" results when an overly dependent child "forces" an older person back into a "parent" role, one which most likely had been given up years before. Here, too, family therapy may be the treatment of choice. At present, despite its potential for elderly couples and their children, it has been virtually ignored for use with older persons (see Gotestam, 1980; Hartford, 1980, for discussions).

DRUG TREATMENT.—Extensive, in-depth discussions of pharmacologic treatment with the aged are available elsewhere (Hicks et al., 1980; Kapnick, 1978). It is probably accurate to say that drug treatment of the aged historically has been too often relied on in instances where other alternatives might have been just as effective, if not more so. It is therefore with the utmost caution that drugs be used with elderly clients. Older persons are particularly sensitive to drug effects; wide individual differences exist regarding response to psychopharmocologic agents. Older persons are not as capable of metabolizing and excreting drugs as are the young. Most drugs (prescription or over the counter) have a longer half-life in older persons; they build up in concentration when fixed dosage intervals are used. Such drugs are not being used by the body and are thus ineffective. This, in addition, makes their interactions with other drugs, antacids, and some foods as well, more likely, producing a variety of side effects that may not only be harmful but may also be misdiagnosed as an irreversible organic brain syndrome (OBS), deemed untreatable by the unsuspecting clinician. Such side effects can range from mild confusion, depression, urinary or cardiac dysfunction, to hallucinations or seizures. Ironically, such symptoms can lead to the administration of *more* drugs to alleviate the condition (which is seen as worsening) for which the drugs were originally prescribed, causing further drug toxicity. One should *always* have an extensive drug history and an accurate record of *what* drugs the elderly person is taking, the *dosage*, and *how often*. *Caution* is the watchword here. While various drugs have been used (major or minor tranquilizers, sedatives, stimulants, hypnotics) to treat depression, paranoia, or schizophrenia, to induce sleep, to lessen fatigue, or to treat symptoms such as confusion or memory loss associated with OBS, their use is often uncritical.

Kapnick (1978) lists simple rules that should guide both the clinician and the lay person in the use of drugs with the aged:

1. Understand the pharmacologic action of the drug used—how it is metabolized and excreted.
2. Use the lowest dose possible that is effective—on an individual basis.
3. Use the fewest drugs the person needs.
4. Do not use drugs to treat symptoms without first discovering the causes of those symptoms.
5. Do not withhold medication on the basis of age per se.
6. Do not use a drug if its effects are worse than the symptoms it was prescribed to cure.
7. Discontinue the use of a drug when it is no longer necessary.
8. Review repeat prescriptions.
9. Encourage the aged person to contact his physician (who should be willing to listen) if he experiences any adverse side effects.

INSTITUTIONAL THERAPY.—Other approaches to therapy involve a variety of treatments that may be useful for some elderly persons in some circumstances: milieu therapy (creation of a "therapeutic" environment involving all staff), remotivation therapy (where the patients' strengths are emphasized, reality is stressed, and sharing, appreciation, and acceptance are reinforced), art therapy, exercise therapy, and dance therapy (Gotestam, 1980; Storandt et al., 1978).

While some literature is not complete enough to provide us with clear answers to questions regarding (1) whether one type of therapy is more effective than another, (2) whether one approach is most effective with older versus younger clients, (3) whether particular therapies are more appropriate for certain disorders, and (4) what kinds of older persons respond best to which types of therapy under what conditions (due to lack of research, or poorly designed studies), several conclusions can be reached. Older persons *are* motivated toward, cognitively capable of, and able to benefit from professional and paraprofessional help. A model of irreversible decrement with age is explicitly rejected by current research (Baltes et al., 1980). Therapy with the aged should always be problem-solving oriented (Gotestam, 1980; Lawton, 1976) and be geared to the person's own goals, strengths, weaknesses, needs, life situation, resources, and particular problem. Thus, whether life review (reminiscence), insight, alleviation of symptoms, resolution of conflict, increasing social skills or self-care behaviors is the goal, it seems clear that the elderly person should be the ultimate concern of the therapist. While family, friends, or staff may benefit, these gains must be of secondary value.

The alleviation of stress may also require intervention at a societal level. Thus, altering attitudes toward the aged, effective use of community, family, and friends, and use of a variety of services (home-based care, outreach, hospice care, foster grandparent program, widow-to-widow programs, enhanced control over institutional regulations, routines and procedures) may prove to be as effective as intervention at the individual level (see Beattie, 1976; Eisdorfer and Stotsky, 1977; and Lowy, 1980 for discussions of social services for the aged and other forms of "social treatment").

The Importance of Evaluation

Whatever approach is used, its effects should be known. It seems obvious that one would want to know whether a given treatment works or not! Thus, assessment of intervention efforts with the aged is critical. Therapy is time-consuming, demanding, and frequently expensive; lives are at stake.

Older persons, as compared to younger ones, are more heterogeneous, as noted above. This fact alone seems to argue for a more individual approach to the outcome problem with the elderly. Those selecting outcome criteria for use with gerontologic populations should opt for measures that are individualized and situationally specific. While a "battery" of such measures for use with elderly samples has been suggested (Levy et al., 1980), these measures are, in many cases, nomothetic (generalizable across persons) in nature, lacking in norms for elderly persons, confounded by the effects of response set (Raskin and Jarvik, 1979), and seem to be, in many cases, pathology-oriented (see Chap. 10). Gatz et al. (1980) recommended the use of multiple perspectives, that is, self, therapist, independent evaluator, significant others, with both an internal and an external focus in evaluating therapy. This, however, disregards the view that much "pathologic" behavior in elderly persons is "context-specific" (Birren and Renner, 1980; Gurland, 1973; Lawton, 1978). While the usefulness of a battery of criterion measures with the elderly must certainly be explored, its value has yet to be empirically evaluated (see Levy et al., 1980 for a description of such a battery).

As has been noted above, poorly developed models of psychopathology and personality dynamics (with reference to the aged) and the likelihood that most efforts at intervention will take place *outside* "traditional psychotherapeutic modalities" suggest that, for evaluative purposes, models of outcome research (both preventive and ameliorative) with the elderly cannot be based on the current efforts in psychotherapy with younger-age cohorts. Both the paraprofessional and the professional should, however, make an effort at evaluation, preferably basing decisions about whether a given intervention technique "works" or not on clinical impression, self-report, and psychometric data.

Many times, the greatest service a therapist can bestow on his or her client is referral to an appropriate agency or individual for treatment. It is extremely important to acquaint oneself with all the agencies available in the community that will render services to an aged client. Knowing where to refer is only part of the picture; equally important is knowing when to refer. For example, many health problems may manifest themselves as psychological disturbances, and to treat such difficulties with psychotherapy alone would be doing a great disservice to the older client. Depression, which is sometimes manifested as a drug effect, will not necessarily respond to psychotherapy alone, no matter how skillfully such therapy is done. When in doubt, the therapist should consult health care professionals about a diagnosis and an appropriate treatment regimen. Referral to a primary care physician or to a psychiatrist is very often appropriate prior to psychological treatment. A great deal of training is necessary before a therapist is capable of proper diagnosis, and referral before treatment begins is often the most prudent course of action to rule out physical causes.

Conclusion

There are occasions in counseling the elderly when common sense overrides one's theoretical orientation. One of the first considerations in counseling an elderly person is whether the individual possesses the necessary information to resolve an emotional problem. Misconceptions about the nature of the problem and misinterpretation of the actions of others often lead to disturbance. For instance, an elderly client might mistakenly believe that a bill received from the hospital must be paid in cash immediately, when in fact an insurance policy will cover the expense.

There are innumerable situations in which the older person reacts to such a misunderstanding by becoming depressed, angry, or anxious, when a simple explanation of the facts will go a long way toward resolving the "problem." Helping the client to reinterpret the actions and intentions of others may be a valuable information-giving service. An example is the elderly person who sees her daughter's attempts to persuade her to enter a nursing home as an effort to "get me out of the way." It may be that serious health problems necessitate such a move, and that reinterpretation of the daughter's intentions would be valuable. Often such misinterpretation of the intentions of others occurs in the absence of communication between the parties in question. It may be advisable to set up sessions in which both parties are present (see discussion of family therapy) so that the therapist can help the two persons reach an understanding. In any case, before complex theories are invoked to explain the disturbed emotions of the client, commonsense alternatives should be explored.

In spite of the diversity of approaches to psychotherapeutic interventions reviewed here, it remains clear that older persons must be counseled on an *individual* basis to avoid harmful generalizations about the ability of older persons to respond to treatment. We can then improve the quality of life for today's elderly, who have long been written off as beyond help. Old age can then be seen as a period of life when continued growth and development can flourish.

REFERENCES

Baltes P., Reese H., Lipsitt L.: Life-span developmental psychology. *Annu. Rev. Psychol.* 31:65–110, 1980.

Baltes P.B., Willis S.: Toward psychological theories of aging and development, in Birren J.E., Schaie K.W. (eds.): *Handbook of the Psychology of Aging*. New York, Van Nostrand Reinhold, 1977.

Beattie W.M.: Aging and the social services, in Binstock R., Shanas E. (eds.): *Handbook of Aging and the Social Sciences*. New York, Van Nostrand Reinhold, 1976.

Beck A.: *Cognitive Therapy and the Emotional Disorders*. New York, International Universities Press, 1976.

Birren J., Renner V.: A brief history of mental health and aging, in Birren J.E., Sloane R.B. (eds.): *Handbook of Mental Health and Aging*. Englewood Cliffs, N.J., Prentice-Hall, 1980.

Birren J., Renner V.: Concepts and issues of mental health and aging, in Birren

J.E., Sloane R.B. (eds.): *Handbook of Mental Health and Aging*. Englewood Cliffs, N.J., Prentice-Hall, 1980.

Birren J., Sloane R.B.: *Handbook of Mental Health and Aging*. Englewood Cliffs, N.J., Prentice-Hall, 1980.

Birren J., Woodruff D.: Academic and professional training in the psychology of aging, in Eisdorfer C., Lawton M.P. (eds.): *The Psychology of Adult Development and Aging*. Washington, D.C., American Psychological Association, 1973.

Blum J., Tallmer M.: The therapist vis-à-vis the older patient. *Psychother. Theory Res. Pract.* 14:361–367, 1977.

Butler R.N.: Psychiatry and the elderly: An overview. *Am. J. Psychiatry* 132:893–900, 1975.

Butler R., Gertman J., Overlander C., et al.: Self-help, self-care, and the elderly. *Int. J. Aging Hum. Dev.* 10:95–117, 1979–80.

Butler R.N., Lewis M.: *Aging and Mental Health: Positive Psychosocial Approaches*. St. Louis, C.V. Mosby Co., 1977.

Davis R., Klopfer W.: Issues in psychotherapy with the aged. *Psychother. Theory Res. Pract.* 14;343–348, 1977.

Donnan H., Mitchell H.: Preferences for older versus younger counselors among a group of elderly persons. *J. Counsel. Psychol.* 26:514–518, 1979.

Eisdorfer C., Stotsky B.: Intervention, treatment, and rehabilitation of psychiatric disorders, in Birren J.E., Schaie K.W. (eds.): *Handbook of the Psychology of Aging*. New York, Van Nostrand Reinhold, 1977.

Ellis A.: *Reason and Emotion in Psychotherapy*. New York, Lyle Stuart, 1962.

Folsom J.C.: Intensive hospital therapy of geriatric patients, in Masserman J.H. (ed.): *Current Psychiatric Therapies*, vol. 7. New York, Grune & Stratton, 1967.

Ford C.V., Sbordone R.J.: Attitudes of psychiatrists toward elderly patients. *Am. J. Psychiatry* 137:571–575, 1980.

Garfield S.: Research on client variables in psychotherapy, in Garfield S., Bergin A. (eds.): *Handbook of Psychotherapy and Behavior Change*. New York, John Wiley & Sons, 1978.

Gatz M., Smyer M., Lawton M.P.: The mental health system and the older adult, in Poon L. (ed.): *Aging in the 1980's: Psychological Issues*. Washington, D.C., American Psychological Association, 1980.

Gotestam K.: Behavior and dynamic psychotherapy with the elderly, in Birren J.E., Sloane R.B. (eds.): *Handbook of Mental Health and Aging*. Englewood Cliffs, N.J., Prentice-Hall, 1980.

Gottesman L., Quarterman C., Cohen G.: Psychosocial treatment of the aged, in Eisdorfer C., Lawton M.P. (eds.): *The Psychology of Adult Development and Aging*. Washington, D.C., American Psychological Association, 1973.

Gurland B.: A broad clinical assessment of psychopathlogy in the aged, in Eisdorfer C., Lawton M.P. (eds.): *The Psychology of Adult Development and Aging*. Washington, D.C., American Psychological Association, 1973.

Hall C., Lindzey G.: *Theories of Personality*, ed. 3. New York, John Wiley & Sons, 1978.

Hartford M.E.: The use of group methods for work with the aged, in Birren J.E., Sloane R.B. (eds.): *Handbook of Mental Health and Aging*. Englewood Cliffs, N.J., Prentice-Hall, 1980.

Hicks R., Funkenstein H., Dysken J., et al.: Geriatric psychopharmacology, in Birren J.E., Sloane R.B. (eds.): *Handbook of Mental Health and Aging*. Englewood Cliffs, N.J., Prentice-Hall, 1980.

Ingebretsen R.: Psychotherapy with the elderly. *Psychother. Theory Res. Pract.* 14:319–332, 1977.

Kapnick P.: Organic treatment of the elderly, in Storandt M., Siegler I., Elias M. (eds.): *The Clinical Psychology of Aging*. New York, Plenum Press, 1978.

Kastenbaum R.: Personality theory, therapeutic approaches, and the elderly client, in Storandt M., Siegler I., Elias M. (eds.): *The Clinical Psychology of Aging*. New York, Plenum Press, 1978.

Knee R.I.: Finance mechanisms affecting mental health services and their delivery, in *Mental Health and Aging: Volume 3—Services*. Washington, D.C., U.S. Department of Health, Education and Welfare, National Institute of Mental Health, 1979.

Knight R.: Psychotherapy and behavior change with the noninstitutionalized elderly. *Int. J. Aging Hum. Dev.* 9:221–236, 1978–79.

Kooken R.A.: *A Stress Inoculation Treatment Procedure for Test Anxiety in Elderly Students,* unpublished research in lieu of thesis. North Texas State University, Denton, 1981.

Lawton M.P.: Geropsychological knowledge as a background for psychotherapy with older people. *J. Geriatr. Psychiatry* 9:221–233, 1976.

Lawton M.P.: Clinical geropsychology: Problems and prospects, in Nygaard D. (ed.): *Master Lectures on the Psychology of Aging*. Washington, D.C., American Psychological Association, 1978.

Lawton M., Gottesman L.: Psychological services to the elderly. *Am. Psychol.* 29:689–693, 1974.

Levy S., Derogatis L., Gallagher D., et al.: Intervention with older adults and the evaluation of outcomes, in Poon L. (ed.): *Aging in the 1980's: Psychological Issues*. Washington, D.C., American Psychological Association, 1980.

Lieberman M.: *Methodological Issues in the Evaluation of Psychotherapy with Older Adults*. Paper presented at the Annual Meeting of the Gerontological Society. Dallas, Tex., November 1978.

Lowy L.: Mental health services in the community, in Birren J.E., Sloane R.B. (eds.): *Handbook of Mental Health and Aging*. Englewood Cliffs, N.J., Prentice-Hall, 1980.

Luborsky L., Chandler M., Auerback A., et al.: Factors influencing the outcome of psychotherapy. *Psychol. Bull.* 75:145–185, 1971.

Maddi S.: *Personality Theories: A Comparative Analysis,* ed. 3. Homewood, Ill., Dorsey Press, 1976.

McGee J., Lakin M.: Social perspectives on psychotherapy with the aged. *Psychother. Theory Res. Pract.* 14:333–342, 1977.

Meichenbaum D.: *Cognitive Behavior Modification*. Morristown, N.J., General Learning Press, 1974.

National Institute of Mental Health: *Mental Health and Aging: Volume I—Research*. Washington, D.C., U.S. Department of Health, Education, and Welfare, 1979.

National Institute of Mental Health: *Mental Health and Aging: Volume 3—Services*. Washington, D.C., U.S. Department of Health, Education and Welfare, 1979b.

Parloff M., Waskow I., Wolfe B.: Research on therapist variables in relationship to process and outcome, in Garfield S., Bergin A. (eds.): *Handbook of Psychotherapy and Behavior Change: An Empirical Analysis*. New York, John Wiley & Sons, 1978.

Raskin A., Jarvik L.: *Psychiatric Symptoms and Cognitive Loss in the Elderly: Evaluation and Assessment Techniques*. New York, Halsted Press, 1979.

Richards W., Thorpe G.: *Behavioral approaches to the problems of later life*, in Storandt M., Siegler I., Elias M. (eds.): *The Clinical Psychology of Aging*. New York, Plenum Press, 1978.

Rychlak J.F.: *An Introduction to Personality and Psychotherapy*, ed. 2. Boston, Houghton-Mifflin, 1981.

Sargent S.S.: Why non-traditional therapy and counseling with the aged?, in Sargent S.S. (ed.): *Nontraditional Therapy and Counseling With the Aging*. New York, Springer, 1980.

Skinner B.F.: *Science and Human Behavior*. New York, Macmillan Publishing Co., 1953.

Smith M., Glass G.: Meta-analysis of psychotherapv outcome studies. *Am. Psychol.* 32:752–760, 1977.

Smyer M., Gatz M.: Aging and mental health: Business as usual? *Am. Psychol.* 34:240–246, 1979.

Sparacino J.: Individual psychotherapy with the aged: A selective review. *Int. J. Aging Hum. Dev.* 9:197–220, 1978–79.

Storandt M., Siegler I., Elias M.: *The Clinical Psychology of Aging*. New York, Plenum Press, 1978.

Sussman M.: The family life of old people, in Binstock R., Shanas E. (eds.): *Handbook of Aging and the Social Sciences*. New York, Van Nostrand Reinhold, 1976.

Wilensky H., Weiner M.B.: Facing reality in psychotherapy with the aging. *Psychother. Theory Res. Pract.* 14:373–377, 1977.

Zimet C.: Development task and crisis groups: The application of group psychotherapy to maturational processes. *Psychother. Theory Res. and Pract.* 16:2-8, 1979.

18

HUMANISTIC HEALTH CARE FOR THE ELDERLY

Roger A. Lanier, Ph.D.

In old age a good physician can be your most valuable ally.

Comfort, 1976

HUMANISTIC HEALTH CARE is a phrase that is becoming increasingly popular in the 80s. The phrase is frequently cited in both professional and lay literature and has evolved to represent an ideal for many health professionals. Three questions, however, are particularly relevant for this new health care movement. Why is there a need for a humanistic health care movement? How does humanistic health care differ from the more traditional approach? Does humanistic health care make any difference? The purpose of the present discussion is to address these three questions.

Why Is There a Need for a Humanistic Health Care Movement?

There is little doubt that there have been major technological advances, tremendous expansions of biomedical research, and the development of specialization and superspecialization in health care during the 20th century. Often, however, the needs and priorities of the health care consumer and those of a highly technological, highly specialized health care delivery system have seemed vastly different (Naughton, 1977). As a result, the quality of health care that is received by the consumer is often less than desirable (Tubesing et al., 1977; White, 1975).

Literature that reviews weaknesses in the current health care delivery system underscores many unmet needs (Andreopoulos, 1974; Beloff and Korper, 1972; Freymann, 1975; Garfield, 1970; Holinger and Westberg, 1975; McNerney, 1975; McWhinney, 1975; Spitzer et al., 1974; White, 1975). Lack of physicians, maldistribution of available physicians, maldistribution of funds, and lack of a holistic preventive form of care have been cited as contributing to this condition (Tubesing et al., 1977; Andreopoulos,

1974; Petersdorf, 1975; Stimmel, 1975). Moreover, deteriorating physician-patient relationships, the loss of credibility of many health professions, and the failures of some institutions providing care, such as hospitals and nursing homes, have been sharply criticized (Berman, 1976; Mendelsohn, 1979). Additionally, some consumers feel they have delegated too much responsibility to the health care system for certain curing and caring functions that should remain the province of the individual (McKay, 1980).

These weaknesses are exaggerated for the elderly health consumer, whose life expectancy has been extended to 72 years, with approximately 80% of all deaths associated with old age. The magnitude of the problem can also be appreciated when considering that 30% of all physician and hospital time and 57 cents of every federal dollar are spent on older people, with projections indicating that provider time will increase to 75% (Butler, 1980). Currently, however, access to adequate health services is a major problem for the elderly. Some of the difficulties involved are inability to drive a car or use public transportation, inability to walk upstairs or sit through long waiting periods in clinics, lack of funds, or just lack of strength to leave the house to see a provider (National Council on the Aging, 1975).

These problems are aggravated by the traditional health system's clear orientation against disability and death. With few positive strategies toward disability or death, patients are often being implored in one fashion or another to get better (Sizemore and Coyle, 1981). Apparently, 69% to 90% of physicians prefer not to tell patients when they are dying (Feifel, 1977). Therefore, patients often go through the period of dying alone, unsupported, or even antagonistic to the aims of treatment (Krantz, 1978).

A recent national survey (Harris and Associates, 1981) found that the majority of respondents indicated they were "beginning to lose faith in their doctors." Substantial proportions of those surveyed criticized physicians for their indifference, poor methods of communication, choice of treatment methods, and overprescription of drugs. Concerns identified by the report also included rising health care costs, excessive waiting times, and anxiety over inadequate care. The report suggested that increasing specialization and depersonalization related to care of the patient were directly related to these attitudes.

The Disease Model of Health Care

The traditional health care system has excelled in the treatment of disease and has traditionally defined health in terms of disease: a healthy person was one who had no physical disability, who had few doctor visits, who rarely missed work because of illness, and who survived a long time (Remen, 1980; Cardus, 1973). Therefore, within the last 50 years, the general goal has been to restore the patient to the status quo ante, the condition prior to the onset of disease (Remen, 1980).

The word "health" was originally the antonym of the word "disease." Yet as inconsistent as it seems, the primary focus of the "health system" has been disease (Cardus, 1973). Physicians and other professionals have been largely trained to think in terms of the disease model; for example, symptoms are obtained, the disease is classified in the appropriate nomenclature, a diagnosis is produced, and treatment is provided (Barbour, 1975). Often, it has even been convenient for providers to view patients as interchangeable or in mechanistic terms and the health professional simply as a biologic repairman outfitted with scientific tools (Garell, 1975).

Within the disease model of health care, the ultimate origin of illness has been limited to within the individual, usually at the microbiologic level. Efforts could then be concentrated at that level and were based on the following assumptions (Hayes-Bautista and Harveston, 1977):

1. An illness has an organic base (Veatch, 1973).
2. The organic base is the result of discrete causal elements (Dubos, 1959).
3. The illness is the involuntary result of an invasion of the host by an overwhelming quantity of causal elements (Veatch, 1973).
4. The appropriate treatment for an illness is an agent that will directly counterattack the causal element and neutralize it (Dubos, 1959).
5. Such an agent can be prescribed and administered only by a technically competent specialist (Parsons, 1951; Veatch, 1973).
6. The knowledge held by the specialist is inaccessible to the lay person; hence the patient must submit to the ministrations of the specialist without interference (Parsons, 1951; Blum, 1960).

Using these assumptions, it has been convenient to divide the individual into turfs, each of which is the province of a set of specialists with extensive knowledge about a single procedure, a single organ, a single tissue, or a single cell (Blum, 1975). Health care was then dispensed according to which fragment of the individual was affected (Simon, 1961). Too often, however, the individual patient has disappeared among the procedures, organs, tissues, cells, or bacteria (Hayes-Bautista and Harveston, 1977).

This approach has been relatively successful for acute diseases where the patient could be quickly assigned to a protocol and returned to his routine. But for chronic diseases or for the emotional components of health care, the approach has been increasingly inadequate (Cardus, 1973; Ardell, 1977; Henig, 1977). Current estimates suggest that approximately 80% of contemporary diseases are classified as chronic (compared to only 30% prior to World War II) and that emotional factors play a significant role in successful rehabilitation for physical disabilities in about 50% of adults and 75% of children (Rusk, 1971; Knowles, 1977; Henig, 1977). Treatment of physical symptoms is no longer enough, particularly for individuals who must live with their disability day after day. In the absence of medical cures, these people are demanding a more humanistic health care approach (Henig, 1977).

This is particularly an issue for the elderly, since chronic illness tends to multiply with age (Comfort, 1976). The elderly are often attempting to live with an average of five diseases (Butler, 1980). Moreover, the majority will die of a terminal illness that will occupy a considerable period of time (Krantz, 1978).

Professional Preparation

There have been a variety of influences on the professional preparation of health care providers; the current approach apparently has not been the result of a linear evolution. Edelstein (1967) notes that since the early Greek period there has been a conflict between physicians who were curatively oriented and physicians who were more philosophically oriented. Hayes-Bautista and Harveston (1977) trace the evolution of this conflict over the past two centuries. Apparently, the dominant system was the one with the philosophical approach. It was more holistically oriented in that causes outside the individual and multiple causation were recognized. This system dominated until the introduction of the germ theory of disease in the late 1860s. At this time, the holistic model was dismissed as a passé, romantic, and naive notion of disease causation. Reinforced by the Flexner report of 1910 and the influence of the basic sciences, medical schools excelled in generating small groups of superspecialists who focused on subhuman elements and organs and intervened with shot, drug, or pill (Bernstein and Lennard, 1973).

The intensive curriculum in many professional schools has been subject to an inevitable degree of failure, however, simply because enough material cannot be taught and assimilated rapidly enough to prepare the future professionals. Also, in the post–World War II era, the emphasis on communication skills and humanistic care, by either conscious or unconscious exclusion, has received a low priority (Naughton, 1977).

There is also a critical need for training related to the care of the elderly. This can easily be justified, based on (1) shifting demographic patterns; (2) increasing use of long-term care facilities; (3) the intensifying role of the federal government to provide better access to health care for the elderly; and (4) growth in the utilization rate and the broadening of types of services offered to the elderly (Comfort, 1976; National Commission on Allied Health Education, 1980). But in spite of differing pharmaceutical responses, the additional need for patient education for the elderly, and the physician's need to examine attitudes related to chronic disease and death, the inclusion of geriatric training within the curriculum is far too rare (Comfort, 1976).

On examination of the medical school curriculum, Berman (1976) queried, "Is it any wonder, however, that a sport that required the tracing of thousands of winding and twisting arteries and nerves and memorizing thousands of bones, muscles and sinuses, would not be surrounded by an aura of scholarship that elicited respect and admiration? Or is it surprising that the personality attracted to this calling responds with the pomposity, over-bearance and sense of infallibility necessary to intimidate and impress patients?"

Former medical students have also noted that even though they had aspirations of being a "country doc," medical school was often found to be very disease-oriented rather than people-oriented. As one former student reported, "People would talk about going down to see the liver in room 301, or the spleen in 429" (Ferguson, 1977).

One possibility for helping to alleviate this problem is for students to witness the provision of humanistic health care by their faculty (Nordlicht, 1977). However, much of the process tends to be left to chance (Remen, 1980; Grayson et al., 1977). Simpson (1972) states that many institutions continue to believe the myth that "merely leaving students around patients for a time is likely to be good for them and they are bound to pick up all sorts of balanced social viewpoints from exposure to the 'splendid animals' by some sort of intellectual osmosis." Recent studies indicate that mere exposure to patients fails to improve student abilities related to the variety of behaviors required for effective practitioner-patient interaction (Barbee and Feldman, 1970; Helfer and Ealy, 1972), and specific training programs have evolved to increase competence in this area (Rasche et al., 1974; Adler and Enelow, 1966; Werner and Schneider, 1974; Pacoe et al., 1976).

Patient Disenchantment

It has been suggested that patients have become more discontented, more critical, and even more hostile as the art of health care has gradually become separated from the science of health care (Remen, 1980). While the value of scientific care must be acknowledged, consumers are increasingly disenchanted with a specialized and very technically oriented health care system that consists primarily of detecting, diagnosing, and treating illness, injuries, and disabilities while ignoring human needs (Grayson et al., 1977; McKay, 1980). Increasingly, there has been pressure to recognize that behind the morass of numbers that identify patients (i.e., social security numbers, hospital patient numbers, account numbers, and specimen numbers) are individual people (Thompson, 1977).

Health care costs and the amount of waiting time have also been sources of patient dissatisfaction (Weeks and DeVries, 1978; Nordlicht, 1977; Pellegrino, 1977). While these concerns are relevant to consumers in most industries, they are of more central importance within the health care system. Adoption of the economic values of the larger society and an almost unionist stance on rights and compensation by some providers (e.g., the growing tendency to adopt short work days and weeks, longer and more frequent vacations, and more regular hours) have been criticized as unacceptable within the health care system (Nordlicht, 1977; Pellegrino, 1977).

Patients are also concerned over such issues as iatrogenesis, that is, the contribution by the health care system toward making sick people sicker (Fink, 1976; Illich, 1976; Henig, 1977). Moreover, the public increasingly tends to question findings which indicated that no great suffering or increase in mortality resulted when only 15% of the hospital beds were occupied at the time physicians went on strike in New York and San Francisco (Berman, 1976).

Pellegrino (1977) points out that consumers have been fearful of health care providers with esoteric knowledge that can alter their lives in ways and by means they cannot fully understand. He reveals that while such power was historically acquired through a special relationship with the spirits, the special relationship is now with technology. He lists several mechanisms that have evolved as the result of these consumer concerns, such as legislative control of quality, costs, distribution, and education related to the health care system; demands for consumer involvement in management, accreditation, and licensing of health institutions; a growing tendency to limit the growth of high technology and research; an increasing number of malpractice suits; and the declaration of a patient's bill of rights. Pellegrino calls for the profession to adopt a more humanistic approach that would narrow the gap between what providers conceive themselves to be, and what consumers expect them to be.

Several authors have also called for a serious reappraisal of the health care professions that would make accountability to society more fashionable and acceptable (Naughton, 1977; Berman, 1976; Mendelsohn, 1979; McKay, 1980; Weeks and DeVries, 1978). Some indicate that while humanistic care has been discussed for years and receives lip service, actual practice fails to reflect substantial changes (Weeks and DeVries, 1978); others propose that "a case can be made for a harsh, cleansing attack in order to prod the doctors into doing something about it" (Berman, 1976); and still others suggest that there is simply a need to relax the concern with "professionalism" so that social and emotional aspects of care receive greater attention (Remen, 1980).

The Physician-Patient Relationship

Certainly an issue that has received much attention in recent years is the deterioration of the physician-patient relationship (Bertakis, 1977). This relationship has been described as a curious and unequal one where the physician "gets respect, adoration, and a handsome fee while the patient, if lucky, gets well" (Berman, 1976).

Several studies have suggested that patients tend to be more dissatisfied with the information they receive than with any other aspect of health care (Duff and Hollingshead, 1968; Korsch et al., 1968; Reader et al., 1957). Apparently, this is largely the result of both the impersonal and technical way in which the information is communicated (Weeks and DeVries, 1978; Bertakis, 1977) and the authoritative stance taken by the physician (Bruhn et al., 1977; Weeks and DeVries, 1978). Effective interaction has also been inhibited by the physician's lack of empathy, failure to provide adequate information, perception of the patient as a disease rather than a person, or general disregard for the dignity, privacy, and comfort of the patient (Gordis et al., 1969; Fisher, 1971; Egbert et al., 1964; Francis et al., 1969; Korsch et al., 1968). Increasingly, patient dissatisfaction with the physician-patient relationship has tended to result in malpractice litigation (Reeder, 1972; Aday and Andersen, 1975).

The effects of specialization have also been criticized as being detrimental to the physician-patient relationship (Miller, 1975; Hanavan, 1977; Tubesing et al., 1977; Pelletier, 1977). Increasing specialization seemed to occur for two related reasons. First, because of the rapid technological advances, specialization was viewed as a method for physicians to remain abreast of specific areas (Tubesing et al., 1977). Second, the compelling logic of the scientific method led to the adoption of therapeutic approaches predicated on breaking down clinical problems into smaller and smaller parts, with intensified problem-solving at this level (Hanavan, 1977). While specialization has many tangible benefits, too often reassembly of the pieces at the conclusion of the health care visit, by moving back up the scale from cell to tissue to organ to the patient, has failed to occur (Hanavan, 1977). Far too often, the coordination of patient care seems left to chance. And in the absence of such coordination, caring, and concern, the physician moves unfortunately close to becoming merely a sophisticated technician (Nordlicht, 1977).

It seems hazardous, particularly for the elderly, to see each of several specialists recommending different and potentially incompatible types of medication or treatment (Tubesing et al., 1977). Since complaints tend to multiply with time, the elderly often receive dozens of medications in a scientific attempt to cover all the bases (Comfort, 1976). Poe and Holloway (1980) have suggested that not a day goes by when a geriatric patient is not seen with symptoms and signs of drug misuse, and they are often found to be on 15 to 20 different medicines. Consequently, unfavorable drug reactions are witnessed for at least one patient in nine where drugs are prescribed. It has been noted that the noninstitutionalized elderly receive an average of 5.6 drugs daily (Krupka and Vener, 1979). Poe and Holloway (1980) say that it is easier for a physician to prescribe than to think, and they are convinced that the overuse, misuse, or abuse of drugs is a major and frequent cause of illness among the elderly. Apparently, from 80% to 85% of the elderly suffer from one or more chronic conditions that can be controlled with the proper use of drugs (Center for Human Services, 1979), but interactions with diet and other drugs must receive adequate attention (Ebersole and Hess, 1981).

Health Care Institutions

While the institutions in which health care is delivered have received less attention than the providers of the care, indications are that they will be increasingly criticized for providing dehumanized care (Thompson, 1977; Berman, 1976; Mendelsohn, 1979; Shem, 1978). Health care institutions share the responsibility (a corporate responsibility) for the care of the patient; that is, when the health care team delivers care within a hospital or nursing home, its members are not in an isolated decision-making context (Pellegrino, 1977). And for the elderly, approximately 70% can expect to die in the institutional environment of the hospital, nursing home, or hospice (Fulton, 1976).

Hospitals have come under much greater criticism recently. For instance, as Berman (1976) points out:

> Hospitals are fine if you're not sick. . . . It's not that comptrollers, accountants, and cost experts lack heart, but like today's string beans or lamb chops, sickness must be carefully weighed, packaged, and paid for, with a little profit for the house. Everything in the hospital from an aspirin to a gargle has a price; except perhaps politeness or compassion, which are unavailable at any price. . . . [It's] show your card, pay in advance, or bleed elsewhere . . . "take-your-number-out-and-wait." . . . Any hospital that wants to make it big in the American Hospital Association must first purge itself of the family physician (or anything else smacking of warmth or common sense).

Symptomatic of the larger problem of nonhumanistic care is the issue related to the administration of heroin or morphine for the care of incurably ill and dying patients (Butler, 1978). Addiction is not a concern for these patients, but relief from pain is. Yet, less than 1% of the hospitals in the United States offer any type of program related to the care of the dying (Butler, 1978).

Nursing homes constitute one of the fastest-growing industries in the United States, with almost 1 billion dollars a year generated in New York alone. But as one Senate report asserts, "They are number one on the list of unsafe places to live," and are often compared with flophouses (Berman, 1976). As Berman (1976) has stated:

> No doubt many doctors have always been dedicated to the aged. Nursing homes are often serviced, supervised, and even owned by physicians. Only licensed M.D.s can supervise the bed sores, malnutrition, and dehydration that are acquired in these homes. In contrast to the inefficient hospitals, nursing homes have long waiting lists and a handsome turnover. According to government statistics, the doctors can do much better in Medicare without budging from their office, so why should they bother with crosstown traffic getting to those smelly places. . . . If these homes nurse anything, it's a profit. . . . The elderly seem to get a better deal with the Sioux Indians who put their elderly out in the forest to gently pass away.

Yet, findings indicate that there are more people over 65 in nursing homes (1.3 million) at any moment than in hospitals (Butler, 1980). For the nursing home industry between 1960 and 1976, there was a 550% increase in the number of employees (from 100,000 to 645,000); a 140% increase in the number of nursing homes (from 9,582 to 23,000); a 301% increase in the number of nursing home beds (from 331,000 to 1,327,358); a 245% increase in the number of patients (from 290,000 to 1,000,000); and a 2,000% increase in revenues (from $500 million to $10.5 billion) (National Commission on Allied Health Education, 1980).

As Thompson (1977) reminds us, however, when discussing the dehumanization of institutions, the easiest thing to do is blame the "system," which is nothing more than a method or plan of arrangements devised by individuals. Therefore, if a system is dehumanizing, it has become so because of the individuals who established it and those involved with it—both providers and consumers.

Patients have bought into the "system" as much as anyone else, and many may be reluctant to change (Fink, 1976). Such change would involve: (1) a redefinition of the sick role and its secondary gains; (2) an examination of health insurance that pays lavishly for illness; (3) a review of the multimillion dollar drug industry and the belief that every illness demands a pharmacologic intervention; and (4) a redefinition of employment benefits that stress sick leave. It is unfortunate, however, that the health care system is currently being challenged from without more than from within, and its evolution is being determined by seemingly disjointed and unrelated events rather than from a central mission and through coordination (Naughton, 1977).

In the traditional system, then, providers see sick people and use their knowledge to treat and return patients to the "normal" state that existed before they became ill (Monaco, 1975). In order to efficiently deliver the quantity of care demanded, patients are generally grouped according to their need, type of illness, and degree of urgency (Thompson, 1977). Within this crisis-oriented system, providers barely have enough time to meet the constant demands for crisis care, while consumers get little attention unless they convince the providers that the ailment is of crisis proportions (Tubesing et al., 1977).

Therefore, while the traditional health care delivery system is technically superior to any known throughout history, the neglected aspects of care call for better communication of health information, better coordination of care, increase in care for the early stages of illness, and a wider variety of patient supports (Tubesing et al., 1977). There seems to be substantial resistance to such shifts, however, because of the major investment in illness that society has incorporated within provider and patient roles and the institutions in which they interact (Fink, 1976).

How Does Humanistic Health Care Differ From the More Traditional Approach?

Today, there is an increasing awareness that contemporary health problems require more sophisticated, complex, multifaceted, and multidisciplinary approaches than the simplistic application of the disease model (Winkelstein, 1972; Fuchs, 1966).

Webster defines "dehumanize" as "to deprive of human qualities, as pity, kindness, individuality, creativity, etc.; make inhuman or machine-like." The most common thread running through the criticisms of traditional health care is that it has become "dehumanized." The humanistic health care movement evolved specifically in response to this identified problem. Obviously, the humanistic health care approach also requires the identification and recording of variables that relate to physiologic function, state of nutrition, genetic background, and body structure and composition, as well as to physical and psychological stress, individual and social behavior, and cultural habitat (Cardus, 1973).

But a major difference lies in a focus on health rather than disease. Illich (1976), for instance, offers the following definition:

> Health is simply an everyday word that is used to designate the intensity with which individuals cope with their internal states and their environmental conditions. . . . Health levels will be at their optimum when the environment brings out autonomous, personal, responsible coping ability. Health levels can only decline when survival comes to depend beyond a certain point on the heteronomous (other-directed) regulation of the organism's homeostasis. Beyond a critical level of intensity, institutional health care—no matter if it takes the form of cure, prevention, or environmental engineering—is equivalent to systematic health denial.

Humanistic health care derives from the concept that human needs should receive the primary consideration in health care and that providers should be humane in attitude, ethic, and behavior (Fink, 1976). A related concept, holistic health care, derives from the idea of wholeness in approaches to giving and receiving health care so that a more comprehensive and better-integrated form of care is striven for than in the traditional delivery system (Fink, 1976).

A frustrating aspect of the humanistic health care approach, however, is that it is still evolving as an area. There are multiple concepts proposed for inclusion; most proposals are a reaction to the problems of the traditional system but most new approaches are not independent of the old system; some of the concepts within the evolving theoretical structure overlap; and there is only beginning to be empirical support which would address the question, "So what?" In fact, it has been suggested that a useful method of approaching the rather amorphous area is to conceptualize it as a social movement (Hayes-Bautista, 1976).

Therefore, at this point in its evolution, the humanistic health care movement seems to be more an attitude than a coherent system (McKay, 1980). Yet, suggestions for a more humanistic form of health care provide a richer framework in which to approach the challenging privilege of caring for patients.

The literature related to humanistic health care seems to reflect five central themes that call for an expansion of the traditional health care system. These themes are:

1. An expanded view of health
2. An expanded view of causality
3. An expanded view of the health consumer
4. An expanded view of health providers
5. An expanded view of alternatives

An Expanded View of Health

Humanistic health care, in an effort to find richer and more personalized ways of conceiving of and delivering care, expanded from a disease model to an educational model (Remen, 1980). This model respects the valid contributions of the traditional health care system but recognizes that medicine and health are not synonymous (Dreissen, 1978). This approach is person-oriented rather than disease-oriented and rejects the restriction of the relationship between provider and consumer to the use of health technology (Dreissen, 1978; Remen, 1980). That is, the approach transcends the treatment of disease or symptom amelioration and concentrates on the relationship between the provider and consumer and on the inner strength of the consumer to accentuate traditional treatment.

Pellegrino (1977) suggests that the phrase "humanistic health care" implies a spirit of sincere concern for the centrality of human values in every aspect of professional activity (i.e., a respect for the freedom, dignity, worth, and belief systems of the individual person and a sensitive, nonhumiliating, and empathetic way of helping). As a result, the view of health is expanded to include the dynamic balance between mind, body, emotions, and spirit (Barbour, 1975). Illness represents an imbalance of these interdependent factors rather than simply the result of pathophysiology.

This model goes further, however, to suggest that individuals can progress beyond a state of health toward a state of high-level wellness. That is, an individual can improve his state of balance through education, growth, and self-actualization (Ardell, 1977). Such concepts significantly alter a view of health in terms of describing the condition on a continuum rather than as a dichotomy; a focus on growth rather than simple avoidance; recognition of a dynamic relationship rather than a static one; encouragement of participation rather than passivity; a greater consideration of subjective values than simply objective ones; and an interest in cumulative and integrated effects rather than independent and fragmented ones (Bruhn et al., 1977). Within this conceptual framework, however, there are currently many assessment difficulties. Perhaps as these difficulties are addressed, the model will become increasingly popular.

An Expanded View of Causality

Humanistic health care, then, must expand its view of causality, and therefore intervention, to include mind, body, emotions, and spirit (Weeks and DeVries, 1978). The patient becomes more than his or her body and therefore more than his or her disease (Remen, 1980). These are important concepts since the traditional view of causality has tended to determine and limit the range of care provided. Such an expanded view of causality, then, offers great potential for richer care results (Miller, 1975).

The medical model has traditionally been disease-oriented; that is the causal element is a specific organic base that is counterattacked and neutralized by a technically competent specialist. Within this framework, patients with similar diagnoses can be treated in similar ways in what has been described as a "replace or repair modality" (Miller, 1975). The humanistic health care model does not reject the involvement of microbiologic elements in the process, but rather it expands the view of causality and therefore concentrates more on health and illness than simply on disease. The personal experience of disease, including the person's attitudes, feelings, thoughts, and values, is considered. As a result, multiple causation and multiple interventions are more often observed and may include elements at the psychological, social, economic, and political levels as well (Hayes-Bautista and Harveston, 1977).

Therefore, humanistic health care attempts to progress beyond isolated symptoms and partial explanations to examine patient complaints in the total context of his environment. Such an approach has been found to be more effective, more scientifically valid, and more cost-effective through the avoidance of the wrong diagnosis, inappropriate diagnostic procedures, ineffective therapy, unnecessary hospitalization, extension of disability, iatrogenic disease, and increased cost (Barbour, 1975).

An Expanded View of the Health Consumer

The role of the health consumer within the medical model has been described as a subservient and passive one, where the individual is expected to abide by medical advice, ask few questions, and be a "good patient" (McKay, 1980). While such dependence can be common in a technologic society where information for rational decision-making is restricted, consumers have become increasingly dissatisfied with their level of participation in an area as sensitive as their health care (Pellegrino, 1977).

The humanistic health care model takes an expanded view of the health consumer by placing the major responsibility for health on the consumer rather than on the professional, and by recognizing the consumer as an active and committed partner in the process rather than a passive recipient (Dreissen, 1978). Indeed, such a mutual participation relationship (Szasz and Hollender, 1956) recognizes the consumer as the primary provider with the other health team members providing counsel and technical assistance for the consumer to make a responsible decision (Fink, 1976).

Comfort (1976) notes that if elderly patients have an effective physician, they will be able to discuss, receive explanations and reassurance, and jointly plan a strategy for any problems related to aging. If, on the other hand, a physician equates infirmity or senility with chronological age, Comfort recommends that the patient change physicians immediately.

Data have always indicated that much health care has been in a preprimary or informal health care system; some studies suggest that as much as 90% of the care occurs in this manner (Alpert et al., 1967; Silver, 1963; White, 1967). In the 1930s, much self-care first occurred due partly to a shortage of physicians but even more to a shortage of money (Ferguson, 1977). Indications are that a trend toward self-care has been steadily increasing (Henig, 1977). Humanistic health care simply recognizes this trend and attempts to involve the consumer as a previously untapped health resource.

Related to this process of activation of the consumer is the creative use of the illness experience to facilitate consumer growth, self-awareness, and self-responsibility (Remen, 1980). Illness, then, may present an opportunity to reevaluate priorities, values, and behaviors, learn new skills, and clarify the importance of human relationships. So the consumer's role is also expanded as it relates to conceiving of the treatment encounter; treatment is no longer limited to symptom amelioration, but includes a focus on how the consumer may improve or become more well.

The above approach also requires that the consumer be viewed in a broader context. Whereas the traditional model essentially allowed like diseases or handicaps to be treated similarly, humanistic health care means that the health problem is viewed in reference to the total life context of the consumer (Barbour, 1975). Accordingly, differential diagnoses are provided for the consumer to assist in clarifying strengths, limitations, and rehabilitation potential (Goldin, Leventhal, and Luzzi, 1974).

Several questions have been suggested for the patient interview to assist consumers in exploring their lifestyles and making appropriate behavioral changes that might not have been systematically included in the past (Tubesing et al., 1977). Four examples are: "What is the aim of your life?" (meaning); "What beliefs and values guide you?" (faith); "What do you choose to spend your lifetime doing?" (commitment); and "What are you willing to let go of?" (surrender).

An Expanded View of Health Providers

Given that humanistic health care provides an expanded view of health, causality, and consumers, it follows that adjustments would also be necessary in the roles of health providers. It has been pointed out (Miller, 1975) that the traditional physician dispenses health in a quick and efficient, authoritative manner as a product rather than as a process. Apparently, this personal style is the result of being trained to accept a number of largely unquestioned authorities, for example the authority of certain journals, some major institutions, certain commanding reputations, and the authority of boards of accreditation and licensure. Pellegrino (1977) suggests that before the humanity of the consumer can be restored, the inequality between provider and consumer must be removed as fully as possible. Through expansion of the role of the consumer and utilization of the health provider as a consultant, humanistic health care significantly reduces this inequality. As the consumer and provider interact more as colleagues, the consumer is encouraged to be aware of his or her choices and to become increasingly responsible for his or her own health, growth, and fulfillment (Barbour, 1975).

The view of health providers must also be expanded because of the expanded view of causality. Given the notion of multiple causation, an interdisciplinary health care team usually provides multiple intervention strategies. This is contrasted with the traditional approach in which a single provider utilizes a single intervention (Hayes-Bautista and Harveston, 1977). In fact, the learning experiences that are provided from this expanded view are often drawn from diverse sources, such as philosophy, psychology, sociology, religion, anthropology, systems theory, literature, and the arts (Miller, 1975). As special efforts are made to gather, integrate, and interpret large sources of data, the treatment encounter becomes characterized by a richness of creative insight seldom experienced in the one-to-one treatment approach (Tubesing et al., 1977).

Such interdisciplinary approaches have produced some interesting research. Notable is the renewed interest in the old concept of the "laying on of hands," when it was found to result in an increase in blood hemoglobin levels (Krieger, 1976).

An Expanded View of Alternatives

The humanistic health care model expands on the alternatives available for treatment or the meaning of various alternatives. Specifically, these include the use of patient education, preventive health care, and the interpretation of such concepts as time, pain, and stress.

The humanistic approach emphasizes patient education and preventive health care because of the expanded view of the health consumer and the definition of health (Beloff and Korper, 1972; Garfield, 1970; McNerney, 1975; Tubesing et al., 1977; Dreissen, 1978). Volunteers and patient support groups are often used to facilitate these efforts.

Patient education is extremely important to humanistic health care since, traditionally, the consumer has lacked much of the essential knowledge needed to make rational health care decisions. Pellegrino (1977) states that the provider's "technical decisions must be congruent with the patient's needs to participate in the choices as freely and rationally as education, time, and the circumstances permit. Disclosure of the facts of the illness; the degree of its gravity, the alternatives open; their relative effectiveness, costs, and dangers; the physician's own experience and skill in comparison with others; and the likelihood of success or failure must all be explicated. Only when the information gap is closed can patients approach truly valid consent, one which permits participation as a human being and enables the patient to incorporate the decision into his/her own value system."

Ferguson (1977) points out that several practical benefits accrue to providers who offer patient education: a decrease in the number of malpractice suits, as a result of increased patient trust and understanding, as well as fewer office and night calls and a much richer relationship with patients.

The interpretation of time also varies between traditional and humanistic models of care. The traditional model can be described as the effective use of a short time interval. A medical history can be taken, diseases diagnosed and alleviated, and even lives saved, all within a 15-minute interval (Miller, 1975). The humanistic model, on the other hand, views the encounter more as a process on an extended time frame than as a brief crisis encounter. For instance, a 30-year-old patient may be viewed more as an individual on a 40-year program of health maintenance and promotion.

The interpretation of pain can also vary between the two models. Whereas the traditional model may view pain merely as something to be alleviated, the humanistic model more often views pain as a potential stimulus or catalyst for patient growth. When pain is conceived as representing a common experience and perhaps one of the first circumstances where the patient does not feel fully in control, the potential to reevaluate major life choices is tremendous (Miller, 1975).

The interpretation of stress may also vary between the two models. The traditional model, for instance, seems more often to interpret stress as a destructive factor to be alleviated. The humanistic model, while accepting the concept that stress can be destructive, recognizes that a certain level of stress may be necessary to facilitate growth (Garell, 1975). As with health and illness generally, stress can only be thoroughly defined within the context of the life span of the individual (Remen, 1980).

Perhaps the most visible aspect distinguishing the humanistic model from the traditional model is the mode of interacting with patients. Remen (1980) has provided an excellent example of an interchange between a patient and a physician that typifies the collaboration and sharing which can occur.

While the specifics of the problem have been omitted, a small part of the example follows:

"Well, you are the doctor," he said.
"Yes, I know. But what are your thoughts about the situation?"
Ted began to consider the facts and formulate a plan of action.
"It looks as if both my lungs are involved. And I need medicine—some antibiotics and cough medicine."
"I'll write the prescription," the doctor said.
"While you're at it, please write something for pain. It hurts me every time I breathe. And I need to be reexamined to see how I'm doing."
"I'll make an appointment in a week."

Such an approach may be, though not necessarily, more cost-effective, particularly since expensive technology is emphasized to a lesser extent (Butler, 1978). Barbour (1975) points out that providers using the traditional model are often caught in a web of multiple organic diagnoses, continued symptomatology, and ineffective drug treatments. He presents one case study in which the patient had made 20 visits over 2 years with 3 hospitalizations, 3 surgical procedures, 4 drug therapies, 17 physicians, 16 different organic disease diagnoses, and 2 psychological diagnoses only for the condition to remain unchanged. The disease model seems to have failed this patient, yet he remains locked into the system as long as diagnoses and treatments are applied and the patient is passive.

Does Humanistic Health Care Make Any Difference?

While the humanistic approach to health care expands on the traditional model to such an extent that significant changes in patient satisfaction, cost-effectiveness, patient compliance, and actual health status are expected, little data are currently available for documentation. One area where substantial evidence does appear to be accumulating, however, is the literature on patient compliance.

It has long been suspected that the practitioner-patient relationship affects patients' adherence to medical regimens (Gordis et al., 1969; Fisher, 1971; Egbert et al., 1964; Francis et al., 1969). Moreover, the transmission of information from physician to patient has been found to affect both the quality of care and the course of treatment (Davis, 1968; Egbert et al., 1964; Francis et al., 1969; Pratt et al, 1957; Waitzkin and Stoeckle, 1972). Patient satisfaction also tends to increase as more information is given (Bertakis, 1977), even though about one third of it may be forgotten (Joyce et al., 1969; Ley and Spelman, 1965).

Noncompliance reportedly ranges from 15% to 93% of patients, with most studies reporting about one third failing to comply (Davis, 1968; Blackwell, 1973; Cohen, 1979; Marston, 1970). Women have been found to default more than men (Morrow and Rabin, 1966), older people more than younger ones (Davis and Eichhorn, 1963), lower more than higher socioeconomic status groups (Donabedian and Rosenfeld, 1964), and those with lower more than higher levels of education (Pragoff, 1962). This wide range in compliance has been generally attributed to the variety of populations studied, various methods of data collection, and different health problems studied (Talkington, 1978). However, confusion in roles and responsibilities can generate noncompliance or illness-producing behavior if the patient rebels against a perceived authority figure (Remen, 1980).

There are few studies of patient compliance specific to the elderly. In one study, however, it was found that 50% of the elderly deviated from the prescribed regimen and, of these, 70% did not comprehend the regimen (Libow and Sherman, 1981). Medication errors and self-medication have also been found to account for 25% to 95% of the noncompliance problem (Gabriel et al., 1977). Compliance difficulties are apparently increased for the elderly because of too rapid or poor explanations, lack of written instructions, environmental hazards (weather conditions, transportation, fear of crime), visual and hearing problems, loss of short-term memory, an inability to open child-resistant medication containers, and a confusion about specific regimens among multiple medications (Ernst, 1981).

It is questionable to what extent physician-patient communication accounts for noncompliance (Berkowitz et al., 1963), yet when the significance of the medical regimen is not clearly conveyed to the patient, a reciprocal failure in compliance is increased (Davis and von der Lippe, 1968). Moreover, patients with long-term illnesses have been found to be more compliant if given careful instructions (Abramson et al., 1961).

Patient satisfaction, however, has been found to increase with the amount of information given to and retained by them. For instance, Bertakis (1977) found that when an experimental group was asked to restate the information provided, following physician feedback, retention increased from 60.8% to 83.5%, as did satisfaction. This total process, including providing the patient with the opportunity to ask questions, added less than five minutes to the average physician-patient interaction.

Even more closely related to the humanistic approach, Talkington (1978) found, is that if four factors were manipulated between experimental and control groups, patient compliance increased from 55% to 73%. These four factors included: (1) establishing good rapport and communication between the patient and physician; (2) providing interaction which results in the patient feeling that his concerns were understood and expectations met, and feeling the health provider was genuinely concerned; (3) encouraging patient understanding of the health problem, causes, treatment regimen, expected outcome of treatment, and consequences of noncompliance; and (4) assuring patient participation in planning the treatment regimen and identification, analysis, and solution of problems that might interfere with compliance. Patients reportedly reacted most favorably to the personal interaction and support provided by the approach. The largest single category related to noncompliance for the control group was disagreement with the physician's recommendations. One patient in the experimental group was quoted as saying, "I'm so suprised that anyone is actually taking time to ask my feelings about things. I'm so used to being treated like an impersonal piece of meat when I go to the doctor."

Presumably, all providers and patients have certain ideas about the kind of relationship they should have and the kind of roles they are expected to play (Mechanic and Volkart, 1960). Talkington (1978) notes that in this era of patient's rights, an emphasis should be placed on the provider assisting the patient to make his own informed decisions, helping to identify and find solutions to problems that may interfere with compliance, and giving support and guidance as needed. She states that "the age of the dictatorial approach to medical care may well be over as patients become more sophisticated and aware through the media." Other evidence suggests that patients who enter lifestyle changes by choice, rather than from another's orders, tend to follow through on their plans (Henig, 1977).

Summary

Humanistic health care expands on the traditional model of health care in its view of health, causality, the role of the health consumer, the role of the health provider, and the use of various health care alternatives. The humanistic model seems to be a reaction to dissatisfaction with the traditional model, but data that may further support the approach are only beginning to become available.

Many patients and providers, however, believe that more of the same traditional system (i.e., hospital beds, operating rooms, nursing homes, and providers) will not address the problems with which we are confronted today (Monaco, 1975). Health far exceeds physiology and such a recognition is essential to clearly address contemporary problems (Remen, 1980).

At another level, however, the concept can be criticized as being so broad, futuristic, and idealistic as to have little practical relevance for health providers. As one author has paraphrased, "When you're up to your derriere in alligators, it is hard to remember that you came to drain the swamp"

(Fink, 1976). Clearly, current incentive systems are structured around the traditional system (Bruhn et al., 1977). Difficulties related to defining problems, developing procedures, allocating personnel, and financing action often relegate to secondary importance humanistic concerns because of necessity rather than by design (Hayes-Bautista and Harveston, 1977).

The simple recognition, however, that "bandaid" health care is being provided may place providers on the path to more humanistic health care (Hayes-Bautista and Harveston, 1977). Moreover, closer inspection may suggest that, despite the new problems, practical methods of getting "out of the swamp (if not to cover one's posterior)" may be inherent in this new approach, such as reduced litigation, increased patient compliance, more responsible patient decision-making, and an increase in patient and provider satisfaction (Fink, 1976). Additionally, the renewed focus on the needs of the patient may have an immediate impact on the quality of services delivered (Hanavan, 1977).

Contrasts between the traditional and humanistic models of health care are of concern to most consumers, but several needs and problems of elderly health consumers further aggravate the health needs and problems of the general population. For instance, there are unique difficulties in accessing health care; specific hazards related to uncoordinated care and medication; a tendency for the number of chronic illnesses to multiply with age; large increases in expenditures of time and money for health care; special difficulties related to compliance; a more critical need for additional if not different types of patient education; the immediate proximity of death and disability; and the need to deal with health stereotypes specific to the elderly. While a humanistic approach to health care is highly desirable for the general population, it is critical for the elderly.

As the impact of humanistic health care continues to grow, it will be interesting to compare the results of the traditional and humanistic systems on a variety of variables (Monaco, 1975). Until then, one might be reminded of Jourard's (1971) statement that "I have come to see sickness as an outcome of not changing when the time for change has come." Certainly, the problems in the traditional system justify some level of change in and of themselves.

REFERENCES

Abramson J.H., Mayet F.G., Majola C.C.: What is wrong with me? A study of the views of African and Indian patients in a Durban hospital. *S. Afr. Med.* 35:690–694, 1961.

Aday L.A., Andersen R.: *Development of Indices of Access to Medical Care*. Ann Arbor, Health Administration Press, 1975.

Adler L.M., Enelow A.J.: Instruments to measure skills in diagnostic interviewing: A teaching and evaluation tool. *J. Med. Educ.* 41:281–288, 1966.

Alpert J.J., Kosa J., Haggerty R.J.: Medical help and maternal nursing care in the life of low-income families. *Pediatrics* 39:749–755, 1967.

Andreopoulos S. (ed.): *Primary Care: Where Medicine Fails*. New York, John Wiley & Sons, 1974.

Angrist A.A.: Humanism and medical ethics. *N.Y. State J. Med.* 77(9):1448, 1977.

Ardell D.: *High Level Wellness: An Alternative to Doctors, Drugs, and Disease*. Emmaus, Pa., Rodale Press, 1977.

Barbee R.A., Feldman S.: A three-year longitudinal study of the medical interview and its relationship to student performance in clinical medicine. *J. Med. Educ.* 45:770–776, 1970.

Barbour A.B.: Humanistic patient care: a comparison of the disease model and the growth model, in Miller S., Remen N., Barbour A., et al. (eds.).: *Dimensions of Humanistic Medicine*. San Francisco, Institute for the Study of Humanistic Medicine, 1975.

Beloff J.S., Korper M.: The health team model and medical care utilization: Effect on patient behavior of providing comprehensive family health services. *J.A.M.A.* 219:359, 1972.

Berkowitz N.H., Malone M.F., Klein M.W., et al.: Patient follow-through in the out-patient department. *Nurs. Res.* 12:16–22, 1963.

Berman E.: *The Solid Gold Stethoscope*. New York, Macmillan Publishing Co., 1976.

Bernstein A., Lennard H.L.: The American way of drugging: Drugs, doctors, and junkies. *Transaction/Society* 10:14–25, 1973.

Bertakis K.D.: The communication of information from physician to patient: A method for increasing patient retention and satisfaction. *J. Fam. Pract.* 5:217–222, 1977.

Blackwell B.: Patient compliance. *N. Engl. J. Med.* 289:249, 1973.

Blum H.: *Factors in the Health Care Delivery System Inhibiting Utilization and What Can Be Done About Them*. Berkeley, University of California (mimeo), 1975.

Blum R.: *The Management of the Doctor Patient Relationship*. New York, McGraw-Hill Book Co., 1960.

Bruhn J.G., Cordova F.D., Williams J.A., et al.: The wellness process. *J. Community Health* 2:209–244, 1977.

Butler R.N.: Meeting the challenges of health care for the elderly. *J. Allied Health* 9:161–168, 1980.

Butler R.N.: Toward a humanistic approach to dying patients. *Am. Pharm.* 18:53, 1978.

Callan J.P.: Holistic health or holistic hoax? *J.A.M.A.* 241:1156, 1979.

Cardus D.: Towards a medicine based on the concept of health. *Prev. Med.* 2:309–312, 1973.

Center for Human Services: *Pharmacy and the Elderly: An Assessment of Pharmacy Education Based on the Needs of the Elderly and Recommendations for Increasing Geriatric Aspects of Pharmacy Curricula*. HRA no. 80-37. Washington, D.C., U.S. Department of Health, Education and Welfare, 1979.

Cohen S.J.: *New Directions in Patient Compliance*. Lexington, Mass., D.C. Heath & Co., 1979.

Comfort A.: *A Good Age*. New York, Simon & Schuster, 1976.

Davis M.S.: Variations in patients' compliance with doctors' advice: An empirical analysis of patterns of communication. *Am. J. Public Health*. 58:274–284, 1968.

Davis M.S., Eichhorn R.L.: Compliance with medical regimens: A panel study. *J. Health Hum. Behav.* 4:240–249, 1963.

Davis M.S., von der Lippe R.P.: Discharge from hospital against medical advice: A study of reciprocity in the doctor-patient relationship. *Soc. Sci. Med.* 1:336–342, 1968.

Donabedian A., Rosenfeld L.S.: A follow-up study of chronically ill patients discharged from hospitals. *Public Health Rep.* 79:228, 1964.

Dreissen J.: Health sharing: Comments on the characteristics of holistic health. *Holistic Health Focus.* 1:4, 1978.

Dubos R.: *Mirage of Health.* New York, Doubleday & Co., 1959.

Duff R.S., Hollingshead A.B.: *Sickness and Society.* New York, Harper & Row, 1968.

Ebersole P., Hess P.: *Toward Healthy Aging.* St. Louis, C.V. Mosby Co., 1981.

Edelstein L., in Temkin O., Temkin C.L. (eds.): *Ancient Medicine: Selected Papers of Ludwig Edelstein.* Baltimore, Johns Hopkins Press, 1967.

Egbert L.D., Battit G.E., Welch C.E., et al.: Reduction of postoperative pain by encouragement and instruction of patient. *N. Engl. J. Med.* 270:825–827, 1964.

Ernst N. (ed.): *Pharmaceutical Interventions and the Aged.* Dallas, University of Texas Health Science Center, 1981.

Feifel H.: *New Meanings of Death.* New York, McGraw-Hill Book Co., 1977.

Ferguson T.: TNP profile: John Travis. *The New Physician* 26:25–27, 1977.

Fink D.L.: Holistic health: Implications for health planning. *Am. J. Health Planning* 1:23–31, 1976.

Fisher A.W.: Patients' evaluation of outpatient medical care. *J. Med. Educ.* 46:238–244, 1971.

Francis V., Korsch B.M., Morris M.J.: Gaps in doctor-patient communication: Patients' response to medical advice. *N. Engl. J. Med.* 280:535, 1969.

Frazer J.G.: *The Golden Bough.* New York, Macmillan Publishing Co., 1972.

Freymann J.G.: Medicine's great schism: Prevention vs. cure. *Med. Care* 13:525, 1975.

Fuchs V.: The contribution of health services to the American economy. *Milbank Mem. Fund Q.* 44:65–101, 1966.

Fulton R.: The traditional funeral and contemporary society, in Pine V., et al. (eds.): *Acute Grief and the Funeral.* Springfield, Ill. Charles C Thomas, Publisher, 1976.

Gabriel M., Gagnon J.P., Bryon C.K.: Improving patient compliance through the use of a daily drug reminder chart. *Am. J. Pub. Health* 67:968, 1977.

Garell D.: Some principles of a health policy for the future, in Miller S., Remen N., Barbour A., et al. (eds.): *Dimensions of Humanistic Medicine.* San Francisco, Institute for the Study of Humanistic Medicine, 1975.

Garfield S.R.: The delivery of medical care. *Sci. Am.* 222:15, 1970.

Goldin G.J., Leventhal N.A., Luzzi M.H.: The physical therapist as "therapist." *Physical Ther.* 54:484–485, 1974.

Gordis L., Markowitz M., Lilienfield A.M.: Why patients don't follow medical advice: A study of children on long-term antistreptococcal prophylaxis. *J. Pediatr.* 75:957–968, 1969.

Grayson M., Nugent C., Oken S.L.: A systematic and comprehensive approach to teaching and evaluating interpersonal skills. *J. Med. Educ.* 52:906–913, 1977.

Grinker R.R.: *Psychosomatic Concepts.* New York, Jason Aronson, Inc. 1973.

Haberle R.: *Social Movements: An Introduction to Political Sociology.* New York, Appleton-Century-Crofts, 1951.

Hanavan F.V.: Restoring the focus on patient needs: The role of interpersonal relations. *J. Allied Health* 6:72–73, 1977.
Harris L., and Associates: A Survey of Public Attitudes Toward Medical Care and Medical Professionals. Chicago, American Osteopathic Association, 1981.
Hayes-Bautista D.E.: Deviant delivery systems. Paper presented at Conference on National Health Policy Issues. San Francisco, Western Consortium for Continuing Education for the Health Professions, 1976.
Hayes-Bautista D., Harveston D.S.: Holistic health care. *Soc. Policy* 166:7–13, 1977.
Helfer R.E., Ealy K.F.: Observations of pediatric interviewing skills. *Am. J. Dis. Child.* 123:556–560, 1972.
Henig R.M.: Do-it-yourself medicine: The patient as physician. *The New Physician* 26:19-23, 1977.
Holinger P.C., Westberg G.E.: The parish pastor's finest hour—revisited. *J. Rel. Health* 14:14, 1975.
Illich I.: *Medical Nemesis: The Exploration of Health*. New York, Random House, 1976.
Jourard S.M.: *The Transparent Self*. New York, Van Nostrand Reinhold, 1971.
Joyce C.R.B., Caple G., Mason M.: Quantitative study of doctor-patient communication. *Q. J. Med.* 38:183, 1969.
Knowles J.: *Doing Better and Feeling Worse*. New York, W.W. Norton, 1977.
Korsch B.M., Gozzi R.K., Francis V.: Gaps in doctor-patient communication: Doctor-patient interaction and patient satisfaction. *Pediatrics* 42:855–870, 1968.
Krantz M.J.: Death with dignity, in Seltzer M., Corbett S., Atchley R. (eds.): *Social Problems of the Aged: Readings*. Belmont, Calif., Wadsworth Publishing Co., 1978.
Krieger D.: Healing by the laying-on of hands as a facilitator of bioenergetic change: The response of in vivo human hemoglobin. *Int. J. Psychoenergetic Systems* 2:121–129, 1976.
Krupka L.R., Vener A.M.: Hazards of drug use among the elderly. *Gerontologist* 19:90–95, 1979.
Ley P., Spelman M.S.: Communications in an out-patient setting. *Br. J. Soc. Clin. Psychol.* 4:114, 1965.
Libow L., Sherman F.: *The Core of Geriatric Medicine*. St. Louis, C.V. Mosby Co., 1981.
Marston M.V.: Compliance with medical regimens: A review of the literature. *Nurs. Res.* 19:312, 1970.
McKay S.: Wholistic health care: Challenge to health providers. *J. Allied Health* 9:194–201, 1980.
McNerney W.U.: Educating the public about health: The missing link in health services. *J. Med. Educ.* 50:11, 1975.
McWhinney I.R.: Family practice in perspective. *N. Engl. J. Med.* 293:176, 1975.
Mechanic D., Volkart E.H.: Illness behavior and medical diagnoses. *J. Health Human Behav.* 1:86–94, 1960.
Mendelsohn R.S.: *Confessions of a Medical Heretic*. New York, Warner Books, 1979.
Miller S.U.: Professional education for humanistic medicine, in Miller S., Remen N., Barbour A., et al. (eds.): *Dimensions of Humanistic Medicine*. San Francisco, Institute for the Study of Humanistic Medicine, 1975.
Monaco A.J.: Holistic medicine. *Hosp. Topics* 53:10–11, 1975.

Morrow R., Rabin D.L.: Reliability in self-medication with isoniazid. *Clin. Res.* 14:362, 1966.
National Commission on Allied Health Education: *The Future of Allied Health Education: New Alliances for the 1980s*. San Francisco, Jossey-Bass Publishers, 1980.
National Council on the Aging: *National Policy Concerns for Older Women: Commitment to a Better Life*. U.S. Government Printing Office, 1975.
Naughton J.: Medical ethics, humanism, and preparation of the modern physician. *N.Y. State J. Med.* 77(9):1448–1451, 1977.
Nordlicht S.: Teaching humanity-oriented medical ethics. *N.Y. State J. Med.* 77(9):1452–1454, 1977.
Pacoe L.V., Naar R., Guyett I.P.R., et al.: Training medical students in interpersonal relationship skills. *J. Med. Educ.* 51:743–750, 1976.
Parsons T.: *The Social System*. New York, Free Press, 1951.
Pellegrino E.D.: Humanistic base for professional ethics in medicine. *N.Y. State J. Med.* 77(9):1456–1462, 1977.
Pelletier K.R.: *Mind as Healer, Mind as Slayer*. New York, Dell Publishing Co., 1977.
Petersdorf R.G.: Health manpower: Numbers, distribution, and quality. *Ann. Intern. Med.* 82:694, 1975.
Poe W.D., Holloway D.A.: *Drugs and the Aged*. New York, McGraw-Hill Book Co., 1980.
Pragoff H.: Adjustment of tuberculosis patients one year after hospital discharge. *Public Health Rep.* 77:671–679, 1962.
Pratt L., Seligmann A., Reader G.: Physicians' views on the level of medical information among patients. *Am. J. Pub. Health* 47:1277, 1957.
Rasche L.M., Bernstein L., Veenhuis P.E.: Evaluation of a systematic approach to teaching interviewing. *J. Med. Educ.* 49:589–595, 1974.
Reader G.G., Pratt L., Mudd M.C.: What patients expect from their doctors. *Mod. Hosp.* 89:88, 1957.
Reeder L.C.: The patient-client as a consumer: Some observations on the changing professional-client relationship. *J. Health Soc. Behav.* 13:406–412, 1972.
Remen N.: *The Human Patient*. Garden City, N.Y., Doubleday & Co., 1980.
Remen N.: Humanistic patient care: Toward a contemporary synthesis of the art and science of medicine, in Miller S., Remen N., Barbour A., et al. (eds.): *Dimensions of Humanistic Medicine*. San Francisco, Institute for the Study of Humanistic Medicine, 1975.
Rusk H.A.: *Rehabilitation Medicine*. St Louis, C.V. Mosby Co., 1971.
Shem S.: *The House of God*. New York, Dell Publishing Co., 1978.
Silver G.A.: *Family Medical Care: a Report on the Family Health Maintenance Demonstration*. Cambridge, Mass., Harvard University Press, 1963.
Simon H.: Ideas, germs and society. *Stanford Med. Bull.* 19:88–96, 1961.
Simpson M.A.: *Medical Education: A Critical Approach*. London, Redwood Press Ltd., 1972.
Sizemore M., Coyle J.: *Social and Psychological Aspects of Aging*. Dallas, University of Texas Health Science Center, 1981.
Spitzer W.O., Sackett D.L., Sibley J.C., et al.: The Burlington randomized trial of the nurse practitioner. *N. Engl. J. Med.* 290:251, 1974.
Stimmel B.: The Congress and health manpower: A legislative morass. *N. Engl. J. Med.* 293:68, 1975.

Szasz T.S., Hollender M.H.: A contribution to the philosophy of medicine. *Arch. Intern. Med.* 97:585, 1956.

Talkington D.R.: Maximizing patient compliance by shaping attitudes of self-directed health care. *J. Fam. Prac.* 6:591–595, 1978.

Thompson D.D.: Are hospitals dehumanized? *N. Y. State J. Med.* 77(9):1451–1452, 1977.

Tubesing D.A., Holinger P.C., Westberg G.E., et al.: The wholistic health center project: An action-research model for providing preventive, whole-person health care at the primary level. *Med. Care* 15:217–228, 1977.

Veatch R.M.: The medical model: Its nature and problems. *Hastings Cent. Rep.* 1:58–76, 1973.

Waitzkin H., Stoeckle J.D.: The communication of information about illness: Clinical, sociological, and methodological considerations. *Adv. Psychosom. Med.* 8:180, 1972.

Weeks L.E., DeVries R.A.: Wholistic health centers: Where are they going? *Inquiry* 15:3–9, 1978.

Werner A., Schneider J.M.: Teaching medical students interactional skills. *N. Engl. J. Med.* 290:1232–1237, 1974.

White K.L.: International comparisons of medical care. *Sci. Am.* 17:233, 1975.

White K.L.: Patterns of medical practices, in *Prevention Medicine*. Boston, Little, Brown & Co., 1967.

Winkelstein W.: Epidemiological considerations underlying the allocation of health and disease care resources. *Int. J. Epidemiol.* 1:69–74, 1972.

INDEX

X